Praise for

THE CHRONIC PAIN SOLUTION

"A superb book! At once medically precise and warmly accessible, *The Chronic Pain Solution* wages a successful frontal assault on pain, perhaps the greatest obstacle to wellness in our society. A must read for patients—and their doctors."
—Mehmet Oz, M.D., Columbia-Presbyterian Medical Center, author of *Healing from the Heart*

"Dr. Dillard's work offers a welcome focus on the 'whole person' in describing the many diseases that produce chronic pain, the extraordinary range of treatment options, and the movement to integrate complementary therapies into mainstream pain management."
—Russell K. Portenoy, M.D., Chairman, Department of Pain Medicine and Palliative Care, Beth Israel Medical Center

"A fine, useful, and highly readable guide to the important field of integrative pain treatment."
—James S. Gordon, M.D., Director, the Center for Mind-Body Medicine; author of *Manifesto for a New Medicine*

"Probably the most comprehensive book of its type I have seen in the past decade, and should be part of your patient library."
—Professor John D. Loeser, M.D., American Pain Society Bulletin

"I highly recommend this wise and practical book to the millions who live with pain."
—Christiane Northrup, M.D., author of *Women's Bodies, Women's Wisdom* and *The Wisdom of Menopause*

THE CHRONIC PAIN SOLUTION

Your Personal Path to Pain Relief

James N. Dillard, M.D., D.C., C.Ac.
with Leigh Ann Hirschman

BANTAM BOOKS

Grateful acknowledgment is given for permission to reprint the FACES Pain Rating Scale: D. L. Wong, M. Hockenberry-Eaton, D. Wilson, M. L. Winkelstein, P. Schwartz, *Wong's Essentials of Pediatric Nursing,* ed. 6, St. Louis, 2001, p. 1301. Copyright by Mosby, Inc. Reprinted by permission.

THE CHRONIC PAIN SOLUTION
A Bantam Book

PUBLISHING HISTORY
Bantam hardcover edition published August 2002
Bantam trade paperback edition / October 2003

Published by
Bantam Dell
A Division of Random House, Inc.
New York, New York

Illustrations by Nancy Heim

Book design by Laurie Jewell

Library of Congress Catalog Card Number: 2002023225

ISBN 0-553-38111-3

Manufactured in the United States of America
Published simultaneously in Canada

BVG 10 9 8 7 6 5 4 3 2

FOR POLLY

CONTENTS

ACKNOWLEDGMENTS

I would like to thank my wonderful agent and friend, Jill Kneerim, who believed in me and in the importance of this work. Without her faith and support, this book would not have been possible. For her gifted writing and eternal patience, Leigh Ann Hirschman deserves a tremendous debt of gratitude. My thanks also go out to my extraordinary editor, Toni Burbank, for her invaluable contributions and her belief in this project. Many thanks to Irwyn Applebaum, Barb Burg, and the whole Bantam team for their enthusiasm and drive.

A number of people contributed by reviewing technical content, and by contributing thoughts and suggestions, including Sekhar Upadhyayula, M.D., Maureen McSweeney, Ph.D., Todd Wilkowski, P.T., O.C.S., Adriane Fugh-Berman, M.D., Kenneth Gorfinkle, Ph.D., Joseph Loizzo, M.D., Ph.D., Tieraona Low Dog, M.D., Barbara Bezdicek, M.D., Steven J. Scrivani, M.D., D.D.S., Fredi Kronenberg, Ph.D., Harriet Bienfield, L.Ac., Kathleen Madigan, L.P.N., and Josephine Musto, M.S., R.N. Though their help has been tremendous, final responsibility for any inaccuracies in the work will rest with me.

I would like to acknowledge the inspiration and teaching of Dr. Michael Lerner, Dr. Rachel N. Remen, and Dr. Andrew Weil for leading the way. They have had a profound influence on my thinking and approach to this topic. I also have learned much from my mentors through the years, including Ted Kaptchuk, O.M.D., L. John Faye, D.C., Scott Haldeman, M.D., Ph.D., D.C., William Prensky, O.M.D., Assibi Abudu, M.D., Michael L. Weinberger, M.D., Stanley J. Myers, M.D., James S. Lieberman, M.D., Russell K. Portenoy, M.D., and Alexander Mauskop, M.D.

My wonderful lawyer and friend, Russell Smith, has been a constant source of support and wise council during the project. My many water dog friends have been wonderful and helpful. They put up with me working every day on this book during a windsurfing trip, without throwing my laptop into the sea. And Caroline Gillespie has been endlessly helpful with proofreading, various reality checks, and helping to keep my life on the rails. I send out much thanks to all.

INTRODUCTION: THE CHRONIC PAIN SOLUTION

Diana, a makeup artist in her late twenties, came into my office toting a shopping bag. She heaved the bag up onto my desk and then slowly eased herself into a chair. She explained to me that she suffered from severe endometriosis, a painful disorder in which uterine tissue implants itself in other areas of the body, and that she had seen several doctors in her search for relief. When I opened the shopping bag, I saw that it was filled with prescription bottles. "Every time I see a doctor, I bring in my bag and he adds another to my collection," she said, obviously expecting that I'd do the same. I looked at the labels; she had been regularly downing a dangerous combination of pills. Still, Diana was in terrible pain. She could drag herself through work, but at night all she could do was lie on the couch with a heating pad on her abdomen. "It sounds trivial," she said, "but the worst part is that I'm lonely. I've been so depressed and exhausted from the pain that no one wants to talk to me." She sighed and ran her hand down the side of her face. "I guess I can't blame them. I'm not the person I used to be. Since the pain started, I'm just not myself anymore."

A few years ago, Victor, a fifty-four-year-old lawyer, developed arthritis in his left hand. His doctor told him to take Tylenol, and when that didn't help, Victor decided he'd just have to live with the pain. At first he hurt mainly before a change in the weather, but now his hand had begun to ache every day. He could still force himself to type documents at his computer, but he wondered if he'd need to fire his longtime secretary and hire a new one who could take shorthand. Sometimes the pain woke him up at night, especially in winter. It was even getting hard to pull on his socks. "Tell me if this is something I'm just supposed to put up with, and I will," he said. "But there's got to be more I can do."

I could tell at first sight that Jacob's life was governed by pain. He shuffled through the door with his arms held close to his sides. I offered him a seat, but he winced and remained standing. In a barely audible monotone, he told me his story. Three years ago, Jacob had injured his back at work; despite two surgeries and long periods of total bed rest, he had not recovered. In fact, he was in agonizing pain every hour of the day. He couldn't work, couldn't relax—he couldn't even sit down—and the doctors who signed off on his workers' compensation payments wouldn't renew his prescription for the only painkillers that had given him any relief. His wife had stuck by him so far, he told me reluctantly, but the marriage was precarious. He summed up his life with pain: "I spend all my time trying to protect my back. I can't even go downstairs to pick up the mail or help with the dishes. I'm afraid to. There's no way I'll risk making the pain worse."

If you suffer from chronic pain, you are not alone. At the pain clinic where I work, the waiting room fills up every morning. Some patients, like Jacob, are obviously disabled, confined to wheelchairs or unable to sit down. Some are more like Diana and Victor; they don't look much different from the patients in any other doctor's office. They sit and read the paper, sip coffee, or work on laptops. If I stop in the hall to watch them, however, I'll usually notice a detail that belies their steady exterior: a hand that reaches up to rub the back of the neck, an arm that never moves from its carefully arranged position on the chair, or maybe just a facial expression that's a little more irritable than that of the average New Yorker with an early morning appointment. Although there are great differences in the degree and kind of suffering, everyone in this room hurts. And there will be another group in an hour, and the hour after that, and for the rest of the day and every day this week. Chronic pain—pain that has lasted longer than six months—afflicts nearly fifty million Americans. It's the third most common health care problem in the United States, behind only heart disease and cancer.

If you ask healthy people to imagine what it's like to live with chronic pain, they will usually draw on memories of painful but short-lived injuries. In a genuine attempt at sympathy, they will supply a list of adjectives that describe the physical qualities: *throbbing, aching, stabbing, burning*. To a certain extent, they're right. But they miss the essential point: Chronic pain does more than hurt. It takes control over the way you live.

Ongoing pain has a way of separating you, sometimes subtly, from the things and people you enjoy. A bad knee can keep you from playing tennis or chasing after your children. Arthritis in your hands may prevent you from cooking or holding a book. You may have told yourself to keep things in perspective: Without tennis, life does go on. But if tennis has been important to you—as a source of socializing, relaxation, fitness, or pure enjoyment—life goes on in a significantly different way. You may not see your friends nearly as much, and without the regular exercise, you may find that you've gained weight or that you can't handle stress the way you used to. The quality of your life is measurably lower. The same goes for cooking, reading, playing with children, or any other favorite activity.

On a more intimate level, pain sufferers often feel they've lost control of their personalities. Constant low-level pain can turn normally pleasant people into snappish malcontents. Pain that is more intense can leave you withdrawn, sullen, or angry. Add the sometimes stupefying effects of pain medication to the mix and you may find yourself saying, along with Diana, "I'm not myself anymore." These shifts in mood can strain professional and personal relationships—sometimes to the breaking point. Because pain is invisible, well-meaning friends and family who are supportive at first may eventually come to doubt the sufferer. They may wonder aloud whether your pain is real, or perhaps suggest that you've "created" the condition in an unconscious bid for extra attention or time off work. You may even feel some of the same doubts yourself. It's not unusual for people in moderate to severe pain to ask me, in all seriousness, if I think they're crazy.

All too often, the treatment process itself only intensifies pain's hold on your life—lunch breaks spent on the phone with the insurance company, meetings missed because the specialist is running late, dignity injured when a pharmacist levels an accusation of faking pain to get drugs. Some people have physicians who treat them like competent adults with a rightful say in their own health care—for any disorder *except* pain. When patients visit these doctors with a pain complaint, they are expected to submit quickly and quietly to whatever treatment is proffered, even when no explanation of it is forthcoming.

Ultimately, only you know what it's like to live with your pain. I can hazard some guesses, but no one can truly understand the inner workings of another's agony. What I *can* tell you is this: No matter how much you currently hurt, no matter how much your pain has affected your life, there's an excellent chance that you can regain control. Control over the physical hurt—the throbbing, aching, stabbing, burning. And control over all the other aspects of a life marked by pain: the mood alterations, the time spent inside the health care system, the deprivation of the things you enjoy.

If you've suffered for a long time, the claims above may sound all too familiar. You may have tried several "miracle cures" already, or seen practitioners who've told you that they'll fix you right up. Invariably, these promises disappoint; often, they actually leave the patient with even more pain (and less money). The solution I offer in this book doesn't propose any one-shot cures. Instead, it operates on the principle that pain is a more complicated disorder than most people realize; as such, it often requires a combination of therapies based on your individual needs. This is the idea behind the country's top pain clinics, including the one where I work. Unfortunately, only a very tiny percentage of sufferers are ever referred to such a clinic or live near enough one to make the trip. I've written this book to put the best, most up-to-date information into your hands.

MEDICINE'S BLIND SPOT

Despite the millions of people in pain every day, our medical establishment does not view pain management as a priority. You may find this statement surprising. Then again, if you've spent years going from doctor to doctor, receiving conflicting diagnoses and advice, you may not. Most pain patients receive limited relief at best; at worst, they receive treatment that is shockingly inappropriate—even harmful.

Victor, the attorney with arthritis in his hand, is just one example out of thousands of *under*treated patients I've seen. The doctor prescribes medications that are either ineffective or too strong; when those don't work or produce intolerable side effects, the patient often just assumes that the condition can't be helped, and quits the search for relief.

Other patients are aggressively *over*treated. This is what happened to Diana, who was given a dangerous combination of prescriptions for her pelvic pain, so that her pain "cure" left her in deeper isolation. Despite her suffering, Diana was actually lucky that her doctor didn't recommend a total—and totally unnecessary—hysterectomy. Many surgeons are all too eager to operate. Of course, surgery is sometimes an important part of treatment, but the sad fact is that anywhere between 40 and 60 percent of back surgeries performed in this country are completely unnecessary. When I see back patients, I am often treating them for improper surgery as much as for their original problem.

I first became aware of this medical blind spot long before I went to medical school. I was an acupuncturist and chiropractor before I became a physician; as a practitioner of alternative medicine, I quickly discovered that most of my clients were pain sufferers who hadn't received relief from their doctors. I treated back pain, irritable bowel syndrome, arthritis, and other conditions, often with success—especially when I combined acupuncture and chiropractic with other nonmainstream therapies. It was gratifying to see my patients reconnect with aspects of life they thought were gone forever. But I wanted to know more about the conditions I was seeing, and I wanted to learn the whole spectrum of treatments for pain, not just the few I used. When I began medical school, the reason my patients had so little success with doctors became clear.

In med school, I looked for courses on pain management. None existed. In my classes on spinal anatomy and neural science, I waited in vain for information about controlling the agony brought on by malfunctions of these systems. Soon it became obvious to me that if I followed the average medical school curriculum, I'd *never* learn about pain.

WHY PAIN IS NEGLECTED

Pain is different from most other conditions doctors are trained to treat. For one, *no tool exists that can measure pain.* Doctors can't locate it with an MRI scan or measure it with a blood test. For some painful disorders, such as those of the joints or discs, there are tests to measure the extent of damage—but the amount of damage doesn't always correlate to how much a person hurts. Most people with diseased-looking joints are pain-free, while many people with severe pain have normal test results. There's no way anyone can even verify that you hurt at all. Pain has its origins in the body, but ultimately it is a subjective phenomenon, and there's no way the medical profession can make an objective measure of it.

Another difference is that pain isn't a disease in and of itself. We don't say "I have pain" or "I've just been diagnosed with pain" in the same way we say "I have asthma" or "I've just been diagnosed with diabetes." Instead, pain is classified as a symptom, like a cough. If you go to a doctor with a cough, she will usually be able to figure out the underlying cause, perhaps a cold or bronchitis. The diagnosis gives both you and the doctor a relieving sense of certainty, and you proceed to treatment. But *in most cases of chronic pain, the cause simply isn't known.* Sometimes it's not even possible to pinpoint the body tissue that's hurting. If you have pain in your abdomen, belly, chest, head, or muscles, the pain may simply be called "generalized," meaning that its exact location within the region is unclear.

Western medicine rightly prides itself on its adherence to precision, measurement, and concrete fact. Unfortunately, pain, with its intangible qualities, just doesn't fit with our way of medical thinking. Until recently, few medical schools have had even *one* course in the causes and treatment of pain. During four years of coursework, students may receive only an hour or two of instruction carved out of a lecture devoted to the many uses of narcotic medications.

Most doctors, then, pick up their information about pain management by watching an older generation of doctors making the rounds—a generation of physicians that was also uneducated about pain. As a result, even the best-intentioned doctors may rely on thinking that has been outdated for decades. Specialists may be blinkered by their own expertise. When they are faced with a patient in pain, they tend to fall back on the method they know best. Surgeons operate, anesthesiologists anesthetize, and physical therapists prescribe exercise—regardless of the appropriateness for the particular case. Most of their patients don't know that any other options exist, until their unrelieved pain drives them to a different doctor with a different specialty.

HOPE FROM THE CUTTING EDGE

There are some welcome signs of change. In January 2001, the Joint Commission on Accreditation of Hospital Organizations decreed that to receive their accreditation, hospitals must consider pain the fifth vital sign, as important to measure as blood pressure or pulse. Doctors who dismiss their patients' pain are now at risk for losing their licenses. The commission also ordained that pain treatment *in addition* to pharmaceuticals be available to patients in hospitals.

Many excellent research facilities have zeroed in on pain. Pioneering researchers such as Ronald Melzack and Patrick Wall, as well as clinicians such as New York City's Katherine Foley and Russell Portenoy, have unearthed a great deal about what causes pain and how to treat it. They've discovered new medications and have found better ways to use the old ones. They've learned which surgeries actually make painful conditions worse and have invented new, less invasive procedures that really work. Even if you made the rounds of doctors just a few years ago for your pain, there may now be new discoveries that can help.

KNOW YOUR ALTERNATIVES

One of the most exciting findings from the cutting edge of medicine sounds like bad news at first: Even the smartest conventional treatments may not do enough. Relying solely on medication for pain is like treating heart disease with nothing more than an angioplasty. Like cardiovascular conditions and diabetes, pain is complex. Its biological causes and complications are numerous—*and* it has a give-and-take relationship with your environment and your personality. One-shot treatments are rarely able to address all its factors. It is now common knowledge that treatment for heart disease that involves medication but doesn't also incorporate dietary changes, exercise, and stress control probably won't succeed. The same goes for effective pain treatment; it must take into account all the individual factors that contribute to your pain, and then it must apply a menu of therapies that addresses each of those factors.

Here's the exciting part: Many of those therapies in that menu are from the world of alternative medicine. They are surprisingly gentle, even pleasant. Certain herbs, such as valerian root, can alter body chemistry as successfully as some conventional medicines, but with a lower risk of intolerance or side effects. (That's a gratifying change from pharmaceuticals, which can be awfully harsh for the day-in, day-out treatment of long-term pain.) Many of my patients with abdominal or back pain rely on specialized massage techniques to relieve flare-ups. The massage not only relaxes cramped muscles and relieves stress but actually blocks the pain signals from moving through the body's nervous system. For day-to-day treatment of back pain, however, most people find more relief from yoga than from any other source. This Eastern discipline stretches the muscles, strengthens the spine, and has a potent restorative effect on the mind as well as the body. Acupuncture is another favorite with patients and a growing number of physicians—at Columbia Presbyterian Medical Center, a bastion of conventional medicine, I regularly stick needles into people.

What's the solution to your chronic pain? I'll be honest: It's not a pill or a new high-tech machine or a smelly herb. The solution lies in a smart *combination* of old and new—of the very best pharmaceuticals and other conventional treatments along with an assortment of alternatives. I've seen thousands of patients find their chronic pain solutions, and I'm confident you can, too.

TAKE BACK CONTROL

The goal of this book is to provide you with all the information you need to take your life back from pain. It explains how pain works, guides you through your many options, and then shows you how to take control of your treatment. I have tried to make it easily adaptable to each reader; it is broken down into self-contained sections and chapters so that you can turn to those that best apply to your situation.

- Part I, "Understanding Pain," debunks some popular myths about pain and describes how a sensory impulse travels through your body and is eventually perceived as pain. I find that a simple understanding of pain is often a great source of relief all by itself. This makes sense: When people know what is happening to their bodies, they feel much more in control. This section also discusses why a treatment philosophy that integrates both conventional and alternative medicine is generally so successful.

- Part II, "Take Control of Your Treatment," suggests practical ways to get the best medical care possible. It is essential that readers of this book work with a doctor who can coordinate therapies, prescribe medication if necessary, and monitor their progress. Although many doctors lack a thorough understanding of pain, you may be surprised at how many are willing to work with an educated patient and to assist you in trying new therapies. I will help you choose a coordinating doctor, talk to him or her with greater clarity and confidence, and elicit the help you need. It's possible that you'll also need an alternative practitioner or two. Since alternative medicine is a largely unregulated field, finding and working with the right specialist can be daunting. This section will help you navigate that territory as well. The final chapter in this part shows you and your doctor how to create a plan for pain control based on your individual needs.

▶ Part III, "Therapies," introduces you to the range of treatment options available today, both conventional and alternative. I explain what they do, which ones are best for your individual condition and needs, how they work, what kinds of dosages or treatment times are appropriate, and what kinds of side effects or contraindications may exist. I also offer advice about combining treatments.

▶ Part IV, "Painful Conditions," arms you with information about your particular problem and helps you identify the treatments most likely to ease your pain.

▶ Part V, "Special Considerations," focuses on pregnant women, the elderly, parents of children in pain, and people who are terminally ill. There's also a chapter for loved ones of pain sufferers to help them understand what you're going through and how to give you support without straining your relationship. The book concludes with stories from people who found meaning—even transcendence—in their pain; they've taught me a lot about the role of grace and human spirit in the chronic pain solution.

There are many ways to read and use this book. Some people may be fascinated by the theoretical material in Part I. Others may prefer to turn directly to the chapter in Part IV that directly addresses their particular disorder. Some readers will want to flip through Part III, looking for new treatment ideas. Many of you will simply want to use this book as a reference, to look up therapies recommended by your doctor. It is now *your* book, to be employed in the manner you find most helpful. It is my deepest hope that it will bring you relief.

PART I

UNDERSTANDING PAIN

1.

SIX MYTHS THAT CAN KEEP YOU FROM HEALING

MYTH #1: YOU JUST HAVE TO LEARN TO LIVE WITH IT

This is a line most chronic-pain patients have heard at some point from a doctor or caregiver. It's usually said in an exasperated tone, implying one of two things, or both: (1) the physician has run through all the available options and there is simply nothing more to be done, or (2) the patient is being unreasonable and demanding in the search for pain relief.

In reality, there is an extraordinary number of therapies that can drastically reduce your pain or limit its effect on your life. Take America's preferred method of pain relief: painkillers. If you've tried a conventional drug that worked but gave you intolerable side effects, you don't need to give up. Other drugs in that same class of medications might well have a very different effect on your internal chemistry. Or you can try a drug from one of the other classes of pharmaceuticals. With a half dozen or so classes of pain-modifying medications to choose from, why some physicians give up after trying just one or two is beyond me. You might need to tolerate a little trial and error, but isn't that preferable to just living with it?

Or perhaps drugs aren't the best form of treatment for you. Some form of hands-on therapy, such as acupuncture, massage, or yoga, may ease your pain much more efficiently and pleasantly. The main thing to keep in mind is that there are more pathways to pain control—*many* more—than even your doctor may know.

Let's also debunk the myth that the patient who doesn't accept pain is being whiny or is putting too many demands on the doctor. Now, I'm certainly not going to encourage people to be rude to their physicians. We doctors work hard, and we appreciate consideration and kindness as much as anyone. But one key to getting good relief is persistence. If your doctor makes you feel like a pest for asking about pain control, I strongly suggest you find another one. The impulse to feel better is natural and healing. If you're told that there's no use in trying, you're likely to feel something even worse than pain: helplessness. People who feel helpless tend to withdraw from the world, stop trying to eat right, stop making the effort to see friends or to do the things they love. Their lives become terribly unbalanced, and their natural bodily defenses weaken. They get sicker, and they hurt more. By contrast, a hopeful outlook, or even a stubborn attitude, can go a long way toward improving your health.

MYTH #2: IT'S ALL IN YOUR HEAD

It really hurts to be accused of faking your pain, or to be told that it's solely the result of some psychological problem. Then you've got anger—or worse, guilt—heaped atop your suffering.

This myth persists because pain is invisible. When people have diabetes, doctors can give them a concrete number—one that represents blood sugar—to explain their mood swings, thirst, and other symptoms. If you have heart problems, doctors will say: "No wonder you've been fatigued lately. Your arteries are ninety percent blocked." But if you have pain, no one can legitimize your suffering with a number or a scan or a picture.

This myth is also based on a misperception about how pain works. Most people, doctors included, assume that pain is *always* the result of damage to the body's tissues. They also believe that the amount of pain you feel directly corresponds to the extent of the damage. The fact is that many people with chronic pain don't have any injury or illness that explains the pain's severity. But that doesn't make the pain any less real.

Chapter 3 will talk about the new model of pain. I won't go into the details here, but we now understand that pain is a complex condition that involves many systems of your body, not just the part that's hurting. Your nerves, your neurotransmitters, endorphins and other chemicals, and your mind and brain are all involved as well. If one of these starts misbehaving, you may well have pain, even if you don't have an injury. Yes, bodily pain can be an expression of emotional suffering. That doesn't mean the pain is made up. In these cases, neurons are indeed firing pain signals, chemicals are facilitating that message, and other physical factors are very much present.

Don't let this myth keep you from using the power of your mind. Some people avoid mind-body therapies, thinking that they work only for people whose pain is purely psychic. In doing so, they're denying themselves an important source of relief. Although your pain is real, it, like everything else in your body, is greatly affected by the workings of your mind. Your brain and your spirit are some of your most powerful tools for pain control. Even people with the most obviously devastating injuries—such as soldiers wounded on the battlefield—have been documented using their minds to reduce or even completely block pain.

MYTH #3:
WHY CAN'T YOU TAKE IT?
IT'S JUST PAIN

Hey, it's not like you have ______" (fill in the blank with any of the following: heart disease, pneumonia, a broken neck). People who utter these words believe that you should just dismiss pain and sweep it right out of your mind. They don't understand that pain goes beyond a mere physical sensation; they don't see that pain has the power to change your relationship to the world, to grip your mind and soul.

Let me make an exception here. Sometimes pain can wind people up so tightly that they stop thinking about anything else. They become exclusively focused on their disorder. In these cases, it can be helpful to say, gently, kindly, "It's just pain." This is a compassionate act of putting pain in perspective for a person who's fallen into a downward spiral, who has come to equate pain with the worst possible of human experiences. From time to time you may need to remind yourself that it's not death, it's not the loss of a loved one; life will indeed go on, even if it's not the life you had before. In the end, *you* decide how much quality there is to that life.

MYTH #4: IF I HURT, MY BODY MUST BE IN DANGER

Pain is one of the most powerful of human experiences. It's meant to get our attention: to pull our hand out of the fire, pry the splinter loose from our foot, rush to the hospital to have our appendix removed. It's natural, and life-preserving, for us to feel that pain signals danger—and that the more pain there is, the graver the danger. The reality is that when pain is chronic, all bets are off. Of course, many progressive diseases such as muscular dystrophy and cancer produce continuing damage that's quite painful. But as I've pointed out above, pain doesn't *always* represent ongoing physical harm. It may be the result of a nervous system firing off erroneous messages, or of your body's inability to produce its natural painkilling substances—to name just two possibilities. This is especially likely for people whose pain has inexplicably continued after an injury has healed, or whose level of discomfort seems inappropriate for their disorder.

The fear of damage and illness that naturally attends pain may alter your nervous system so that you hurt even more. That tense state of "pain alert" can also give you headaches, insomnia, digestive troubles, and other woes. Knowing that pain is not actually harming your body may not eliminate it. But if you can disconnect anxiety and tension from the hurt, you're on the path to significant relief.

MYTH #5: THERE IS ONE SPECIAL DOCTOR/PILL/HIGH-TECH PROCEDURE/ALTERNATIVE METHOD OUT THERE THAT WILL STOP MY PAIN

This is the magic-bullet theory of pain relief, and its refrains go something like this: "I have to keep trying new doctors until I find the one that will fix me once and for all." "There's an herb that's supposed to take away pain. I'm sending in my money today." "This painkiller doesn't work. I took it and I still feel some tenderness in my muscles."

For most of our lives, we go to see doctors when we're sick. They give us a pill or perform a procedure, and we feel better. If we have a bacterial infection, we get an antibiotic. If we have a blockage in our arteries, a surgeon performs an angioplasty to reopen the blood vessels. We've grown accustomed to this one-to-one correspondence: one illness, one treatment.

But chronic pain isn't like other disorders. In most cases, there isn't one single problem we can point to, such as a bacterium or a blockage or a malfunction in enzyme production. That makes diagnosis difficult and sometimes even impossible. Chronic pain is usually the result of several things going awry—mechanical, chemical, and neurological—and it also is affected by the state of your soul. There's rarely one simple solution that can penetrate to all the layers of pain. If someone promises you a cure-all for pain or tries to sell you a "miracle" potion, I'd advise you to run the other way (and alert the Better Business Bureau).

The solution this book offers is integrative medicine, the combination of conventional and alternative therapies. Each of your treatments will have an aspect of your pain written on it. But just as the alchemy of baking transforms ordinary flour, sugar, butter, eggs, and heat into a glorious birthday cake, a group of well-chosen therapies is more than the sum total of massages and injections and breathing exercises. There's a synergy among the treatments that adds up to something bigger—to your very own chronic pain solution.

MYTH #6: A LIFE WITH PAIN ISN'T WORTH LIVING

The goal of this book is to help you control pain. I have every confidence you can do it; I've seen it happen for thousands of people. The techniques and knowledge exist. But it's possible that your pain won't completely disappear. Lots of programs promise a "pain-free life" or say that they will cure your pain. You may have tried them, and if so, you know that they don't fulfill those promises.

I think it's important to ask yourself at the outset: What will you do, and how will you feel, if your pain doesn't completely disappear? It may be that you can cut your pain by three-quarters or one-half. The quality may change from an unbearable piercing sensation to a more tolerable ache. Or you might go from having pain all the time to having periodic flare-ups. But you may still have some pain.

A good strategy when you're faced with pain is to break the experience into two parts: the pain itself, and the suffering, the havoc pain wreaks on your life. Pain causes suffering when it takes away your focus, your ability to perform tasks, and your control over your emotions. After experimenting with the therapies in this book, you may still have some physical pain. But your *suffering* may be nearly eliminated. Maybe you'll be able to play with your grandkids again, or attend parties, or make your bed in the morning, even though once those activities were out of the question. Maybe you'll feel more like your old self again. When these things happen, your life is significantly better and more satisfying. That's the ultimate goal of treatment.

2.

THE YOGI AND THE ANESTHESIOLOGIST: INTEGRATIVE MEDICINE IN ACTION

The scene is a small examination room, the kind you might find in any doctor's office. There's a table, a row of cabinets, a sink, a framed photograph of a calla lily, a window hung with white metal blinds. What sets this room apart is the activity inside it. As a woman in street clothes lies on the examining table, a man stands above her, working a slender silver needle into the base of her left wrist. The patient breathes deeply, slowly, as if she's asleep. The acupuncturist then repeats the procedure on the right hand, and then both ankles. When he is done, he covers his patient with a blanket, turns off the lights, and sits by her side in the darkness.

In a room down the hall, an anesthesiologist is outfitted in blue radiation gear. Her patient lies facedown on a table, with a small section of his back exposed. Directly above him, a fluoroscope, a type of X-ray machine, projects a continuous image of his spine onto a nearby monitor. The doctor studies the screen, and once she is satisfied, she fills a syringe with a combination of liquid anesthetic and anti-inflammatory medication and guides the syringe into the patient's back. Slowly, she taps the needle down deep into the spine, relying on the image to show her when she's reached the pocket of space near two painful discs. When the monitor shows that her needle has reached the precise location, the doctor pushes gently down on the syringe, sending the anesthetic flowing out around the discs, coating the inflamed nerves.

In a third room, two men sit on the floor together. The doctor demonstrates a yoga pose called *paschimottanasana:* He extends his legs straight out in front of his body, feet flexed, and gently bends his torso forward, his arms reaching toward his toes. The patient imitates the position, and the doctor gently makes a few corrections. Once the patient understands the pose, he holds it and relaxes quietly. In the meantime, the doctor writes out a prescription for a painkiller.

On any day of the week, this is a set of scenes you might find in the office where I work. This clinic, along with several others across the country, offers top-notch conventional care for pain—scans and X rays, physical therapy, medications, injections, and so on—alongside alternative approaches such as acupuncture, herbalism, and yoga.

To many health care practitioners, this kind of practice amounts to blasphemy. As you might expect, there are plenty of conventional doctors who can't stand the thought of mind-body or energy healing being given the same legitimacy as "real" medicine. But some alternative healers also find this kind of clinic upsetting. They see the willingness to prescribe pharmaceuticals or perform injections as treason against the world of holistic medicine. What's humorous is that these two sides, whose advocates probably wouldn't even sit down to dinner together, actually have something in common. They each believe that there exists one true path to healing and that all other practitioners are simply lost in the woods, with darkness fast descending.

But I've found that people with pain have no such ax to grind. Most of us know the stereotype of the alternative-medicine consumer, the guy who eats nothing but sprouts and algae, who downs thousands of dollars' worth of supplements, and who wouldn't go to a hospital even if he were sporting a gaping head wound. In my experience, most people who try alternative medicine—and almost half of Americans have—actually possess a much more balanced philosophy. These people may practice tai chi or take herbs, but they're also dubious about throwing away centuries of hard-earned Western medical knowledge. If you've been thinking that neither conventional nor alternative medicine holds the single key to health, you're absolutely correct. Fortunately, medical research is catching up with common sense, and now the best pain doctors are integrating the two approaches, with impressive results.

What to call this combination of alternative and high-tech medicine is still a matter of debate. You may hear the term *complementary* or *CAM,* which is an acronym for "complementary and alternative medicine." The U.S. government, which is sponsoring several research centers to explore this old-but-new medicine, uses the latter. Many practitioners, including me, find this term misleading: It suggests that alternative medicine is only a minor adjunct to "real" medicine. Andrew Weil, M.D., has proposed the term *integrative,* which implies that both kinds of medicine have equal footing and that they can be woven together into a sensible combination. *Integrative* is the term I'll use throughout this book.

In an ideal world, everyone in moderate to severe pain would live near one of these integrative clinics and have no trouble getting both a referral and insurance coverage for the treatment. But one of the reasons I wrote this book is that getting treatment at such a practice isn't possible for most people. If you have relatively minor pain, it might not even be worth the extra effort. Without a clinic, you can still derive great benefit from an integrative approach. You can supplement your conventional treatment with gentle self-care, or you can work with your doctor for a more comprehensive approach, pulling in other healers to create your own integrative pain team.

No matter how you integrate alternative and conventional treatment, it's important to understand just what each has to offer. This chapter is a consideration of the strengths and weaknesses of both.

CONVENTIONAL MEDICINE: A CORNERSTONE OF THE CHRONIC PAIN SOLUTION

It's Western research that's given us our best understanding of pain, along with diagnostic techniques that can determine which disorders may underlie the hurt. MRI and CAT scans, X rays, and even the old rubber-hammer reflex test can tell us a lot about your condition and help determine the most appropriate course of therapies. Someone who's suffering from a lifetime of wear and tear in the back will get a radically different set of treatments than someone whose back pain is generated by a neurological disorder, and we can best diagnose these different causes with traditional office exams or high-tech equipment.

Conventional drugs and procedures, when properly applied, can function as the border pieces of the pain-management puzzle: When you've sorted through your conventional options and found the ones right for you, it may be easier to see how alternative treatments fit into your program. People who know my background sometimes assume that my interest in gentle, holistic medicine presupposes a fear of or distaste for pharmaceuticals. But when it comes to tough pain, the accuracy and precision of Western medicine is tough to beat.

ANDERS'S STORY: HIGH-TECH MAKES THE DIFFERENCE

Anders is a Norwegian painter who suffers from Ehlers-Danlos syndrome, a rare disease that produces joint and muscle pain that's very difficult to bear. Anders was reluctant to take the morphine his doctor had prescribed, which made him unacceptably sleepy and drugged. By the time I met him, his pain was incapacitating. He couldn't sit in a chair and work or even carry on a long conversation. I convinced him to try morphine again, but this time using a different delivery system: an implanted pump that sent the drug directly to his spinal cord. Because this method bypassed the brain, Anders remains alert and wakeful. Now he's much more comfortable, but he's also fully himself, thanks to a combination of pharmaceuticals and technology.

Recent years have seen a boom in new drugs for pain. If you haven't seen a pain specialist lately, you may be surprised at what the latest drugs can do for you. For example, there's a new class of drugs that can help relieve the inflammatory pain of arthritis and other conditions without the same risk to your stomach posed by medicines such as aspirin and ibuprofen. We've also learned that many existing drugs can be put to new use treating pain. We've discovered that epilepsy medications are very effective at treating neuropathic pain, a deeply frustrating condition in which the nerves become hypersensitive and fire even in the absence of a painful stimulus. Certain kinds of antidepressants, when used in extremely low doses, can help people with pain-related insomnia, often without affecting their mood or mental state. And if you suffer from anxiety or depression related to pain, there are many pharmaceuticals that can give you a helping hand, so that you are in a better position to deal with the physical component of your problem. If the total effect of drugs on your life is that they make you more able to function the way you'd like to, then they are a valid and important part of your treatment.

Pharmaceuticals aren't the only game in conventional pain medicine. One procedure that's made news in the past few years is intradiscal electrothermal annuloplasty, or IDET. Early studies indicate that this outpatient technique relieves select kinds of disc-related back pain *70 percent* of the time. Nerve blocks, a kind of deep injection performed by an anesthesiologist, can cool the fierce visceral pain caused by some chronic illnesses. Joint replacements can let arthritic knees manage stairs again. I could go on and on . . . and you can read more about the cream of conventional medicine in Parts III and IV.

IF CONVENTIONAL MEDICINE IS SO EFFECTIVE, WHY DO I STILL HURT?

Despite its remarkable advances, conventional medicine alone just doesn't provide adequate relief for most people. The numbers tell the story: Even though conventional medicine is the first place Americans turn to for help, fifty million of us are still in chronic pain. I believe there are three major reasons for this deficit.

1. ***Conventional medicine is reductionist.*** By "reductionist" I mean that patients are too often treated not as people but as composites of physical units to be attended piecemeal. Our medical schools teach young doctors to think of the body as a machine—a beautiful, intricate machine, but a machine nonetheless. That makes the physician a kind of mechanic or handyman, someone who is called in to fix broken gears or replace faulty pieces. In this scenario, we are reduced to body parts, to the ankle, hip, or muscle that's bothering us—we become "the appendix in room nine" or "the pinched nerve in room one-oh-two."

This philosophy works very well when the body is in a state of acute crisis, such as after an accident or other physical trauma. If someone in my family had a stroke or a broken bone, I'd get them to the emergency room as fast as possible. The doctors there would treat the blocked blood vessel or set the bone. They keep a very narrow, very intense focus on the body part that's been damaged, and it's that technical precision that sees the patient through the crisis.

But the reductionist approach doesn't work very well for chronic pain. If you have a sore hip and your doctor thinks of you as "the hip in room twenty-one," looking only at your hip when diagnosing and treating you, she's going to miss out on the big picture. As I'll explain in more detail in Chapter 3, pain doesn't exist solely in the part that hurts. Your experience of pain also involves your nerves, brain, neurotransmitters, hormones, emotions, thought patterns, relationships, and life history—all the things that make you a unique, whole human being. Medicine that doesn't look at how all these systems work together just isn't optimally equipped to handle pain.

Take stress. Difficult emotions and troubling personal situations can contribute to pain; so, too, can pain create stress for its sufferers. No matter which comes first, the two are notorious for feeding each other. Treatment that doesn't take into account your fear of the next surprise visit from pain or the family crisis that's been hounding you is going to be incomplete at best.

So is treatment that reduces your pain but ignores your quality of life. If a medicine makes you constipated and irritable and forces you to wake up in the middle of the night to take your dose on time, leaving you sleepless until morning . . . well, it might lower your pain level, but it's making your *life* worse.

2. ***Conventional treatments can be too harsh or invasive.*** Let's look at medications first. While I believe that pharmaceuticals have much to offer the person in pain, they also have very real and sometimes intolerable side effects. I know very few people who want to take pills that make them groggy during the day. Other common side effects such as dizziness, constipation, and dry mouth are no fun either. Most worrisome is how casually and exclusively our society relies on drugs—either prescription or over-the-counter—that can produce frightening, even fatal effects.

NANCY'S STORY: WHEN NSAIDS TURN NASTY

Nancy, a forty-nine-year-old mother of three, has been suffering from back pain for years. Nancy can always feel at least a little pain, which she had been controlling with an over-the-counter pain reliever. This medication is from a class called non-steroidal anti-inflammatory

(continued)

drugs, or NSAIDs for short. It's one of the most commonly prescribed classes of drugs in the world, and most of us are familiar with the over-the-counter brand names: Advil, Motrin, Bayer, and others. Many people rely on them just to get through the day.

A few weeks before I saw her, Nancy's pain flared up. Where it once had been bothersome but controllable, it was now nearly paralyzing. She couldn't go shopping, make meals, or take care of her younger children. To get through this rough patch, Nancy increased her daily dose of the NSAID, taking more than was advised on the package. The pain in her back dropped some, but soon Nancy's stomach began to hurt. She consulted her doctor, who immediately recognized the symptoms: The NSAIDs had burned away some of her gastrointestinal tract's outer lining, and blood from this wound was collecting in her stomach.

Nancy's fine now. She went to the emergency room, where doctors used a gastroscope to pinpoint the traumatized area and then cauterize it to stop the bleeding. Nancy was able to go home after a couple of days, but she's going to be weak for a while, which will make her back pain and the rest of her life harder to deal with. And the danger was real. The NSAID could have done its damage just where an artery entered her stomach. When that happens, it's very difficult to stanch the bleeding. More than sixteen thousand people die from NSAIDs every year, approximately the same number as those who die from AIDS. Still, I have hopes that Nancy's finding her way to a chronic pain solution. She's now taking drugs that won't hurt her stomach, and she's learning meditation and breathing exercises to help her take the edge off a flare-up.

I'm not telling you this story to scare you away from NSAIDs (although there may be some other options worth your consideration). Almost every therapy that works also carries some risk; informed risk taking is part of good treatment—and part of life itself. What concerns me is that too many people are led to believe that NSAIDs are completely harmless. Even when they are informed of the risks involved, no one advises them about the gentler therapies available. If you've been relying on NSAIDs, I can help you discover some alternative treatments that will reduce your need for pills, along with your chances of developing this frightening side effect.

Surgeries are a second pillar of conventional pain management. Although surgery is often the wisest option for *acute* pain that's caused by a blood clot or a shattered bone, surgical intervention for *chronic* pain has an extremely poor track record.

BRENT'S STORY: THE FAILED BACK SYNDROME

Brent was a delivery man for a food supply service in Atlanta. Every morning, he'd load his truck and then go on to his rounds of bars and restaurants. At each drop-off point, he would unload some of the cases from the truck and cart them into the kitchen. He was young and healthy, and the intense physical aspect of his job had never been a serious challenge. One day, though, as he was lifting a carton of salsa bottles, he felt something give way in his back. Brent dropped the carton. Some of the bottles broke, and when he tried to stand and fetch a mop, he found he couldn't straighten up.

After a few weeks of rest, Brent still hurt. He went to the company doctor, who referred him to a specialist. The specialist, an orthopedic surgeon, delivered the bad news first. Brent's back required surgery. The good news was that the surgery would fix the problem, and that afterward Brent would be pain-free. Brent agreed to the surgery—it seemed his only option—but the operation did not deliver the promised results. Instead, Brent's first sensation upon coming out of anesthesia was of a blaring pain in his low back. Before his eyes could even focus on his wife, Sandy, seated beside him, he knew something had gone terribly wrong. Not only had the surgery failed, it had made his pain worse.

Instead of making his delivery rounds, Brent spent the next year on the pain circuit, going from doctor to doctor, hoping to find someone who could fix him. He received disability payments, but the checks were only about three-quarters of what he was making previously. Money had been tight before, and now there were medical co-payments and high deductibles to pay. Sandy had to go back to work full time while taking care of him and their children during her off hours. Brent had another surgery to ease the pain caused by the first,

(continued)

this time the last-resort technique of fusing the bones of the spinal column together with metal rods.

Again, the surgery seemed to only make things worse. This time the pain was so intense that Brent would scream whenever he moved. Sandy tried to hang in there with him, but a lifetime of caring for a depressed invalid who was either in a state of rage or a narcotic stupor was more than she could face. By the time Brent arrived in my office, he was divorced and had moved north.

I can't always tell how much people hurt just by looking at them. I have to talk to them, ask them questions, and examine their bodies before I have a clear picture of their suffering. But Brent's pain was a tangible presence in the room. When he walked from the chair to the examining table, he grabbed on to the furniture in agony. His face was pinched, with a dogged look, the kind you might see on veterans of brutal wars. At this point, Brent was thirty-two.

"This isn't right," I said. "There's something off here."

Brent gave me an expressionless stare. Of *course* this wasn't right.

Despite his difficulty moving, Brent allowed me to perform a series of tests, including a bone scan as well as flexion and extension studies. It was hard for me to tell Brent my conclusion. His second surgery, the one he'd undergone to remedy the first, had not been performed correctly. The fusion of the bones had not taken, and the rods were still loose. Every time Brent moved, the metal in his body was scraping against his bones.

Unfortunately, the only solution to this problem was a third surgery. I sent him to a very fine surgeon, who corrected the fusion, and after the surgery Brent's gripping pain was gone. He still had the same pain that was present before the first surgery, however. The third operation had simply corrected the first two.

Brent's case demonstrates two of the problems I have with many surgeries for pain. For one, many of them simply don't address the causes of pain. Brent's symptoms were not, and never had been, those of someone with severe neurological losses, a condition that usually *does* require an operation. There was no indication that surgery would help him. Why, then, did the surgeon operate—and why do so many others continue to operate in similar circumstances? My guess is that these surgeons are caught up in the metaphor of body as machine. They sincerely believe that they can fix it by taking the body apart and putting it together again. They just can't see that such a "fix" isn't always what's best for the patient.

The second problem is that surgeries are invasive procedures by nature, with a much higher risk factor than almost any other pain treatment available. When they go wrong, the consequences can be dire. According to some estimates, as many as 40 percent of spinal fusions and disc removals result in chronic, debilitating pain—pain like Brent's, that's ratcheted up from a dull throb to a piercing scream. There's even a name for this phenomenon: the failed back surgery syndrome. Other risks are present for *any* surgery: infections, bleeding, a bad or even fatal reaction to anesthesia, and other complications. Not to mention that surgery is a highly stressful event that requires a long recovery time.

Once again, I don't feel that operations should *never* be considered for pain. But I do think that conventional medicine relies far too heavily on aggressive treatments such as pharmaceuticals and operations. As you'll see, Brent might have been spared a lot of sorrow if someone had introduced him to gentler medicine as a first course of action, rather than as a last resort.

3. ***Conventional medicine fosters passivity and dependence.*** This is an outgrowth of the body-as-machine idea, the notion that every so often we have to haul ourselves in for repair. We've been conditioned to think that only outside measures—drugs or shots or surgery—performed by professionals can have an effect on us. When we go to the doctor, we submit ourselves to treatment and expect that much of its workings will remain incomprehensible to us. After all, the doctor is the expert. What do we know?

I submit that we actually know a great deal about what our bodies and minds need in order to flourish. Unfortunately, many of us have lost touch with this innate healing intelligence. We've lost faith in our own ability to restore ourselves. We don't trust our bodies when they tell us they need exercise or rest or better food or a break from heavy medication. We start believing that health must be purchased at great cost to our pocketbooks, our dignity, and sometimes our greater well-being.

THE WORLD OF ALTERNATIVES

Perhaps you've already resigned yourself to living with inadequate pain relief or disruptive side effects. If so, I think you'll find that alternative therapies have a great deal to offer you.

Alternative medicine is a staggeringly broad category that encompasses, by definition, health practices that are not taught in Western medical schools. They include folk remedies from American and western European culture; these easily accessible and sometimes even free therapies have been pushed aside by the influence of pharmaceutical companies on our medical schools and by our emphasis on high-tech procedures. Alternative medicine also draws on health systems from other societies, which offer radically different ways of thinking about the body, spirit, health, and disease. In this book I've included only those modalities that have a growing amount of research on their side (some, such as biofeedback, have so much proof that the National Institutes of Health have endorsed them for certain conditions) or that I can vouch for personally, because I've witnessed their clinical effectiveness. Here are four of the reasons you may want to consider including alternative therapies in your pain-relief plan.

1. ***Alternative medicine advocates gentle, natural therapies.*** This quality is especially important in pain management, because people in pain generally need to keep up their treatment for several months or even years. That's a long time to use medications that are harsh or that deliver strong side effects. Gentle treatments are also appealing to people who have other health problems and who feel that their bodies are already flooded with synthetic chemicals.

DESIRETTE'S STORY: A GENTLE TREATMENT FOR PAIN-RELATED INSOMNIA

I met Desirette when she was in the hospital, dying of metastatic breast cancer. She was receiving high doses of conventional pain medicine, but they left her agitated and uncomfortable, unable to sleep at night or even rest comfortably. The hospital staff had suggested she try some sleeping pills, but her brother resisted that option, as he suspected she'd only end up feeling worse. He asked me if there was anything else that could help.

(continued)

I sat at the foot of Desirette's bed and performed reflexology on her feet and hands. Reflexologists massage specific points on the hands and feet that are believed to effect changes in body organs that correspond to those points. (In this respect, it's a little like acupressure or acupuncture.) Soon her body visibly relaxed, and she was breathing deeply and evenly. I taught Desirette's brother how to massage her and also showed him specific acupressure points he could hold to encourage rest and calmness. When I left, Desirette's brother was sitting by her side, stroking her hand gently. That night, Desirette slept soundly for the first time in a week. After she passed away, her brother told me that reflexology made her final days more peaceful. It also comforted him and his family to be of use to Desirette and to stay physically connected to her in the sterile and sometimes intimidating hospital environment.

ARE YOU BALANCED?

The concept of *balance* is important in alternative medicine. How many of the statements below apply to you?

- ☐ I rarely get enough sleep.
- ☐ I live in a city full of noise and air pollution.
- ☐ My work hours are long and hard.
- ☐ I rarely have the time or the taste for a home-cooked meal.
- ☐ I wish I had more warm, personal contact with other people.
- ☐ I'm tired all the time. I don't have the energy I used to.
- ☐ My ideal vacation would be a trip to a deserted island. I'd give anything for a day all by myself with nothing to do.
- ☐ I'm bored. My life lacks stimulation and excitement.
- ☐ I can't remember the last time I got vigorous exercise.

(continued)

If you've checked off any of these items—and many of us would confess to at least two or three—you may be in danger of losing the balance between activity and rest, work and play, stillness and movement, serenity and excitement. What does this have to do with pain?

A healthy, balanced body is stronger and better able to heal itself. An imbalance—whether caused by too little good food, too much work, or constant assaults from the environment—can leave us weak and easily overpowered by germs and injuries. Unfortunately, most of us live in such a way that a healthy balance, in which we're able to ward off contagious illness and debilitating painful conditions, is hard, if not impossible, to maintain.

Alternative medicine attempts to strengthen your body, to improve its resilience and healing power. It does this by restoring you to a state of balance. If you are overwhelmed and overworked, an alternative practitioner may prescribe a quiet therapy, perhaps massage or meditation. If you haven't moved your muscles in a while, yoga or swimming in a tank of warm water may be more in order.

2. ***Alternative medicine treats the whole patient.*** Hippocrates wrote, "It is more important to know the patient than to know the disease that the patient has." A key component of most alternative therapies is the time a practitioner spends getting to know just who you are. During your first appointment, you can often expect a long interview with personal questions that go far beyond the usual "Where does it hurt?" Alternative practitioners take stock of the whole person. They'll ask you how you're sleeping, if the problem is affecting your work or your marriage. Expect questions about your diet, exercise, sources of tension and stress. And if they're truly respectful of your whole being, they'll work with you to find therapies that fit into your schedule, your budget, and your way of life.

3. ***Alternative medicine may not cure your pain—but it sure could heal your life.*** Good alternative healers don't see themselves as warriors against disease; instead, they look back to the word *heal,* which means "to make whole." When we feel fractured and damaged by disease, they want to help us be whole again, to reduce our suffering and stress, to bring our bodies and minds back into alignment. Since pain takes a terrible toll on emotional and psychic well-being, therapies that employ the power of the mind can be quite healing.

MEGAN'S STORY: A PERSON, NOT A HEADACHE

Megan was a graduate student, visiting her parents in their rural home during winter break, when she was suddenly struck by a migraine headache of such enormous force that it literally blinded her, leaving her completely unable to function. "My mother would have to bathe me, and she would have to hold me while I sat on the toilet, because the pain was so bad that I had no balance," she says. She began to worry that something more serious than a migraine was at work.

Her mother drove her to the doctor, who took one look at Megan and announced, "I can tell from looking at her eyes that she doesn't have a brain tumor." With that brisk consolation, he wrote out a prescription. The entire encounter lasted no more than fifteen minutes.

The medication reduced the pain a little, but the migraine continued . . . for seventeen days. For thirteen of those days Megan was completely blind. During the remaining four, she slowly recovered her vision.

Migraines, as you know if you've ever had one, are like earthquakes. There are some rumbles of warning, the big hit, and smaller tremors afterward. You get a migraine, it goes away, and then you get a few smaller ones in the following days or weeks. The bigger the initial migraine, the stronger the headaches that trail them. In Megan's case, the aftershock headaches were as strong as an initial migraine might be for someone else. By mid-January, she had experienced a series of them, each of which laid her up for several days at a time. At this point, she had returned to school. In hopes of better care, she went to her university's health service, which was generally regarded as the gold standard for student-care systems.

"They really couldn't help me," Megan says. "They just couldn't figure out what was wrong. I basically became a guinea pig for migraine drugs. And anytime I took those drugs, I was completely knocked out. For days." She hated the effects of the drugs so much that she discovered her own partial solution. She taught herself how to recognize the warning signs of a migraine—the "rumbles" that precede an earthquake—which for her were a dull pain in her neck

(continued)

followed by lights that flashed in front of her eyes. If she took a double dose of an over-the-counter pain reliever, Megan found, she could often stop the migraine before it overwhelmed her. Nevertheless, the problem didn't completely go away.

A few years later, Megan's studies in political science took her to South Africa, where she was to research her dissertation on the street gangs there. This was high-stress work: Not only did she have to handle the usual pressures of academia, she also had to venture into some of the most violent townships in the country, where it was not unusual to hear gunfire in the streets. One day she was driving alone from Cape Town to Johannesburg. This ten-hour trip across the desert must be made straight through; friends had warned Megan that for a woman alone, there were no safe opportunities to stop. Soon after her trip got under way, Megan's neck began to hurt, and she saw lights flashing. She had forgotten to bring any pain relievers with her, so she had to keep driving, navigating as best she could around the splotches in her vision field. She arrived safely, but the trip had been grueling.

By this point in her life, Megan had nearly given up on doctors for pain relief. But after her frightening cross-country experience and several more days with the migraine, she decided to make an appointment with her housemate's physician.

The South African doctor was like none other that Megan had ever encountered. According to Megan, "He sat down and he started to ask me about my medical history in a way that no doctor really had. He *literally* sat down and we had a conversation. He asked question after question." He asked her not just about her symptoms but about her entire life, even those things that might not obviously connect to her headache. He asked Megan about her childhood—what sports she'd played and whether she'd even been in any accidents. They also talked about her life in the present—what she did for a living, the way she sat in her chair, the kind of computer screen she used, what she did for relaxation and exercise, and so on. This stood in stark comparison with her previous experiences, when doctors would spend no more than twenty minutes at a time—if that—with her, even during the initial consultation.

The doctor's conclusion came as something of a surprise, but in the way of most revelations, it quickly began to make sense. He told

(continued)

her that she wasn't suffering from migraines at all. Instead, he suspected that her problems dated back to a serious car accident Megan had been in when she was sixteen. She had had whiplash at the time, but she had been living on an island without access to good medical care, so the problem was never properly understood or treated. Over the years, the pressure had built up in her neck until it began to reverberate up into her head. This pain was identical to that of a migraine.

At first, the doctor prescribed a painkiller for Megan. When that didn't help, Megan expected him to give her a second medication. Instead, he suggested Megan try traction to relieve the pressure on her neck. For some people, the word *traction* conjures up images of skiing accidents, full-body casts, and a sadistic-looking set of wires and pulleys. But in most cases, a traction device is simply used to pull gently on your head and neck, and the therapy can be performed for just a few minutes at a time. It stretches out your soft tissues, opens up spaces between the joints, and allows the discs of the spinal cord to receive more fluid. Megan went in for one traction appointment that afternoon, and by the end of the session, her headache had vanished. She'd never had an initial migraine that disappeared after only a day or two, and certainly none of her headaches had ever stopped on a dime before. The headache did not return, she experienced no side effects from the treatment, and there were no aftershock headaches in the coming months. Megan has now learned to nearly eliminate her debilitating headaches and most of her neck pain by regularly using a gravity table—a device that allows Megan to lie flat with her head at a lower level than her feet—to relieve the compression that builds up in her muscles and bones.

Megan is someone who never let pain get in the way of her life. Aside her from own perseverance, what made the difference for Megan was having a doctor who saw her as a person, not as "the migraine in room four." Her doctor in South Africa—where there is less money for pharmaceuticals but more time to spend on patients—had the wisdom to look beyond the symptoms to the whole life that existed around them. As Megan says, "What makes the difference, what will solve the problem, is to *really* understand the person and their life." That's one of the best reasons to seek out alternative modes of healing.

Although the traction and eventually the gravity table addressed the physical source of Megan's headaches, there's no doubt in her mind that the quiet, meditative time she spent participating in these therapies reduced her stress level and helped keep the headaches at bay.

Brent, who underwent the three surgeries for his back, also discovered that mind-body techniques can be truly healing. His final surgery, which corrected the mistakes of the first two, stopped his worst pain. But he still suffered from a great deal of distress and remained unable to work or socialize. He was isolated, depressed, and frightened about what would happen to him. I prescribed some medication that would help quiet his nerves, which were misfiring and hypersensitive from years of intractable pain, and that helped. But, after much resistance, he also agreed to try some relaxation techniques, including meditation. Brent, who would roll his eyes whenever the subject of alternative medicine came up, found he *loved* to meditate! The quiet focus and contemplation could reduce the pain of a flare-up and his need for medication; when he practiced it on a regular basis, it kept his daily pain down to a quite bearable level. Ultimately, he told me, the mind-body techniques were the most effective pain relievers he'd ever used. They also helped him gain control over the other aspects of his life that had been damaged by pain. He was able to dramatically reduce his anxiety, and he became an easier, friendlier person to be with. He reestablished contact with some old friends and got up the energy and focus to enter a retraining program at work.

Did meditation cure Brent? I don't think so. He still had pain, for one thing, and a lot of credit is owed to pharmaceuticals for his overall success. But meditation may very well have *healed* Brent. That is, it showed him how to take control of his pain, rather than letting it control him and his emotions. It helped make him whole again.

4. ***Alternative medicine encourages you to take responsibility for your health.*** Alternative medicine emphasizes personal responsibility and the belief that you are in the best position to know what's best for your body and your life. Instead of submitting yourself to a professional, you're encouraged to learn about your condition, to do what's necessary to keep yourself well, and to know when you need to call on outside help. During those times, you're expected to be an active partner with your health care provider as you work out a plan to restore your health.

So many pain patients have spent years visiting doctor after doctor, submitting to one treatment after another. When you start working with someone who expects you to be an active partner, your whole perspective can change. Instead of expecting someone else to give you a "fix," you come to expect that healing resides within you—even if, as in the case of Brent, you can't be 100 percent pain-free. Both Megan and Brent learned that relief came more quickly when they brainstormed with their doctors and talked with them about their needs and goals. It's a much more satisfying way to approach your own health care.

BRING YOUR SAVVY WITH YOU

Alternative medicine does have its drawbacks. For one, the sheer number of options is bewildering. Where do you start? With acupuncture or biofeedback? Should you try homeopathy, herbalism, chiropractic, or some form of touch healing? Alternative medicine encompasses an astonishing variety of techniques and philosophies, some of which directly contradict the views of the others. Some therapies are better for certain kinds of problems and certain kinds of people than others. Some are just bad news, no matter who you are. How do you know which are safe and appropriate?

It's also true that the foreign quality of some of the treatments can be intimidating. Acupuncture is probably the most obvious example: Most of us just aren't accustomed to getting stuck with pins. Reiki, a Japanese technique that incorporates the laying on of hands as a means of enhancing a person's energy field, can seem like outright fraud to most Westerners. (I think it's the phrase "energy field" that gets most people snickering.) It can be helpful to remember that these treatments are indeed foreign—but only to us. To millions of Chinese people, for example, acupuncture isn't alternative; it's simply medicine. The same goes for Reiki in Japan. The challenge is to sort out the strange but legitimate from the stuff that's just plain strange.

It's hard to imagine someone suffering severe problems as a result of meditation or therapeutic touch. Nevertheless, some alternative therapies harbor potential dangers or side effects. Herbs are generally safer than pharmaceuticals, but the reason they work is that they contain active chemical products—and any chemical potent enough to make you better is also strong enough to do some damage, especially if mixed with other herbs or conventional medications. Chiropractic techniques have been known to injure people; even yoga can hurt you if you try the more advanced poses before you're ready. And we must always face the sad truth that alternative medicine attracts its share of fraudulent practitioners who have little other than the bottom line—not your health and safety—in mind.

You can avoid many of these pitfalls simply by understanding your condition and becoming an informed consumer. You can learn which therapies are most likely to help you, what to expect from them, how to identify a legitimate practitioner if you need one, and how to work with your doctor to make sure you don't run into trouble. I hope to help you do all these things.

INTEGRATIVE MEDICINE: THE BEST OF BOTH WORLDS

Conventional medicine has excellent diagnostic tools and some of the most effective pain-relieving drugs we know of. Alternative medicine is gentle, empowering, and ideal for treating complicated conditions that involve your whole life. Do you have to choose?

Practitioners of integrative medicine know that conventional and alternative treatments actually make a good team. Each is strong where the other is weak; used intelligently, an integrative practice will bring out the best of each approach. At the very least, integrative medicine for pain greatly expands your options, as doctors and patients have the combined menus of therapies at their disposal. Here are a few of the many ways I've seen people employ integrative medicine for pain control:

- Combining nutrition, exercise, and mind-body medicine for day-to-day pain management, with a pharmaceutical prescription in case of a flare-up

- Taking a milder daily pharmaceutical but adding alternative methods such as massage, acupuncture, or mind-body strategies during times of severe pain

- Using acupuncture, massage, or dietary changes to reduce the side effects of conventional treatments

- Relying on conventional techniques for diagnosis but employing alternative methods for treatment

Many people improve their conditions greatly just by mixing one or two alternative treatments with their conventional medications. But you'll get the most out of integrative medicine when you approach it as an entirely new philosophy of health care. Integrative medicine is a recognition that pain intersects with *all* of you—your body, your mind, and your whole life. It addresses malfunctioning neurotransmitters as well as soaring stress levels. It uses the latest techniques to examine your nerves, your brain, your muscles, your hormones—but it also acknowledges that drugs to cure your physical ills don't do your life much good if they also knock you out. It involves trial and error, because it recognizes that you're an individual whose treatment isn't going to be like anyone else's. It demands more from the patient, who must be educated, active, and responsible, but it also asks the health care provider to treat people in pain as human beings. Above all, it's an art, a skillful blending of therapies and calibration of doses that suits your unique needs.

The most important factor in pain relief is your commitment to healing. That you're reading this book already demonstrates your interest in doing more for yourself. Chapter 3 will help you take the next step. It offers a new perspective on the nature of your pain and how it works its way through your body and your life.

3.

WHERE DOES IT HURT? THE NEW MODEL OF PAIN

When you don't understand how pain works in your body, it can come to seem like a supernatural force—something dark and capricious that can strike at any moment, snatching away your pleasure and productivity at a whim. That pain is invisible both to the casual observer and to the most sophisticated laboratory equipment only enhances this sense of mystery. Like religion, pain has to be taken on faith by your doctors, family, and friends. And in fact I've seen many patients who treat pain as if it's an angry god who must be appeased at all costs. They say things like "I'm afraid to walk down the stairs today. What if my arthritis punishes me with more pain tomorrow?" or "I'm not going to the party. If I stay home, maybe my sciatica will reward me with a good night's sleep." Some people devote their entire lives to keeping this force at bay.

There are some pains that seem especially mysterious. Take David, who put his back out two years ago while moving some furniture for his parents. Repeated scans and tests have indicated that his injury has long since healed, but his pain levels continue to ratchet upward. Then there's Marian, who's felt horrible pelvic pain for several months now. Her doctor has told her there's nothing wrong with her. Both David and Marian, and millions of others like them, live not only with pain but with fear: that they have a serious disorder that's gone undetected, or that they have somehow "made up" their affliction with their minds.

Most people feel much easier once they have a basic understanding of the nervous system and how pain travels through it. This is true no matter what your underlying condition, because knowledge dispels much (although probably not all) of the mystery, giving you more mastery and control. This understanding is especially important if you've been told that you're feeling an inappropriate level of pain, or that there's no reason you should be hurting at all. The information here may relieve your mind. It should also point you toward more-effective therapies.

Later in this book, I will devote a chapter to each of the most common painful disorders. In this chapter, I want to introduce you to the new scientific insights that apply to every painful condition—that is, how an electrical signal sent out by a nerve turns into the unpleasant feeling we call pain. I'm calling special attention to this topic because it's the aspect of pain medicine that is most misunderstood by doctors and others, and it's also the one that offers the most chances for reversing pain.

THE OLD MODEL OF PAIN

Suppose you're walking through the kitchen when you trip over the cat-food dish. You lose your balance and stumble forward. Your first instinct is to steady yourself, and without thinking, you reach out toward the nearest solid object, which happens to be the red-hot stovetop. You feel burning pain. You scream. You pull your hand off the burner.

So where does it hurt? On one level, the answer is clear. The palm of your hand is where it hurts, and no doubt about it.

For centuries, scientists agreed that this was the right answer—and the only answer. Their theory went like this: Pain is the result of an injury to a body part. When you're injured, the nerves of the damaged area send a message of pain up along the spinal cord to the brain, where the message is received and read. In this scenario, the injured part is where the message is written, and the nervous system is just a passive conductor of an electric impulse (the pain message), much like a telephone wire.

The problem with this theory is that it can't account for many common and not-so-common experiences. For instance, a study of Civil War soldiers found that new amputees reported hardly any pain at all, despite having undergone crude operations. Apparently the soldiers were so relieved at leaving the battlefield alive that their pain barely mattered. And it has long been well known that in times of danger, the body can ignore pain. People who are running for their lives down a dark alley might not feel a sprained ankle, at least not until they've made it to safety. This survival mechanism keeps attention focused on the number-one priority, escaping. In both of these situations, it's clear that the pain signal has changed. Somewhere on the way to the brain, the message is altered or stopped.

It doesn't take a life-threatening situation or a battlefield mentality to elicit a modified pain response. Have you ever done any of the following?

- Bitten your lip to temporarily drown out a throbbing headache
- Rubbed a bumped elbow to dull the pain
- Forgotten about your pain while absorbed in a movie or a book
- Noticed your pain feels worse after eating certain foods
- Felt increased pain after a night of insomnia or a hard day at work

This list demonstrates just a few of the ways that pain can change as it moves through your nervous system. In the face of these common experiences, the old theory just doesn't hold. There's more—a lot more—going on than a message passing from one end of a wire to another.

THE NEW MODEL OF PAIN

In the past four decades, many scientists decided the old theory was simply unacceptable, and they began to experiment and lay the groundwork for a new way of thinking. We don't know everything about how pain works, but there's enough information now to make a difference for most sufferers. This new model of pain demonstrates that pain doesn't happen only in the part of your body that hurts. You may have burned your palm, but that's not where your pain really lives. Pain makes its home throughout your nervous system: in your nerves, your spinal cord, your internal chemistry, and your brain. In some instances, very real pain occurs when there's no damage to the body whatsoever. The nervous system generates the pain all by itself.

(It's possible, for example, to feel genuine pain in a body part that's been amputated—try explaining *that* using the old theory.) The question then becomes: How can you use this knowledge to block or reduce pain?

Over the next pages, I'll show you some of the most exciting discoveries, the ones that can help you and your doctor step in and change—or even delete—the pain message. They include:

- The pain gateway—how pain travels through the spinal cord
- Endorphins—the body's natural painkillers
- Neurotransmitters—pain's postal system
- Hypersensitized nerves—how a breeze can feel like a burn
- Spontaneous firing—when nerves yell "pain" without prompting
- The brain—pain, suffering, and your soul

CLOSING THE GATE ON PAIN

The first major breakthrough in our understanding of pain came when two scientists, Ronald Melzack and Patrick Wall, discovered that pain messages can be altered or stopped in the spinal cord on their way to the brain.

The old model of pain implies that there's a designated "pain pathway," a special set of nerves that conducts pain signals to and from the brain. The reality is that different kinds of sensations travel the same path, and how much pain you feel—if any at all—is determined by how they share the road.

Nerves make up this pain "roadway." Most nerves branch out from your spinal cord to your skin and other body tissues. There, they end in microscopic receptors, each of which is sensitive to a specific kind of sensation, not just pain but also light touch, sharp touch, vibration, and so on. When a sensation triggers the appropriate nerve receptor, the receptor translates it into an electrical impulse that shoots along the length of the nerve.

The electrical impulse travels along the nerve and ultimately reaches its first destination, the spinal cord. Here, the impulse meets up with all the other signals that are coming into your body at the same time: information about temperature, touch, vibration, and other sensations.

Different sensations, same pathway. This is where the old model of pain really begins to break down.

Melzack and Wall discovered that at the back of the spinal cord, a structure called the dorsal horn acts as a gateway for all the messages that are trying to pass through. Certain events can open the gate, so that the message passes up the spinal cord to your brain; others will close the gate and stop the signals in their tracks. Since they don't make it up to your brain, you never perceive them. You can learn to control this gate and reduce how much pain passes through.

Certain kinds of sensations travel faster through the nervous system than others. Dull pain travels along the nerve at a relatively slow pace, from half a mile to two miles per second. Sharp or burning pain clocks in at anywhere between five and thirty miles per second. The nonpainful sensation of touch, including pressure and massage, travels fastest: thirty-five to seventy-five miles every second. When we're talking about seconds, any difference can seem trifling. But it turns out that the gating mechanism in the spinal cord is triggered by relative speed. If you have more than one kind of sensation entering your dorsal horn at the same time, the faster one will win out, blocking the transmission of the slower one.

HOW FAST IS A FEELING?

TYPE OF SENSATION	SPEED (IN MILES PER SECOND)
Dull pain or itching	0.5–2.0
Sharp or burning pain	5–35
Touch	35–75

That's why you automatically rub or apply pressure to an injured area: The rubbing sensation travels faster than the painful one and beats it to the gate. And if you've ever tried to stop a throbbing headache by biting your lip or digging your fingernails into your skin, you now know that your actions are backed up by biology: The sharp injury trumps the slower pain from the headache.

There are many ways you can take advantage of this knowledge. Massage therapy can limit the pain of a nasty flare-up and can help you avoid taking a higher dose of pills. Herbal remedies made with capsaicin, the active ingredient in hot peppers, can be applied topically to deliver a slight and even pleasant heating sensation that blocks achy or sharp pain. Many of the therapies described in Chapter 10, "Distracting Your Nervous System from Pain," include those that replace the sensation of pain with something else.

Michael, a Long Island police officer who had suffered a back injury on the job, found a high-tech way to close the gate on pain. Exercises, pharmaceuticals, and acupuncture had helped, but he still had more pain than he could tolerate. His physical therapist suggested transcutaneous electrical nerve stimulation, or TENS for short. In TENS therapy, a device that delivers mild electrical stimulation is positioned at the base of the spine. The electric sensation doesn't hurt, but it does travel faster than the painful sensation. In Michael's case, the TENS unit closed the gate on pain almost completely, even when injections and medications had failed.

ENDORPHINS

While pain signals are traveling up the spinal cord, your nervous system is also sending chemical messages *down*. These messages, which are produced in the brain and released in the spinal cord, have the power to affect the gating mechanism. Usually they reduce the amount of pain you're feeling, but they can also halt it completely. We haven't yet identified every chemical that's involved, and there are many, but the most famous class of substances has a pain-blocking effect that's almost identical to that of morphine. These substances are popularly known as *endorphins,* and their existence proves that we have the ability to produce our own pain relief. (In clinical circles, these substances are known as endogenous opioids, meaning opioids produced in the body, and the word *endorphin* describes just one particular example of those substances. Here, I'll use the word's broader, popular definition.) There's more good news: Unlike morphine, endorphins don't produce harsh side effects such as extreme sleepiness and constipation.

Endorphins work by activating the opioid receptors on nerve cells, reducing pain and lifting mood. They may also block substance P, a neurotransmitter involved in communicating pain. (I'll talk more about neurotransmitters very soon.) We also know that the release of endorphins is associated with certain mental states. A rush of relief or joy can trigger the release of endorphins; it's well known, for example, that people who are in a state of sexual or religious ecstasy simply don't feel pain the way the rest of us do. That's partly because they're too absorbed in their own happiness to be bothered with pain, but also because their brains are producing high doses of endorphins, which block the pain signal in the spinal cord. (This also explains how overwhelming relief stopped the pain of the amputee Civil War soldiers.) More moderate mental states, such as serenity or full engagement in a pleasing activity, can also result in endorphin release.

In fact, when your body is working properly, almost all pain signals are inhibited at least a little bit by endorphins. This is true for minor pain, such as that from cuts and scrapes, and big pain from serious injuries. You can think of endorphins and the other chemicals at work here as a kind of automatic braking system for pain, either slowing it down or bringing it to a full stop. But consider this: If you ride the brakes on your four-thousand-pound sport-utility vehicle every time you go out for a drive, eventually those brakes will wear out and the truck will go barreling down the road at top speed. If your nervous system is overworked by constant pain, its equivalent of brakes—the endorphins and other chemicals—loses its effectiveness. Your pain heads full strength toward your brain.

I've seen this happen to lots of people with ongoing disorders such as arthritis. First, their pain is unpleasant but manageable, but as their braking system wears down, it becomes absolutely unbearable. They also become more sensitive to other kinds of pain as well, and gradually they start to suffer from all kinds of aches that might not have bothered them before.

Other factors can inhibit endorphins, too. Stress, depression, and inactivity—all of which can *result* from pain—will keep you from getting the maximum relief your body can provide. The pain builds on itself, leading to behaviors and mental states that increase your suffering.

Happily, there are many therapies available to help you stimulate endorphin production, even if your braking system has been worn out. I like yoga for its combination of physical motion and stress reduction, which together really get your endorphins going, but a brisk walk in the fresh air can also do wonders. Massage, acupuncture, acupressure, and reflexology are also good choices. You might be surprised to hear that one of the best ways to produce endorphins is to get absorbed in a good story. I know many people who can temporarily block out the worst pain of a flare-up—and avoid taking extra medication—by reading a detective novel or watching a Hitchcock thriller.

WOULD YOU CHOOSE TO BE PAIN-FREE?

Some people are born without the ability to feel pain at all. When you're suffering from chronic pain, this syndrome, congenital insensitivity to pain, can sound like a blessing. That is, until you consider how dangerous everyday life would be if you couldn't rely on pain's warning of danger. Infants with this syndrome may bite their tongues repeatedly, because pain doesn't tell them to stop. Their taste buds can be permanently damaged as a result. Children who hurt themselves while climbing trees or riding their bicycles don't run to their parents for help—they simply keep playing with a broken bone or an open wound. Nor do they ever learn to associate certain situations, such as playing barefoot on sharp rocks or a splintery surface, with pain and injury. Without pain to alert them to danger, it's hard for people to make it to adulthood alive.

NEUROTRANSMITTERS

According to the old model of pain, a message is sent along a wire and then received by the brain. As we now know, that's just not true. Not only do different signals compete along the same path (see "Closing the Gate on Pain," page 32), but the wire along which the message travels isn't like the copper stuff behind the walls of your house—it isn't a solid unit. Instead, it's made up of individual nerve cells. It's literally live wire.

Moreover, none of those nerve cells actually touches the others, so the pain signal has to jump across a gap from one nerve cell to the next, and then to the next, and so on. The signal is aided in this function by neurotransmitters, chemicals that transmit information between two nerve cells. Let's compare neurotransmitters to the postal system in my New York City neighborhood. The nerve cell sends off a neat little package, stamped and sealed, and most of the time the information is delivered to its recipient, the second nerve cell, still looking fresh and tidy. But sometimes the message is changed en route. The neurotransmitters—the postal carriers—may choose not to deliver the message at all. Or they may deliver it in such a way that it's unrecognizable—beat-up, rained-on, squashed—as the package that the first neuron sent out. They may even speed up the message and present it with a flourish and extra attention. (Okay, so they're not *always* like the postal system.) If the message is pain, you'll want to encourage neurotransmitters to "lose" the message, just as postal carriers can "lose" packages that federal agents later find in their basements. If the message is one that blocks pain, you'll want that message delivered loud and clear and as quickly as possible.

NEUROTRANSMITTERS AND PAIN

Below are four neurotransmitters that appear to have significant roles in pain, along with some ways you can encourage them to "lose" pain's message or to enhance a message of relief.

NAME	HOW IT AFFECTS PAIN	WHAT INCREASES IT	WHAT DECREASES IT
Serotonin	May reduce perception of pain; a deficiency can cause insomnia, depression, and anxiety	Certain foods, medications, mind-body techniques, sleep, exercise	Inherited deficiency; lack of sleep; mood disorders
GABA	Inhibits pain; encourages relaxation and sleep	Exercise, sleep, medications	Inherited deficiency; lack of exercise; lack of sleep
Substance P	Promotes pain	Nerve receptors signaling unpleasant sensation	Dietary therapy; herbs; massage and other physical contact; medications; mind-body techniques
Dopamine	Decreases pain in some cases	Medications; possibly exercise	Possibly, profound physical stress (as in surgery) and lack of sleep

When neurotransmitters are thrown off balance and start producing more or less than they should, they can prevent normal, short-term pain from fading away. This is an important point: Neurotransmitters can help create a message of pain *even after an injury has healed or when there's no injury at all.* And they can intensify the pain of an existing injury or illness. As you can see from the chart, they may also contribute to some of the most frequent side effects of pain—insomnia and depression—which in turn make the pain feel even worse.

HYPERSENSITIZED NERVES

I was the fourth doctor Rick had seen. He'd gone to a general practitioner, an anesthesiologist, and an orthopedic surgeon, but no one had been able to figure out what made his back hurt so much. He'd thrown it out while doing some chores, but that was a year ago. Now the smallest of motions felt like a punishment. Sometimes even the touch of his shirt against his skin sent him into agony. Rick was terrified he might have a bone infection or a pinched nerve, maybe even a tumor, but every scan and X ray had come up negative.

Rick's case is by no means unusual. The frustration and fear Rick experienced were due to his quite understandable assumption that the intense pain in his back must indicate a serious injury to that area. I agreed that something was terribly wrong, but the problem was not in his back—nor was it all in his head. Simply put, Rick's nerves had rewired themselves in such a way that they transmitted erroneous messages of pain. If you have pain that doctors find mysterious, or if your pain is more severe than seems appropriate for your condition, it's possible that your problem is at least partly the result of nerves that have been hypersensitized.

This points to another way in which the nerves are not like telephone wire: Because our wiring is made up of living units, it can actually change—sometimes for short periods of time, sometimes for years. (Scientists call this *plasticity*.) Sometimes the nervous system changes in such a way that it feels *less* pain: As you saw at the beginning of this chapter, it can ignore body damage such as a sprained ankle when you're running for your life. But your nervous system can also be altered so that it becomes overly sensitive. This is what happened to Rick. Normally, our bodies can easily distinguish between low-intensity stimuli, such as light touch or low-grade pain, and high-intensity ones, such as muscle damage. Rick's nerves could no longer make that distinction, and now his nerves confused movement or the touch of fabric with massive injury.

Although we don't yet fully understand how nerves become hypersensitized, we do know people with nerve damage are at risk. But so are people who've simply received a long-lasting blast of acute pain. It appears that after a severe injury or other lengthy encounter with pain, some cells may die off, while others lose their old connections and make new ones that are less appropriate. Some activate new chemical messengers that make them more sensitive to pain. There may be more contact at the gaps between the nerve cells (this is one reason neurotransmitter release, which occurs in these gaps, sometimes goes awry), and the mechanisms that normally keep pain at a proper level are blocked.

All of these changes mean that the signal going up to the brain is greatly amplified. It's as if you've turned the dial on your stereo to a low volume—say, 2 or 3—but your speakers are booming out at 9 or 10. You can turn the dial all the way down, or you can even try unplugging your stereo, but the speakers just keep going. The pain may spread across a larger area of the body. In extreme cases, a person with rewired nerves may find it painful to make any movements at all, or even to breathe.

We are just beginning to understand the role of emotions in hypersensitization. We can't say for sure yet, but there's some evidence that high levels of panic, fear, or anger—all of which are natural reactions to severe pain—contribute to alterations in the nervous system. This probably makes some evolutionary sense: In effect, your brain senses so much danger from the pain that it tells the body to keep the pain signal coming. It's a way of keeping the whole system on high alert. For some unfortunate people, though, this sensitized nervous system is unable to return to its normal state after the crisis has passed.

The most effective therapy for hypersensitization pain is a solid understanding of it. Most people feel great relief at learning they are neither crazy nor terribly ill. Over time, this calmness can be instrumental in returning the nervous system to normal. There are pharmaceutical options, including low doses of anticonvulsants and tricyclic antidepressants, for handling this kind of pain; many people have also found that breathing exercises or meditation helps them tune the shrieking sound of nerve noise down to a quiet background hum.

WHAT'S YOUR PAIN TOLERANCE?

The test below demonstrates that pain is a changeable sensation, one that different people feel in different ways. Take it only if you're in general good health and don't have a serious medical condition or any disorder that disturbs the nerves or blood vessels. This includes conditions such as diabetes, Raynaud's disease or phenomenon,

(continued)

heart disease, peripheral vascular disease, and collagen vascular disease.

To test your tolerance for cold pain, you'll need a large basin, cold water, ice, a thermometer, and a timer. Fill the basin with the water and ice until the water temperature reaches 32 degrees Fahrenheit.

Set the timer for two minutes. Then immerse your arm in the cold water. Note when you first begin to perceive the cold as pain; this is known as your *pain threshold*. Then see how much time elapses before you need to pull your arm out; this is your *pain tolerance*. Do not keep your arm in longer than two minutes, or you'll risk harming yourself.

How long did you keep your arm in the water? A famous study has shown that some groups of people have different pain thresholds and tolerances from others. For example, female college students had a pain threshold of sixteen seconds and a tolerance of thirty-seven seconds, but female ballet dancers, who have daily experience with pain, went three times as long before either feeling pain or hitting their tolerance. If you have friends or family members who are game, ask them to try the experiment and compare notes. Most likely, you'll have very different thresholds and levels of tolerance.

Once you've written down your initial set of times, you might want to try some techniques that can change how you feel cold-water pain. Do any of the strategies below extend your pain threshold or tolerance? (Let at least an hour go by before repeating the test, as the blood vessel changes produced by the cold water can last for a while.)

- ☐ While one arm is in the water, have a friend vigorously rub or scratch your other arm.
- ☐ Focus on your breathing. Breathe in to a count of four, hold the breath for four counts, breathe out for another four counts, and then wait for four more counts until inhaling again.
- ☐ Put on a headset and listen to your favorite music.

SPONTANEOUS FIRING

Just as nerves can become hypersensitive to events that are normally not painful, they can also broadcast pain messages in the absence of any stimulus whatsoever. This cruel phenomenon is known as spontaneous firing.

Phantom limb pain is an extreme example of spontaneous firing. A person has a body part amputated, either by accident or by surgical procedure, and then begins to feel pain that seems to be located in that missing part. Phantom limb pain is *not* the normal pain that's felt at the point of severance. Instead, a person with a missing arm may report an unbearable burning sensation in the second knuckle of her first finger, or in her elbow.

According to the old model of pain, this just doesn't make sense. How can you hurt in a part that doesn't exist? Because phantom limb victims didn't fit into that model, it was assumed that their pain was purely psychological, an expression of grief for the missing body part. But if you know that pain is created in places other than the part that hurts, you can see how phantom limb pain is possible. It seems that when a nerve's original destination is gone, two things can happen. First, the part of the brain that's set up to control the amputated part goes a little crazy. Without normal sensory signals from the missing hand or foot coming in to govern them, the brain cells that are dedicated to that part may start acting like a roomful of unruly kids without a teacher, activating spontaneously. Second, the nerves that once led to the missing part don't just fizzle out and lie dormant. Instead, they try to form new connections, sometimes in such a way that they confuse themselves and send out pain signals for no real reason. Even nerves that are cut off in the amputation can come back from the dead—and like all good ghosts, they spend lots of time wailing and rattling their chains.

You don't have to be an amputee to experience spontaneous nerve firing. Anyone with nerve damage can fall victim. People with trigeminal neuralgia, postherpetic neuralgia, kidney disease, and spinal cord disorders are candidates; nerve damage can also result from chemotherapy drugs and other medications, gunshot wounds, and major accidents, among other things. This kind of nerve-generated pain, which doctors call neuropathic pain, has a distinctive and horrific quality: It burns, sears, and shoots—and some people choose to take their own lives rather than face it on a daily basis.

Not so long ago, neuropathic pain was considered impossible to treat. Very recently, though, pain doctors have been getting good results with drugs traditionally meant to block seizures in people with epilepsy. These drugs settle down nerves that squawk, sometimes to the point where they stop misfiring altogether. Many people with neuropathic pain have also found that they can use mental disciplines to drown out the hurt. As you'll see, it's also important to subdue the alarm bells that pain sets off in the mind. This is a task that's easier to accomplish once you understand that nerve pain isn't signaling danger. It's just an incorrect message.

THE BRAIN: WHERE PAIN GETS PERSONAL

The brain holds the final—and potentially most important—pieces of the new pain model. Let's say that you've sustained a minor injury, perhaps a paper cut from turning a page of this book. You don't have any nerve damage or hypersensitivity, so everything works normally: The sharp-pain receptors in your finger send signals to the nerves attached to them, and those nerves and their neurotransmitters conduct the sensation up to the spinal cord. Because you're not experiencing any other major waves of sensation right now, the sharp-pain message passes through the gate with no trouble. It travels up the nerves of the spinal cord and into the thalamus.

But do you feel pain?

Pain's not a given once the signal enters your brain. The thalamus routes the pain signal to multiple sites, each of which influences how we respond to it. The brain can also choose to ignore the signal entirely. If you've ever seen children playing out in the cold, packing snowballs without their mittens and rolling around in slushy puddles for hours, you know how joy and excitement can check pain. Professional athletes routinely play on ripped muscles and fractured bones. Their practiced focus allows them to feel less pain than you or I might. And you've probably heard of monks who walk over hot coals as a way of testing the mind's control over pain.

How much pain you feel and how much it bothers you are determined to a large extent by mental processes. I've already mentioned several ways that mental states can enhance or diminish physiological responses that affect pain. Runaway stress apparently has the power to reduce endorphins and reset your nervous system entirely. Serenity and mental engagement can stimulate pain-blocking endorphins, and mind-body techniques can alter your levels of neurotransmitters. You can also follow the lead of those athletes and fire-walking monks, who learn mental disciplines to help turn their attention away from pain.

SUFFERING

Suffering is often used as a synonym for *pain,* but the two are actually quite separate. Pain is the physical hurt. Suffering is the human experience of pain, the degree to which it affects your quality of life. Your fingers or neck might ache or burn—that's pain—but if that achiness or burning sensation makes you frustrated, sleepless, or fearful of the next flare-up, you *suffer.* There are people who feel pain without suffering much. It hovers constantly in the background, and it's not pleasant, but it doesn't control their moods or their actions.

Ironically, the people who don't let pain get to them are often those who have the most devastating disorders. When the novelist and poet Reynolds Price was hit with spinal cancer and resulting paralysis, his pain was at a level that's unimaginable to most of us. But, as he recounts in his book *A Whole New Life,* he eventually developed an attitude toward pain that allowed him to write, sleep, paint, teach, and enjoy his friends. He actually increased his artistic activity. His pain is always there, but it no longer dictates the terms of his days.

I'm confident that you'll find therapies to reduce your pain, maybe even eliminate it. But I also hope you'll pursue techniques to reduce your suffering. Many of them are cheap and readily accessible, and the majority of them draw on the immense power of your mind.

The Limbic System

When you feel pain, your limbic system is automatically activated. The limbic system is the oldest and most primitive part of the brain, and it controls your feelings as well as the actions of your involuntary nervous system. At the receipt of the pain signal, your limbic system kicks out a powerful array of emotions, making you feel panicked, angry, scared, or sad. The limbic system also triggers the release of hormones that affect your physical state. Your heart beats faster, your blood pressure skyrockets, your muscles tense up, and blood is diverted from your digestive system to your arms and legs. These changes—in conjunction with the strong emotions—are known as the fight-or-flight response, and they help us run, fight, or otherwise spring into action. When pain is acute, this response gives us the ability to lift concrete pipes off a trapped leg, jump out of a burning building, or run for medical help.

But when pain is chronic, there is no fire that's burning your back, no concrete pipe that's mangling your limbs and making you hurt. In short, there's nothing you can escape from. As you have seen, the pain message sometimes doesn't even signal bodily damage; it may well be the result of rewired or misfiring nerves. Even when chronic pain *is* the result of injury or illness, the limbic system's response becomes counterproductive once you're under good medical care.

The limbic system's reactions are meant to be temporary. When they don't go away, or when they occur repeatedly, they begin to wear you and your body down. Most people in pain develop secondary problems as a result of the mind's response, including:

- Depression or anxiety
- Rage or irritability
- Fatigue
- Insomnia
- High blood pressure
- Digestive troubles
- Headaches, neck aches, backaches, or other pains from chronic muscle tension
- Weakened immune functioning

And so chronic pain can beget a seemingly endless downward spiral. You have nagging arthritis pain, your limbic system triggers a continuous stream of aggressive hormones, and now you have arthritis *and* headaches and insomnia. This extra pain and body weakness affects your production of endorphins and neurotransmitters and even begins to make some changes to your nervous system. Soon your arthritis pain feels much worse than it ever did, and on top of everything else, you're too worn out and cranky to socialize anymore. Your friends stop calling. More than anything else, this cycle can send your life spinning out of control.

One of the best ways to lessen your suffering is to tone down your limbic system's response to pain and other forms of stress. People who have certain kinds of damage to their limbic system report that although they can still feel painful stimuli, the pain itself doesn't really disturb them. They're aware when they receive a wound, but it's a cool, distant knowledge, without the panic or fear that we usually associate with such situations. The pain is there, but it has no control over their feelings or their lives; that is, they don't *suffer*. You wouldn't want to feel this way about pain in *all* circumstances—you need to feel panic or alarm if you've hurt yourself and require medical attention—but when it comes to chronic pain, learning to manage your emotional response can change your life.

It's not possible to turn off your limbic system. But with some practice, you can use age-old mental techniques to cultivate a sense of distance from your aches. Pharmaceuticals, herbs, aromatherapy, massage, and other treatments can also help. Although you might still have pain, it'll have less power to drive you crazy. And because the brain's processes are plugged into your internal chemistry as well as your spinal cord and nerves, standing back from your pain can actually reduce the pain signal.

ELLEN'S STORY: "I'M A FRAIL PERSON NOW"

The way you *think* about pain is as crucial to the experience as the way you *feel* about it. If you can take control over your thoughts about pain—that is, if you can change what pain means to you—you can reduce your suffering. Ellen's story is a good illustration of this concept.

Ellen's problems began with a mild ache in her left shoulder. After a few weeks, the constant soreness had extended itself down along the left side of her back, and whenever she tried to pick up a laundry basket or lift one of her small children into her minivan, she felt a stabbing sensation that took her breath away.

Over the course of several visits to the doctor, Ellen was diagnosed with a sprained rotator cuff. She waited several weeks for the injury to heal, as her physician advised her, but still the pain didn't go away. Finally, her doctor said to Ellen, "I know you hurt, but I'm afraid you'll just have to learn to live with it."

(continued)

Ellen's family suggested that she follow the doctor's advice, so the next weekend Ellen made up her mind to grit her teeth and push through her pain. She spent an entire afternoon gardening—a task she loved but had given up since the injury—pulling up weeds, carrying bags of soil, and laying down mulch. She felt a sense of satisfaction she hadn't had in months. But that night, her entire left side, not just her shoulder and back, felt as if they were on fire. In the morning, she could barely move.

After this experience, Ellen's life changed. She wasn't a complainer, but she quietly began to protect her shoulder at all costs. She stopped gardening, of course, and she no longer went for her regular evening bicycle rides with her husband. She arranged for her carpool partners to take over driving duties, as she was afraid to hoist the smaller children into her van. Even her laundry ritual was affected: In order to avoid lifting a basket full of clothes, she'd fold each piece, place it into the basket, and then wait for her husband to carry it up the stairs.

By the time I saw her, Ellen was no longer the vivacious young mother she'd once been. Instead, she was bored, weak, and sleepless. Despite her carefulness, her pain was still there.

"I'm a frail person now," she told me. "I don't like it, but I've come to accept that I have to be extremely careful of what I do and how I move. If I let my guard down, things could get even worse."

As I talked with Ellen during this first visit to my office, I expressed my confidence that together we could greatly reduce the severity of her shoulder and back pain. I wanted to change her prescription painkiller, which seemed too mild for her, and I immediately thought of several alternative therapies that might work. But I knew that first we needed to address the way her thoughts about the pain were actually making it harder to live with.

To Ellen, the pain wasn't just pain. It was a sign that she was vulnerable and weak. That's an entirely understandable interpretation, but it wasn't really accurate. Her pain was real, but it flared up only under easily identifiable circumstances: those that involved heavy use of her shoulder. I agreed that gardening wasn't a good choice of activity for her, as it stressed the body part that hurt her most. But I thought it was too great a leap to go from avoiding gardening to avoiding *all* activity. She could go on bike rides and pick up the laun-

(continued)

dry basket. If she got the kids to use a stepstool, she could help navigate them into their car seats.

Ellen thought about this for a moment. "Won't movement trigger deeper damage to my shoulder? Don't I risk tearing up the joint again?" she asked.

No one had explained to Ellen why the pain wasn't going to rip her muscles apart or condemn her to a lifetime in a sling. It certainly *felt* that way to her. I told Ellen that although her rotator cuff had definitely been injured at one point, it was healed now. The continuing pain was likely caused by a combination of rewired nerves, stress, secondary muscle tension, and a badly worn-out pain braking system. Moving her shoulder might hurt, but it wasn't really doing any harm to her. In fact, it was most likely her nearly total *lack* of exercise, combined with the boredom and isolation she felt, that led to the insomnia and that made her feel so weak.

Ellen felt frustrated that her body was giving her amplified pain signals, but she was relieved to have someone explain, in terms that made sense, why her pain didn't signal terrible bodily harm or illness. Over the next few months, she redefined the meaning of pain in her life. Instead of thinking of pain as a message of dire consequences, she began to think of it as a broken alarm. The alarm was and is hard for her to live with, but it was better than living with a self-image of frailty or the fear of disability. Ellen increased her activities, and whereas she once rested every few hours for fear she'd overexert herself, she now took breaks only when she truly felt tired. She quickly reported an increase in energy and better sleep . . . which is to say that she no longer *suffered* so much from her pain.

Changing her thoughts didn't miraculously cure Ellen. But her quality of life richly improved, and after a while, her pain levels began to drop. This often happens to people who employ the power of the mind. They learn to let pain bother them less, and soon physical changes occur. Increased amounts of serotonin and endorphins are available, to begin with. More important, perhaps, is an effect that integrative medicine seeks to induce: Life becomes more balanced and enjoyable. From this healthy position, the body and mind are in an excellent position to heal pain—and to take the best advantage of all the therapies available.

What was true for Ellen isn't true for everyone. Not everyone with an achy shoulder suffers from a sprained rotator cuff, for one thing. I also know many people who respond to pain not by overprotection but by ignoring it. Their refusal to face the problem can keep them from receiving proper care. Your response and your treatment should be tailored to your individual needs, and you must get a good diagnosis before you make any assumptions about the nature of your disorder. The point here is that your thoughts about pain can affect your life dramatically, so you'll want them to be based on an accurate understanding of your condition.

PAIN AS AN EXPRESSION OF THE SOUL

I've talked about the problems created when Western medicine tries to reduce pain to a mechanical problem. But what about the view from the other side, that some pains are purely psychological or spiritual? Can pain be explained in terms of repressed anger and anxiety, of unnamed fears and desire for social gain?

It is ill-advised to draw a neat line connecting pain with a given psychological state. "You have headaches because of your mother" or "This patient's endometriosis is caused by a neurotic focus on her career" are statements that are insulting and even unimaginative, given how they diminish the human experience. It can't be said too often: Pain is rarely caused by just one factor, mental states included. However, it is undeniable that physical pain and psychological pain occupy interlocking spheres. Our bodies can hurt our spirits, in that chronic pain can make us depressed or anxious. So can spiritual maladies lead to pain in the body.

Sometimes physical pain is connected to a need for more careful observation of the spirit. If we listen to pain, it might tell us that our lives are out of balance: too many tight deadlines, family tensions, isolation, too many items on the to-do list. It's trying to teach us something, and we'd be smart to listen.

For some people, ongoing pain brings certain benefits: avoidance of a hated job, attention from others, or income from a lawsuit. Are these people purposely protracting their pain? Having examined many of them, having seen their unmistakable despondence, I don't think so. But it is well documented that people with pain-related lawsuits pending do not heal as quickly as others. One idea to contemplate is this:

Perhaps when we have something significant to gain from pain, the mind is prevented from fully dedicating itself to mending the body.

As odd as it may sound, pain may even serve a protective psychological effect. Pain can give us a socially acceptable reason not to see people who hurt us. It can allow us necessary time to think over a difficult problem and to rest. In his book *The Creative Malady,* George Pickering suggests that many great historical figures, including Charles Darwin and Florence Nightingale, developed illness in order to cordon off enough quiet, isolated time to create their most important works—for Darwin, his *Origin of Species,* and for Nightingale, her instructions for overhauling the fatally unsanitary conditions of British military hospitals. Neither person is accused of faking the sickness; instead, body and mind may have created it together to address a genuine creative need. And the lives of generations have been enriched for it. That's a paradox worthy of our consideration, and it illustrates how complicated it is to unravel anyone's psychology or to pass judgment on it.

But if you sense that your pain is linked to difficulties at home or at work, or that your pain has an existential dimension, the courage to examine these connections, to bring them out into the light, will serve you well. If you believe that your pain may be in part a physical expression of a psychological wound, you might try to think of your pain as useful, as a device for drawing your attention to the matter. And while you perform the difficult work of examining what this hurt might mean for you, you should of course pursue methods for easing or stopping the pain.

I hope that this chapter has helped you begin a new relationship with your pain. Most people have been left in the dark about their problem. When they learn about the new science of chronic pain, they already begin to feel more control—and more hope.

PART II

TAKE CONTROL OF YOUR TREATMENT

4.

EVALUATE YOUR PAIN

Pain sufferers often tell me how much anxiety and frustration they feel in doctors' offices. Much of this unpleasantness stems from the vague and invisible nature of the disorder. Pain is difficult to talk about, especially with health professionals, who have been trained to value the concrete and precise and to dismiss the intangible.

This chapter will try to ease some of those tensions by helping you perform a complete self-evaluation of your pain. The tools here, many of which are used by pain specialists, are designed to help you talk to your doctor with greater clarity and confidence.

I believe they will help you outside the doctor's office as well. It's a fundamental principle of integrative medicine that you become a partner in your health care. That's easy to say, but it can be hard to turn into a reality. Self-evaluation is an excellent place to begin. When you know—*really* know—your pain, how it affects your life, and what you want most out of your treatment, you're more likely to zero in on those therapies that will help you the most.

TIP: KEEPING A PAIN FILE

If you're not already keeping a file on your condition, it's a good idea to start one. In this file, you can keep your self-evaluation material and records of doctors' visits, along with the tracking system I'll discuss in Chapter 6, "Create a Plan for Pain Control." If you prefer, a notebook with pockets or a three-ring binder would work just as well.

YOUR PAIN HISTORY

"Tell me the story of your pain." A few weeks ago, I saw a colleague of mine make this request of a patient. The patient, who had crippling back trouble, had been examined a dozen times and by several doctors in the past couple of months. He was clearly irritated and impatient. His jaw was tensed, and his fingers played nervously on his knees. He sighed at the thought of hauling out the details, which were old news to him. My colleague urged him on, though, and sat silently as his narrative progressed. By the time the patient had finished, his face had grown softer, and his manner was calm. "Thanks for listening," he said, and he meant it. A simple request—*tell me your story*—had a visibly healing effect.

Telling your story can be therapeutic in itself. Getting the details down on paper can also help you see connections between changing circumstances and treatments and the amount of pain you've felt. I suggest that you find a half hour or so (longer if you need it) when you'll have some privacy and quiet. Turn off the phone, lock your office door, or do whatever it takes.

Prepare for writing your story by considering the following questions:

1. What was your life like before the pain?
2. When did the pain start?
3. What did you do about it?
4. Has the pain altered over time? In what way?

5. How has the pain changed your life? Be specific here: Has it made you sleepless or moody? Does it keep you from playing sports or walking the dog?

6. What has pain kept you from doing that you would most like to do again?

After you've contemplated these items, start writing. Let your story unfold naturally. It doesn't matter if you're not a born writer. Just keep going, and don't worry about spelling or grammar or sticking to a certain format. If your condition keeps you from writing or typing, you can dictate your story into a tape recorder.

When you're done, set the story aside in your folder. After a day or two, come back to it and read it over. Is there anything you'd add or delete? Are there any relationships between pain and other parts of your life that weren't obvious to you before?

This story is helpful in itself, but it can also assist you as you communicate with your doctor. I don't recommend that you hand her your story, or that you tell it in its entirety, as there are more profitable ways to spend the limited time of an office visit. But you *can* highlight the portions of your story that are the most important and relevant, and use them as a guide for talking to your physician.

KEEPING A PAIN DIARY

The pain diary is the most effective tool for discovering which kinds of foods, stresses, activities, and other factors make you feel better and which make you feel worse. This knowledge can point you in the right direction for treatment.

The pain diary has another advantage. Pain can sometimes feel like a black hole that consumes everything in its path. When people track the presence and level of their pain, they are often surprised to find that it is not all-encompassing. Instead, it rises and recedes, can be altered under certain conditions, and may at times be quite bearable.

On pages 57 and 58, you'll find a sample diary sheet that's been filled out, along with a blank diary page that you can photocopy. Determine three times during the day when you'll make entries in your diary, and then stick to that schedule. It's important that you keep making entries even when you're not in pain, or when you feel so bad that you'd rather just go to bed. Regularity is the key to the diary's success.

You should keep it for at least a week before you see your doctor, although some people find it so useful that they keep it longer. It's also a good idea to return to the diary whenever the level or quality of your pain has changed or is changing.

Pain level. The pain diary asks you to record your pain level at three different times during the day. You can do this by ranking your pain on a scale from 0 to 10, where 0 is absolutely no pain, 5 is moderate pain, and 10 is the worst pain you've ever had. For women who've had children, labor is a good way to establish what a 10-level pain feels like; others should think back to their most painful experience—often a broken bone—and use that as a guide. Don't worry about how other people might rank the same kind of pain you're feeling. All that matters is how the pain feels to *you,* relative to *your* experience.

0	1	2	3	4	5	6	7	8	9	10
NO PAIN					MODERATE					WORST PAIN

It may take some time for you to feel comfortable with the scale and to feel that you're using it consistently. That's fine. Keep in mind that you're not trying to justify your need for treatment or prove the existence of your pain to anyone. You're simply establishing a baseline against which your future pain will be measured. Say your pain tends to fall somewhere between 5 and 7. If your pain suddenly spikes to a 9, you and your doctor will know that something unusual is going on. If after a series of acupuncture treatments your level goes down to between 3 and 5, then you'll know the acupuncture is working.

Quality of pain. This section of the diary asks you to describe the kind of sensation you feel. Is it burning? aching? shooting?

Try to resist the temptation to always rank your pain at the highest end of the scale. Even women undergoing natural childbirth experience dramatic fluctuations in their pain levels. If you find that your entries consistently come in at 9 or 10, you may benefit from mind-body treatments that help you change your relationship to pain. (See Chapter 8 for more information.)

PAIN DIARY

DATE/TIME	PAIN LEVEL	TYPE OF PAIN	RECENT ACTIVITIES/CONDITIONS	ACTION TAKEN (IF ANY)
Date:				
Time 1:				
Time 2:				
Time 3:				
Date:				
Time 1:				
Time 2:				
Time 3:				
Date:				
Time 1:				
Time 2:				
Time 3:				
Date:				
Time 1:				
Time 2:				
Time 3:				
Date:				
Time 1:				
Time 2:				
Time 3:				

PAIN DIARY (SAMPLE)

THE IMAGINARY AUTHOR OF THIS SAMPLE IS A WOMAN WITH TENSION HEADACHES.

DATE/TIME	PAIN LEVEL	TYPE OF PAIN	RECENT ACTIVITIES/CONDITIONS	ACTION TAKEN (IF ANY)
Date: 9/16				
Time 1: 7 A.M.	5	Lancing	Just woke up	Took 3 aspirin
Time 2: 1 P.M.	2	Aching	At desk all morning	None
Time 3: 11 P.M.	5	Throbbing	Reading	3 more aspirin
Date: 9/17				
Time 1: 7 A.M.	4	Sore and aching	Woke up	2 aspirin
Time 2: 1 P.M.	3	Aching	Working at computer	Walked to bank and back
Time 3: 11 P.M.	5	Aching and throbbing	Watching TV	2 aspirin
Date: 9/18				
Time 1: 9:30 A.M.	4	Aching	Just woke up (slept in)	None
Time 2: 1 P.M.	8	Lancing	Couldn't do ANYTHING	3 aspirin
Time 3: midnight	?	Tight	Out to dinner—had some drinks	None (do drinks count?)
Date: 9/19				
Time 1: 8:30 A.M.	8	Splitting	Went to brunch—had coffee	Coffee (??)
Time 2: 1 P.M.	1	Dull	Shopping <u>and</u> visited friends	
Time 3: 11 P.M.	5	Aching	Reading	2 aspirin
Date: 9/20				
Time 1: 7 A.M.	5	Throbbing	Just woke up	None
Time 2: 1 P.M.	0		3 cups of coffee in A.M.	See coffee (left)
Time 3: 11 P.M.	4	Tight	Writing letters	2 aspirin

WORDS THAT HURT

"English," Virginia Woolf wrote, "which can express the thoughts of Hamlet and the tragedy of Lear, has no words for the shiver or the headache. . . . The merest schoolgirl when she falls in love has Shakespeare or Keats to speak her mind for her, but let a sufferer try to describe a pain in his head to a doctor and language at once runs dry."

Here's a list of adjectives that may help you describe your pain as precisely as possible. It was inspired by Ronald Melzack's McGill Pain Questionnaire, a tool used by many pain physicians and clinics.

ACHING
BEATING
BLINDING
BORING
BRIEF
BURNING
COLD
CONSTANT
CONTINUOUS
COURSING
CRAMPING
CRUSHING
CUTTING
DRAWING
DRILLING
DULL
FLASHING
FLICKERING
FREEZING
GNAWING
GRIPPING
GRUELING
HEAVY
HOT
INTERMITTENT
JUMPING
KNIFING
LANCING
MOMENTARY
NAGGING
NAUSEATING
NEEDLING
NUMB
PENETRATING
PERIODIC
PIERCING
PINCHING
POUNDING
PRICKING
PULLING
RHYTHMIC
PULSING
RADIATING
RASPING
SCALDING
SEARING
SHARP
SHOOTING
SICKENING
SMARTING
SORE
SPLITTING
SPREADING
STABBING
STEADY
STINGING
SQUEEZING
SUFFOCATING
TAUT
TEARING
TENDER
THROBBING
TIGHT
TIRING
TINGLING
TRANSIENT
TUGGING
WRENCHING

Recent activities/conditions. Under this heading you'll describe your recent or current situation at the time of writing. Did you just wake up or finish lunch? Were you climbing the stairs or talking with your boss? This section will help you see how certain aspects of your life may be linked to your pain.

Action taken. If you're feeling pain at the time of the entry, describe any action you've taken to try to ease it. You may have taken medication, for example, or tried to distract yourself by getting involved in your work.

Results. Use this column to list how the action you've taken has affected you. Perhaps it has taken away your pain but made you sleepy, or maybe it's changed the quality of pain from wrenching to pulsing.

OPQRST

Once you've written your story and kept the pain diary for a few weeks, you're in a good position to complete OPQRST, a mnemonic device doctors use to diagnose pain. Answering these questions will sharpen your knowledge about your pain, and it's an excellent way to prepare for your doctor's visit. In contrast to the longer exercises above, you should try to make your answers here as clear and succinct as possible.

Onset. When did the pain start?

Provokes. What provokes the pain—that is, what makes it worse? And what makes it better?

Quality. What does the pain feel like?

Radiates. Does the pain travel, or does it stay in one place?

Site. Where do you feel the pain?

Timing. When do you get the pain (morning, evening, weekend, the menstrual cycle), and how long does it last?

SET GOALS FOR TREATMENT

Mrs. Douglas was a very proper elderly widow who prided herself on her independence. But her self-reliance had been greatly compromised by osteoporosis, which left her with a number of small fractures in her spine. Arthritis compounded the pain. She could still cook for herself and crochet sweaters for her young granddaughters, but she was unable to move around for any length of time. When I asked her what she wanted to get out of treatment, she told me, "I want this pain to go away."

I can't help admiring people who hope for the best. But I was worried that Mrs. Douglas was setting herself up for disappointment, which might make her feel unhappier and lead to even more pain. So I asked her what bothered her most. Her answer was prompt: She couldn't walk to the corner grocery by herself. Every time she needed an egg or a quart of milk, she had to call either a neighbor or one of her children. Often she felt so humiliated at the prospect that she simply did without.

So we decided that one of the goals for Mrs. Douglas's treatment would be to walk to the store on her own, even if it caused her some pain. I tailored her treatment with that goal in mind. She began some gentle exercise training, and a specialist at the clinic fit her for a low back brace, to be used specifically for going to the store. I also taught her some meditation and breathing techniques to use just before she left the house, to help her handle any pain that arose.

I'd like you to set three goals for your treatment. You might start by trying to bring your pain level down a few points, maybe from an 8 down to a 5. (You can always lower the number further as you progress.) You can also look back at the story of your pain, especially your responses to the questions about how your life has changed since the condition began, and see what you'd most like to be able to do again. Perhaps the lost sleep bothers you most. A goal for you, then, might be to get six good hours of sleep a night. Again, you can change these goals as you begin to feel better.

Write down these goals and put them in the front of your file, where you can see them often.

THREE GOALS FOR TREATMENT (SAMPLE)

1. Walk to the grocery store.
2. Reduce average pain level from 7 to 4.
3. Find a therapy that brings down my stress level.

In the next chapter, I'll discuss how to work through these goals with your doctor.

5.

BUILD YOUR PAIN-MANAGEMENT TEAM

Because pain is so complex, most people need more services than their regular physician can provide. They need a pain-management *team,* one that consists of professionals who can address the problem from different angles. That team may consist of just two people, or it might involve several practitioners.

Although a pain team might sound expensive, it is quite possible to get the best care without draining your time and pocketbook. Here are some tips for navigating the health care system and assembling your pain team. You'll also find some suggestions for speaking to your doctor about two difficult topics—pain and alternative medicine—with greater ease.

HOW TO FIND A DOCTOR

Your pain team needs a leader, one qualified person who can rule out underlying conditions, prescribe medication if necessary, and coordinate treatment. This is especially important when you're using alternative therapies, as you need to make sure they won't aggravate your condition or combine poorly with your existing treatment. For this task, you'll want a conventionally licensed physician. It's best if you can find someone who actively practices integrative medicine or who is at least interested in it.

YOUR OPTIONS

Pain clinics. If you suffer from moderate to severe pain and live near a pain clinic that is practicing integrative medicine, you should make an effort to get there. At the clinic, you'll be assigned to a doctor who will coordinate your care among the other health professionals on staff, and who may also refer you outside the clinic when necessary.

A pain clinic, also called a pain center, is simply a group of health care professionals devoted to pain diagnosis and management, and almost every moderate-size city has at least one. How effective that clinic is depends on the quality of its professionals and the range of services they offer. Call a local medical school and ask if they have a pain center; if not, ask if there's one in the area that they'd recommend. If you do hit on a clinic that's within a reasonable distance, you still need to do a little investigation. Most pain clinics feature doctors who are more open to integrative medicine than general practitioners, but some are little more than anesthesia mills, in which the doctors perform injections and not much else. So you should call the clinic itself to find out how many different treatment options and/or specialists are available. At the very least, a clinic should employ three specialists: a coordinating doctor who specializes in pain, a physical rehabilitation expert, and a psychologist or psychiatrist. This variety indicates that the clinic recognizes the complexity of pain and the importance of multidisciplinary treatment. If the clinic has a massage therapist, acupuncturist, and chiropractor on staff, even better.

Pain specialists. Officially, the medical community does not recognize a single specialty known as "pain medicine." Instead, doctors who focus on pain usually come from one of four existing specialties: anesthesia, rehabilitation (also known as physiatry), neurology, and psychiatry. You should check that anyone who calls himself a pain specialist has a board certification in one of these specialties *and* that he limits his practice to pain treatment. As a very general rule, pain specialists tend to be more aware of integrative medicine than other physicians, because their field has seen so much success with it.

To find a pain specialist, you may need to ask around. Since integrative practitioners within a single community tend to know one another, you might ask a respected chiropractor, osteopath, or acupuncturist for recommendations. You can also talk to your internist and to other practitioners, or you can call medical schools and teaching hospitals.

Internists and family physicians. You may not be able to find a pain clinic or a pain specialist, especially if you live in a small town. This is by no means a disaster. What matters most is that you have a competent physician, someone who makes you feel comfortable and who is willing to work with you. Since you'll be practicing integrative medicine, it's nice if you can find a conventional doctor who's knowledgeable about alternatives. Again, word of mouth is your best bet here. However, a doctor who is actively excited about integrative medicine isn't absolutely necessary. All you need is a doctor who will handle your conventional care while making sure the other therapies you want to try are safe for you.

Doctors of osteopathy. Doctors of osteopathy (D.O.) are fully licensed physicians. What differentiates most of them from other doctors is a special interest in the body's structure, along with the practice of bone manipulation to maintain wellness and heal certain diseases. As you might expect, these doctors are often open to alternatives. If there's an osteopathic college near you, call it for recommendations. You can also ask chiropractors and acupuncturists.

Dentists. This option is limited to people with dental and facial pain. A surprising number of dentists practice holistic or integrative medicine; ask around for recommendations.

WHEN TO SWITCH DOCTORS

- ☐ The office is unclean or disorganized.
- ☐ You feel dismissed or ignored.
- ☐ The doctor is so rushed that you don't have time to ask a reasonable number of questions.
- ☐ The doctor will prescribe only one form of treatment—medication, injections, physical therapy—and refuses to consider anything else.
- ☐ The doctor spends more time talking to you about money than about your condition.
- ☐ The doctor seems competent enough, but you just don't feel comfortable talking to her.

TIPS FOR WORKING WITH YOUR DOCTOR

A lot of doctors, especially general practitioners, are uneasy with chronic-pain patients. They haven't been trained to handle the disorder, and they're uncomfortable with its vague, invisible qualities. To be fair, many pain patients themselves can be pretty tough. They've usually been bouncing around the system for a while, which makes them frustrated or contentious—not to mention that unrelieved pain doesn't exactly encourage a sweet disposition. Whether this applies to you or not doesn't matter: There's likely some prejudice against you, just because you're in pain.

If you run into a doctor who gets irritated when you bring up your pain, it's time to move on. But when it comes to most physicians, there's a lot *you* can do to coax out the best attitude and treatment. Here are some strategies to get the most from your visit:

▶ Start a professional relationship with the nurse. Often nurses know more about the practical aspects of pain control than doctors do; many are also more open to alternative therapies. As you get to know the nurse, you can begin to take advantage of her knowledge.

▶ Be prepared to answer OPQRST. (Details about this diagnostic tool are in Chapter 4.)

▶ Bring your pain diary. (Also in Chapter 4.)

▶ Bring in a list of medicines and other treatments you've tried. At the very least, bring in the bottles with their labels. It's helpful if your list includes how long you tried each treatment and what your reactions were.

▶ If you've had scans or tests run, bring copies of the results with you, or have them sent over ahead of time.

▶ Allow your doctor to begin the appointment on her terms. Let her ask questions and complete the physical exam. Most physicians reserve the end of the appointment for more detailed discussion, so use that time to ask your questions and fill in any other information you think is relevant.

▶ Respect the doctor's time. You deserve to have the doctor hear about your symptoms and answer your questions. But reality dictates that you confine yourself to the relevant information. You don't need to rush, but you should share the *edited* version of your pain story—that is, just the material you've selected and highlighted from Chapter 4.

TALKING TO YOUR DOCTOR ABOUT PAIN

Because most doctors don't have a deep knowledge of chronic pain, you may find yourself in the position of teaching your doctor about your condition. This isn't as scary as it sounds, since most doctors are quite willing to learn more about disorders and their treatment. The best approach is to make a specific request and then back it up with a solid resource. For example, you could say, "My current prescription isn't working for me, and I'd like to try some other drugs. I've read about other classes of medications. Do you think any of these would work?" You could then bring this book, with the relevant information clearly marked. Or "I've read about nerve pain. The predominant symptom is a burning, shooting quality, which is exactly what I feel. What do you think?" Again, you could bring in the appropriate backup information, either from this book or perhaps from one of the resources listed in Appendix F.

Many people instinctively make a connection between an event or circumstance and the cause of their pain. If your doctor doesn't ask you what brought on the pain, you may need to introduce the subject yourself: "When I kept my pain diary, I noticed that I always feel worse after a bad day at the office. Do you think tension or my chair might have something to do with my pain?"

Note that in each of these cases, the request ends with a deferral to the doctor's opinion. This sounds a professional note and is most likely to get the best results. Most physicians will agree to study material at a later time and get back to you. If your doctor simply refuses to read anything or to take your request seriously, then you need to find someone else.

TALKING TO YOUR DOCTOR ABOUT INTEGRATIVE MEDICINE

Introducing the subject of integrative medicine requires a slightly different tactic. If you ask a question such as "Will Reiki help my condition?" you might hear something like the following in response: "It won't make much of a difference." "I don't care for treatments like that." "Might as well spend your money on a lottery ticket."

Don't expect most conventional doctors to enthusiastically embrace integrative medicine. They're simply not trained in it. But you don't need your doctor to love alternatives; you just want him to make sure what you're doing is safe for you. Instead of asking for your doctor's endorsement, try asking if he has any *objections* to a specific treatment: "Would you have any problem with my using acupuncture treatments?" "Is there any reason I shouldn't take yoga classes?" "I want to take glucosamine. Is it safe to take along with my current medications?"

TWO ONLINE RESOURCES FOR YOU AND YOUR DOCTOR

The National Institutes of Health (NIH) now include a National Center for Complementary and Alternative Medicine (NCCAM). This government organization subjects alternative therapies to rigorous testing and then posts the results. If you and your doctor would like to visit this site, go to http://nccam.nih.gov. And even the stodgy main body of NIH has taken a serious look at some alternative treatments for chronic pain and its cousin, insomnia. It has concluded that many of those therapies, including acupuncture and certain mind-body treatments, are effective for these conditions. To see the consensus statements on these topics, visit http://odp.od.nih.gov/consensus/cons/pain.htm.

THE PAIN TEAM

You've identified a therapy you'd like to try, and your doctor has given you the all-clear. In most cases, the next step is to find a qualified practitioner of that therapy. When it comes to conventional medical specialties such as anesthesiology or orthopedic surgery, things are pretty straightforward. Your pain-team leader can usually make a recommendation, and you should look for the same qualities in a specialist as you would in a regular doctor. If you're about to undergo a complicated procedure, you might wish to ask the specialist about her educational and professional background. Most offices have copies of a printed biography on hand.

When it comes to hiring an alternative practitioner, you're faced with a more difficult decision. Most of the alternative specialties are still developing professional standards, and the lack of licensure and certification procedures means that this field attracts more than its share of crackpots and charlatans. Nevertheless, a few basic guidelines, along with some common sense, will help you find responsible healers. In Part III, I'll outline in more detail what to expect from specific types of alternative practitioners.

NATUROPATHY: ONE-STOP ALTERNATIVE CARE

Naturopathy is a healing profession with an appealing philosophy: The body has the power to heal itself. Naturopaths attend a four-year postcollegiate training program that gives them the credential N.D. (doctor of naturopathic medicine) and teaches them a variety of natural methods to support this healing process, including many that are featured in this book. It's up to the individual practitioner to decide exactly which therapies she will offer, but most practice dietary, herbal, and manual healing treatments, and a great many use acupuncture, homeopathy, and others. If you are going to use several alternative therapies, and if you live in a state where naturopathic physicians are licensed, you might find that a good naturopath saves you time and provides you with continuity of care (since you won't have to visit one person for acupuncture, another for massage, another for homeopathy, and so on). Your naturopath should have attended one of the five accredited naturopathic colleges in North America: Bastyr University in Seattle; Canadian College of Naturopathic Medicine in Toronto; National College of Naturopathic Medicine in Portland, Oregon; Southwest College in Scottsdale, Arizona; and the University of Bridgeport College of Naturopathic Medicine in Bridgeport, Connecticut. You will still need a conventionally licensed doctor (an M.D., D.O., or D.D.S.) to serve as leader of your pain team.

WHAT TO LOOK FOR IN AN ALTERNATIVE PRACTITIONER

▶ A license, if one is available from your state for this particular field. Call your state's licensing board. Remember that a license is a *minimal* requirement, not a guarantee of quality.

- National certification, where available. As of this writing, acupuncturists and chiropractors all must pass national exams before they may practice. There is a national exam for massage therapists, but it's not required in states that require their own examinations.
- Membership in an accreditation society, if there is one. Accreditation societies are listed in Appendix E.
- Referrals. Ask your doctor, your nurse, other alternative practitioners, or professional schools and organizations. If you see the same name come up repeatedly, you've probably found a winner.
- A clean, organized office or workspace.
- An up-front approach about how much the treatment will cost and how many sessions will be required.

WHEN TO RUN FROM AN ALTERNATIVE PRACTITIONER

- Your state regulates this field, but the practitioner doesn't have a license.
- You hear words like *miraculous* or *sure-fire,* or claims of 100 percent success rates.
- The office is dirty.
- The practitioner is more concerned about your money than about you.
- The practitioner is not forthcoming about the length of treatment or its cost.
- The practitioner wants to initiate several different therapies at once. (How will you know which is working?)
- You've given a therapy a fair trial and it just hasn't worked for you—but the practitioner is unwilling to give it up. She may be trying to jack up the bill.
- The practitioner refuses to speak with your doctor.
- You just can't afford it, even if the practitioner is competent.

SELF-CARE

You're a member of the pain team, too, and not just because you do the hiring and firing. This is especially important if you're on a limited budget. You may not be able to afford regular massage or expensive supplements, but there's a lot you can do on your own. Some of the most effective techniques are also the cheapest: Mind-body therapies such as meditation and guided imagery require absolutely no financial investment and can dramatically reduce pain. There are other options, too. You can take a few yoga classes and then do the poses at home, or buy some aromatherapy oils for a few dollars. Even if you don't need to save money, self-care is important: It exercises your innate healing powers, and it gives you back your sense of control.

6.

CREATE A PLAN FOR PAIN CONTROL

In the coming weeks and months, you'll consider your options for pain control, make priorities, and test out therapies. In other words, you'll undertake an experiment in your own healing. Such an experiment can become a source of pleasure in itself. When a therapy works, the thrill of discovery will be yours. As you learn more about your body and mind and how to make them feel better, you'll develop an even deeper satisfaction. It definitely beats placing yourself at the mercy of the medical system and hoping for the best. And, of course, you won't be working alone. You'll have a safety net formed by health professionals.

How will you know which therapies to try? You can start by looking through this book. Keep in mind that your treatment should be customized for your body, your mind, your financial situation, and the day-to-day realities of your life. Happily, there are a great many options available—enough that, with a little patience and willingness to experiment, there's an extremely good chance you'll find a combination that makes you feel much better. Below are tips and tools that can help you hit on that combination as quickly as possible.

PUT SYNERGY ON YOUR SIDE

Chronic pain is too complex to treat with only one therapy. Pain builds on itself; it threads its way into your mind, your nerves, your muscles, your digestive system, your internal chemistry, and so on until it becomes an intricate web, with your life entangled in its center. But healing builds on itself, too. Certain treatments lend support to one another, and the best combinations unleash a powerful synergy, in which the whole is greater than the sum of its parts.

Perhaps you have back pain that stems from an old sprain. Since the injury healed years ago, you wonder if you're suffering from misfiring nerves. With your doctor's approval, you might decide to try medication to quiet them down. Certainly, that therapy alone may help. But say that you've noticed two other dimensions to your pain. For one, your lower back muscles seem awfully tight; you find yourself rubbing your hand across your back frequently during the day. Second, you know that the pain escalates when you're under fire at the office.

If you add regular massage therapy and some stress-reducing breathing exercises to the daily medication, you'll have addressed three different dimensions of your pain. Moreover, those therapies will be more powerful together than they would have been on their own. The breathing will help relax your muscles and keep your nerves from misfiring, the massage will enhance stress reduction, and the medication that quiets nerve pain will give you less reason to tighten your muscles and to succumb to work stress. You'll have created synergy for reducing your pain and improving your life.

As a way of helping you make decisions, I've separated the therapies listed in Part III into seven major categories. Each category represents a different strategy for controlling pain. For example, "Move or Be Moved: Physical Therapies" seeks to reduce pain by physically manipulating bones and soft tissues. The therapies in "Distracting Your Nervous System from Pain" work on the nerves, spinal cord, or brain to shift their attention away from pain signals. In "Mind-Body Medicine," you'll find ways to employ the mind's healing power. And so on.

I like to draw on therapies from at least three of the seven categories, so that the treatment plan is coming at pain from several different angles. In case that number seems overwhelming, be assured that many therapies, such as meditation or aromatherapy, are easy to use and are even pleasurable. Nor does every therapy have to be used every day—far from it. Many work on a weekly, monthly, or as-needed basis. Keep in mind, though, that there is no magic number. You may need more therapies, or you may need fewer.

TRUST YOUR HEALING INSTINCT

When I began practicing alternative medicine, I was surprised at the power of the healing instinct. Time and again, I'd see how people are drawn toward those therapies that help them the most. "I don't know why," they'd say, "but I just had a feeling that acupuncture [or chiropractic, or acupressure, etc.] would work for me." This pattern continues in my office today. How can I account for this wisdom of people untrained in medicine? Maybe the healing instinct is simply a yearning for balance. Just as plants grow toward the light, we seek out those things that naturally restore us to a state of equilibrium. A typical example is a patient, his body and mind in knots, who tells me that he'd like to take yoga or get a massage. I tell him that his instinct is impeccable: Both therapies will unkink his muscles and calm his mind, making him stronger and more resistant to pain.

This phenomenon also demonstrates the importance of the placebo effect, in which our beliefs and hopes increase the effectiveness of a therapy. The term "placebo effect" is often used in a derogatory manner, as if people who benefit from it are dupes. But there's a growing movement to think of the placebo effect as testament to the power of the mind. Why not harness these powers by choosing treatments that appeal to you? Your good feelings may give those treatments an extra boost. (Of course, use your good judgment as well as your instincts when considering therapies, and always check things out with your doctor.)

INFORM YOURSELF ABOUT YOUR DISORDER

Fibromyalgia, headache, back pain, peripheral neuropathies, and more ... Part IV of this book reviews the most common painful conditions. Each chapter opens with a description of a particular condition, including its symptoms and causes, and the tests your doctor should run. It then proceeds to a list of the best therapies.

For each condition, I've listed the therapies that have either been scientifically proven to help or that have strong anecdotal evidence in their favor. If you read the chapter on neck pain, for example, you'll see that muscle tension and poor posture are two of the most likely causes, so you'll want to try postural techniques and muscle-relaxing therapies. Postherpetic neuralgia, also known as shingles, is basically a nerve disorder, so if you have it, you should look at therapies that address nerve malfunction and help you turn down its persistent wail.

You might be surprised at how many options are at your disposal—you might even wonder where to begin! With that in mind, I've highlighted those therapies that should be your first choices. These usually include customized elements of good nutrition, exercise, and relaxation, which are inexpensive and easy on the body. You may also see certain pharmaceuticals or other treatments highlighted as well.

The remaining therapies—the ones that aren't highlighted—also have a good record for your problem, but they may be riskier or appropriate only for a particular set of needs. Or perhaps they are simply excellent runner-up therapies. As you're making choices, listen to that healing instinct: The therapies that appeal to you are the ones most likely to help.

CONSULT YOUR DOCTOR

Your doctor may have some suggestions for tailoring a plan to your needs; at the very least, she can tell you whether a therapy is contraindicated by your current treatment or even if it's dangerous for you. See Chapter 5 for tips on how to approach your doctor about introducing new therapies.

PUT YOUR PLAN ON PAPER

When you're ready to make a plan, begin by listing the therapies you'd like to try. Use the tips above to help you get started; look for those treatments that seem best suited to your condition or that hold an appeal for you. Once you've done that, assign each therapy a priority. You'll want to introduce just one new therapy at a time—otherwise, you won't know what's working, or what's causing a side effect. With the exception of very simple therapies like meditation, breathing, and changing to a more healthful diet, you should check with your doctor about each therapy to make sure it's safe for you.

You'll also need a system for tracking your results. A good tracking system will minimize the time you spend looking for pain relief, because it helps you proceed in an orderly fashion and helps make clear which therapies are working. On page 76, you'll find a blank form you can copy and use to stay on top of the therapies you're currently trying as well as those you'd like to try, the dosages and time frames of treatments, and the results.

THE ADEQUATE TRIAL

You know about your right to a fair trial. Your pain therapies deserve one, too. Medical researchers like to talk about "the adequate trial." That means that you should give a therapy an adequate chance to work—it should be tried at the correct dosage or frequency and for an appropriate amount of time. With acupuncture, for example, it can take several sessions to find the right number and placement of pins, and for the treatment to take full effect. The same goes for prescription medications: If you get the wrong dosage or don't give the pills time to work, the trial isn't fair. So use this book or your practitioner's advice to determine a reasonable dosage and time frame for each treatment you want to try. (Of course, if you have a severe reaction to a therapy or discover that you can't afford it, it may be time to give it up. Make sure to contact your doctor before going off any prescription medication.)

I also recommend that you look back on therapies you've already used and rejected. Is it possible that some of them weren't given fair trials? If so, you might want to give them another chance.

MAKE BASIC WELLNESS YOUR NUMBER-ONE PRIORITY

When your life is balanced—in other words, when you're in good mental, physical, and spiritual condition—you're more resistant to pain. That's because your body is performing with minimal effort, making more energy and attention available for warding off challenges to its health.

Unfortunately, pain makes everything harder, including taking care of yourself. That's part of the downward spiral. You hurt, you stop

THERAPY TRACKING SYSTEM

THERAPY	GOAL OF THERAPY	DOSAGE TAKEN OR FREQUENCY USED	LENGTH OF TRIAL	RESULTS	SIDE EF

THERAPY TRACKING SYSTEM (SAMPL

THIS SAMPLE IS FILLED OUT AS IF FOR A PERSON WITH FIBROMYALGIA.

THERAPY	GOAL OF THERAPY	DOSAGE TAKEN OR FREQUENCY USED	LENGTH OF TRIAL	RESULTS	SIDE EF
Elavil (tricyclic antidepressant)	Reduce muscle soreness; improve sleep	20 mg	4 weeks	Soreness down a few notches— sleep still not great	None
Elavil	Same	50 mg	2 days	Pain scale down by 4	Unacceptable—slept for 15 hours!
Elavil	Same	25 mg	4 weeks	Pain scale down by 3; sleeping soundly	Metallic taste and sometimes dry feeling in mouth
Meditation	Decrease stress, cope with pain	20 minutes daily	1 week	None	Hate sitting still
Tai chi	See above	2 classes/week	3 weeks	Less stress and soreness, great sleep	None
Homeopathy (rhus tox)	Reduce muscle soreness	30x/day	4 weeks	Not sure— seems about the same	None

exercising and start indulging in junk food, you hurt more, and on and on. So if you're not already following a basic wellness program, I suggest that you make doing so your number-one priority. This is true even if you're very sick or elderly, or if your ability to move around is limited. By following the strategies here, you'll give yourself a helping hand out of that spiral.

Get moving. You need a balance between motion and rest, and most of us need to tip the scales toward more movement. Exercise increases endorphins as well as the neurotransmitters serotonin and GABA. It reduces pain from muscle tension and stiffness in the connective tissues and can ease many of pain's secondary effects—fatigue, insomnia, depression, anxiety, and digestive woes. Suggestions for exercise can be found in Chapter 7, "Move or Be Moved."

Eat well. When you hurt and your activities are limited, potato chips start looking like your consolation prize. But poor dietary choices—too much red meat and junk food, too few fresh fruits and vegetables—increase pain. They encourage inflammation, and the added pounds put extra stress on your joints. A simple pain-control diet can significantly reduce pain and improve your sense of well-being. Chapter 9 lays out the pain-control diet and explains the role of foods in pain.

Reduce stress. Pain causes stress, stress causes pain ... get trapped in this cycle, and soon you're so far off balance you can't remember what relaxation feels like. Mind-body therapies and other soothing treatments, which help you manage stress and cultivate distance from your pain, can dramatically limit your suffering. You probably know your favorite methods of stress relief, so give yourself permission to use them. Carve out some alone time, get a massage, or meditate in your backyard. Learn breathing exercises to use at the office, on the bus, or whenever you need a thirty-second break. Most of us can benefit from additional techniques as well, so read Chapter 8 for more suggestions.

Stay engaged with life. Pain is isolating. Too many sufferers spend long hours by themselves, bored and dispirited, watching television or playing video games. Although these activities may take your mind off the pain, they don't really provide the mental and social stimulation necessary for health. In the end, they leave you more drained than refreshed. If this sounds like you, look for ways to increase your involvement with life: Join a support group, take up a hobby, do volunteer work, or get back in touch with old friends.

PART III

THERAPIES

7.

MOVE OR BE MOVED: PHYSICAL THERAPIES

THE ALEXANDER TECHNIQUE / CHIROPRACTIC AND OSTEOPATHY / EXERCISE / HEAT AND COLD THERAPIES / THE FELDENKRAIS METHOD / MASSAGE / PILATES / ROLFING AND HELLERWORK / TRACTION

"You have freedom when you're easy in your harness," Robert Frost wrote. People in pain tend to sigh a little when they hear these words, because ease and freedom seem so elusive.

I believe that you *can* achieve more ease and freedom. Maybe not the kind you had when you were eighteen, but the kind that lets you take your mind off your pain and get things done. Some of the best ways to get this feeling are described in this chapter. Most of them adjust your "harness"—your bones, muscles, tendons, and ligaments—so that you stand taller, feel less pinched, and move more easily. Many of them have subtler neurological benefits as well. They improve your mood, help you sleep, and make you forget your pain, even if just for a short while.

As you read this chapter, try to find forms of both *touch* and *movement* that appeal to you. I want to discuss touch first, because most of us just don't get enough of it. Before drugs and high-tech procedures came on the scene, one of the primary healing techniques used by doctors and nurses was touch. They knew that simply by laying their hands on the sick—whether in the form of massage, diagnostic poking and prodding, or hand-holding—they could offer a patient deep, primal comfort. In some cases, this physical attention may have sped up recovery by stimulating the immune system.

Today, doctors and nurses are pushed to their limits by brutally tight schedules. They'd like to take the time for touch, but they simply can't. The same goes for the rest of society. It's one of the ironies of the current age that as the world gets more and more crowded, as we ride bumper to bumper and stand shoulder to shoulder, we feel more physically isolated.

People in pain tend to be especially touch-deprived. This may be a result of the pain itself. The physical limitations and the isolation, as well as the depression and anxiety, can build a wall between you and everyone else. But as with so many aspects of pain, there's a vicious circle here, because touch deprivation can also *intensify* the hurt. When you aren't cared for or nurtured on a regular basis, your body will let you know it. Sometimes it sends that message in the form of tension and pain.

CLAUDIA'S STORY: A BRIDGE BACK TO LIFE

Claudia, an elegant woman in her sixties, came to see me about neck pain. She insisted on prescription medication, but she was so tight and sore—when I brushed the skin of her back with my hand, she actually jumped—that I suggested she try massage in addition to pain relievers. She was reluctant, but after several visits, she finally agreed. At our next appointment, Claudia looked calmer and more relaxed than I'd ever seen her. She told me that as she was receiving the massage, it occurred to her that she hadn't been meaningfully touched since her husband had died years ago. She was starving for the physical contact with another human as much as for the therapeutic manipulation of her muscles. From this point, Claudia's progress was remarkable. Soon she was playing sports she'd avoided for years, including tennis, horseback riding, and even downhill skiing.

I realize that massage therapy isn't right for everyone. It can get expensive, and some people feel vulnerable getting skin-on-skin contact from strangers. This chapter covers many other therapies, including the Alexander Technique and heat and cold therapies, that have some of the benefits of touch; they tend to emphasize the manipulation of tissues—your "harness"—over the more subtle neurological effects. Look through them to see if any appeal to you. I'd also like you to consider ways to get more touch outside the therapeutic setting. You could learn some of the home massage techniques listed in Appendix B and trade off giving and receiving massages with a loved one. Volunteer to give infant massages at your local hospital's neonatal intensive care unit or to hold the hands of residents at a nursing home. Or consider adopting a pet: The touch of a warm animal can envelop you in the give-and-take of a nurturing relationship.

Most people know that exercise is an essential component of staying healthy and of recovering from illness . . . but, as with touch, we just don't get enough of it. To live without exercising and stretching is a mistake that leads to increased pain. If you don't move, you're feeding your pain. You're stiffening up your muscles and joints, you're impairing the proper regulation of neurotransmitters, and you're increasing tension and stress. With the right exercise, you can *decrease* pain on all its levels. Even better, you can increase your mobility and your functioning, which means that you can participate in life again.

I want you to look for one touch therapy and at least one form of exercise that you can manage on a regular basis. When you have an appropriate program of touch and movement in place, you'll soon feel pain's burden growing lighter. Even if you're elderly, disabled, or on a budget, you can create a program that fits your needs. Following are some suggestions to help you decrease your pain and increase your enjoyment of life.

POINTS THAT TRIGGER PAIN

Many people in pain, no matter what the underlying cause, develop something called "trigger points"—knots or taut bands of muscle that feel tender when pressed. These points also send pain radiating to another part of your body, so that a point in your shoulder may cause pain in your neck or head. Several treatments described in this chapter, including specialized massage techniques, can release these trigger points. For more information, see Chapter 24, "Myofascial Pain Syndrome."

THE ALEXANDER TECHNIQUE

Do you poke your head forward when you walk or read? Do you tense your shoulders at the computer? Posture mistakes such as these are a frequent cause of pain and restricted mobility. The

Alexander Technique (AT) is a system of instruction that teaches its students how to hold themselves more naturally and to move with greater efficiency and freedom.

The Alexander Technique was developed in the late 1800s by F. M. Alexander, a Shakespearean actor who suffered from voice loss. Through a period of long and detailed self-observation, he concluded that his posture, especially the movements of his head, neck, and upper back, put too much strain on his vocal cords and failed to give proper support to his breath. As he changed his posture, his voice improved, along with his mood, breathing, and general health. He developed a following, first of similarly afflicted actors and then of people with respiratory problems. Now, the Alexander Technique is widely used to break unconscious and damaging habits of movement.

Although its instructors claim that the technique can improve the health of almost anyone, I have found it most effective for people with upper-body musculoskeletal pain—meaning head, neck, shoulder, and upper back problems. I often recommend it when I see people who jerk their head and neck when they move, or who seem to be clenching those muscles tightly, or who have generally poor posture that they can't seem to correct. The Alexander Technique is extremely gentle, incorporates the benefits of light touch, and is about as low-risk as therapies can get.

I tried Alexander myself a couple of years ago. My neck and shoulders were aching, and I felt like one big cramp. During the lessons, my teacher, Tom Lemens, observed me as I performed the most basic of motions—standing, walking, and so on—and soon isolated one pattern of movement that seemed especially troublesome. It turned out that I was tensing my neck and shoulder muscles whenever I got up out of a chair, forcing them to do an unusual amount of work. Tom had me sit down and get up dozens of times. He'd place his hand on my chin or my back to guide me into better form, and then he observed as I tried the movements on my own and offered suggestions. I found the classes pleasantly absorbing and somewhat challenging; it took more mental work than I would have thought to relearn basic movement patterns. Frankly, it was also a little odd to think so hard about sitting down and getting up. Soon, though, the neck and shoulder pain eased up quite a bit, and the movements I'd learned became second nature.

Your instructor should be certified by the North American Society of Teachers of the Alexander Technique, which requires a minimum of sixteen hundred hours of training. (Contact information for this organization can be found in Appendix E.) Some teachers approach AT as a series of repetitive drills; much better are those who lead you to insights about *why* you should change your motions. Ask your teacher about his philosophy and get some recommendations before signing up.

When I tried AT, it took about six sessions for me to feel that I'd corrected my movement enough to reduce my pain, and I decided to stop treatment there. This goes against what most Alexander teachers will tell you, which is that you'll need one thirty- or forty-five-minute lesson every week for at least six months. My feeling is that limited problems like mine need less treatment, while more complicated and deeply ingrained ones may well need the full duration. It's your decision, and one you should base on a trial of at least five or six sessions and on how you feel afterward. Classes are usually private, although a few teachers offer classes for small groups.

CHIROPRACTIC AND OSTEOPATHY

Although in many respects chiropractors and osteopaths are quite different—to begin with, osteopaths are fully licensed physicians who can prescribe drugs and perform surgery—when it comes to pain treatment, both rely principally upon spinal manipulative therapy, or SMT.

In SMT, a highly trained practitioner uses quick, directed thrusts to move a joint to its anatomical limit. This is the motion that produces the characteristic cracking or popping sound of chiropractic. (By contrast, a physical therapist will move a joint only through its current range of motion, or just a little past it.) Although we're not precisely sure why SMT works so well, there are two promising explanations. The first is that the action normalizes the microrange of joints, allowing you to move more freely. The second is that it resets neurological patterns, perhaps affecting muscle tone, the function of the involuntary nervous system, and the way pain signals are processed in your spinal cord. In all likelihood, both reasons come into play. SMT also delivers the benefits of hands-on healing. The term *chiropractic* is derived from Greek words meaning "done by hand," and a good practitioner will communicate a strong, physical sense of caring, much the way the old-fashioned family doctor used to do.

Spinal manipulation is at its best when used for stiffness and pain along the body's central axis (the spine, neck, and head), and when it comes to handling an acute episode of low back pain, it's one of the most effective therapies around. I was a chiropractor before I became a physician, and when I was a medical resident, the staff physicians who were clued in to the benefits of SMT often called me into the emergency room to treat acute, disabling episodes of low back pain. After manipulation therapy and a little rest, the person was usually able to walk out of the ER with a straight back. I still use manipulative techniques nearly every day in the office. After treating someone, I can feel the difference with my hands. The spine or neck feels looser, spongier, and more mobile. Unfortunately, the long-standing antagonism between chiropractic and conventional medicine has prevented most hospitals from keeping spinal manipulators on staff to treat such problems, despite quality research that proves its efficacy. It's not crazy to suggest that every emergency room should have someone who is trained in SMT on hand twenty-four hours a day.

This brings me to the problem of chiropractic's reputation. In much of the world, especially Western Europe, spinal manipulation therapies are a standard aspect of health care. In the United States, chiropractors are suspected of being unscrupulous quacks. I'm sorry to say that this reputation is sometimes—but by absolutely no means always—justified. A few decades ago, it wasn't unusual to find chiropractors who were quick to make unrealistic claims for their technique, telling patients that it would cure multiple sclerosis or irritable bowel syndrome. (It can't.) Now, thanks to better training and regulation, you won't run into this problem very often. Today, if a chiropractor is going to be unethical, it'll be in the area of pricing. Chiropractors are notorious for ordering too many expensive X rays or for prescribing overly long courses of frequent treatment—and making you pay up front for the privilege. Some will try to sell you hundreds of dollars' worth of supplements at the end of the visit.

But a great many chiropractors are of sterling character, and it is well worth seeking them out. These caring, educated people offer an excellent method for treating pain and a few other disorders. You can find them by asking your doctor or nurse or a practitioner of another alternative therapy. Your chiropractor should be a licensed graduate of an accredited chiropractic college and should take continuing-education classes. She should also be willing to work with your doctor and even allow your doctor to observe.

When you arrive for chiropractic treatment, expect to fill out the usual paperwork, answer questions about your medical history, and receive a diagnostic examination. This exam will focus on the neuromuscular system, so the practitioner will check your reflexes, range of motion, strength, and so on. She will also examine your spine and posture, feeling for areas of tenderness. In most cases, you should receive SMT in the same visit as your initial exam. If your chiropractor wants to take X rays, ask why. Legitimate reasons for X rays include a suspicion of a serious abnormality in the area, such as a dislocation or fracture if you've had an accident recently, or a tumor. If your chiropractor says that she needs to check for "bones out of place," ask if she can treat you without X rays. If she agrees, then you should proceed to treatment. If not, take your business elsewhere.

When you receive SMT, it's normal to feel some pain. After all, you're pushing the joint out of its comfort zone. You may even feel some discomfort a few hours or even days afterward, but it should not be a serious problem for you. After the chiropractor finishes SMT, she should give you some stretches and exercises to practice at home. You really must perform these exercises; without them, SMT will improve your condition for only a short period of time, rather than over the long term. She may also offer other kinds of therapies, including hot or cold packs, electrical stimulation, or dietary advice.

A visit to an osteopath will follow similar lines. The diagnostic workup will look more like that of a conventional physician, and you may be given some manipulation of the arms and legs in addition to your spine. As fully licensed physicians who have completed medical internships and residencies, osteopaths are in a better position to give you fully integrated medicine. They can prescribe medication, look for underlying diseases, and talk to you about other therapies. Osteopaths do not have the same reputation problem as chiropractors, and they're much less likely to oversell you on treatments, X rays, or products. They can be hard to find, however, especially in small towns. And you should make sure that the practitioner actively practices manipulation therapy and is trained to do it properly, as some osteopaths eschew manipulation in favor of strictly conventional medicine.

If you have acute lower back pain, you can expect to notice a significant difference after your first treatment, but you will probably need to go back for a total of four to six visits over the course of two weeks. For chronic pain along the spine and head, you should be able to tell after six or eight treatments whether SMT is right for you. After that, you may need to receive continuing treatment for as little as six weeks or as long as four months. Insurance providers will usually cover osteopathic treatment, since osteopaths are physicians, and most plans have some degree of chiropractic coverage.

Contraindications: Do not use spinal manipulation if you have a bone fracture or break, any kind of bone cancer, an inflammatory joint disease such as lupus or rheumatoid arthritis, osteoporosis, or serious infection.

Contact information for professional chiropractic and osteopathic organizations can be found in Appendix E.

EXERCISE

One of the country's top anesthesiologists, who has performed upward of forty-five hundred deep injections for pain, once told me why he believes in what he does. You'd think that he'd cite the pain-numbing quality of anesthetic drugs, but he didn't. "I do injections to get the person mobilized," he said. For him, injections are helpful only insofar as they get someone comfortable enough to exercise and start using the painful area. The same is true for many other treatments. Here's the bottom line: If you don't exercise, you won't get optimal pain relief.

I've already discussed the pain spiral, in which you first experience a relatively moderate amount of pain but then become increasingly debilitated as the physical and emotional responses to it send you sliding faster and faster downward. Reducing exercise as a response to pain is one of the surest ways to start that spiral in motion. When you don't exercise, your body reduces its output of serotonin and endorphins, and it's less able to produce GABA, a neurotransmitter that inhibits pain and lets you sleep. Your muscles and bones become more vulnerable to knots and weakness, and you're not as able to fight off illness. You become moodier. And if you stop using the painful area completely, the lack of normal sensory input may result in nerves that misfire or become hypersensitive.

That said, I realize that pain can make regular exercise extremely difficult. In Appendix A you'll find some gentle stretches and strengthening exercises. They're appropriate for everyone, and they can get you mobile enough to start a more comprehensive program.

GIANNI'S STORY: "I'M TOO OLD AND ACHY TO EXERCISE!"

"I'm not in Naples anymore!" said Gianni, an Italian gentleman in his seventies who always wore a neatly pressed suit and tie to the office. I had been seeing Gianni every week or so to give him injections for degenerative arthritis in his lumbar spine, and I was trying to convince him that if he got some exercise, he wouldn't need to come in so often. "I'm too old," he told me with a wave of his hand. "When I was young, I could climb mountains, I could chase girls—even when they were on bicycles! But now it hurts too much."

I explained to Gianni that I wasn't asking him to go hiking or to jog down the street. I wanted him to ease into a routine that was appropriate for his age, ability, and pain level. Finally—after a little more good-natured griping—Gianni agreed. His body was weakened from pain and decades without exercise, so he started by walking in a warm-water tank we have in the office. The first two times he came in to use the tank, he'd shake his head when he passed me, as if to say, "I can't believe I let you talk me into this!"

But after his third exercise session, he stopped in to see me. "You know, I've got to tell you: I actually feel a little better. I thought exercise would make me feel worse. But I don't feel so stiff anymore."

Within a few weeks, Gianni was strong enough to perform some exercises on land, much like those you can find in the back of this book, and he began to lift light weights under the guidance of a physical therapist on staff. He became such an enthusiastic advocate of exercise that he convinced his wife to take long walks after dinner with him (Gianni may not be in Naples anymore, but I suspect he's still a ladies' man). Now he's gone for several months without an injection. Sure, he may still need an injection every once in a while for a flare-up—but for day-to-day relief, he is able to manage his pain by himself, at home.

PHYSICAL THERAPY: MAXIMIZING RELIEF, MINIMIZING PAIN

I can't imagine my pain practice without the physical therapists on staff. Every day, I write prescriptions for physical therapy (PT), and every day, I see patients who credit their pain relief to hardworking, compassionate physical therapists.

Physical therapists administer many of the services discussed in this book. They can massage your sore neck, put a hot pack on your knee, and fit you for devices such as TENS and braces. But they do all these things in the interest of getting you moving again—and so they'd *love* to help you learn gentle, customized exercises that will make you stronger and more limber. They can even reduce the pain of exercise by applying heat and cold therapies, massage, or electrical stimulation.

If it's been a while since you've worked out, or if you're in a lot of pain, a physical therapist can design an exercise plan to suit your needs. Your doctor will probably be happy to write you a prescription for PT—most physicians are overjoyed when their patients show a serious interest in exercise. Just be sure that your physical therapist is experienced in pain or orthopedics (since some specialize in other problems, such as stroke), and watch out for "schlock therapy," in which the therapist substitutes a passive treatment such as a quick rubdown and hot pack for the real work of reconditioning your body.

WHEN IT HURTS TO WORK OUT

"Exercise? Ugh!" some of my patients say. "It hurts just to get out of bed in the morning! Can't you just give me a nice little pill?"

The fear of exercise pain can stand in the way of your chronic pain solution. Like Gianni, you'll soon discover that appropriate exercise feels *good*—but you should prepare yourself for some mild muscle fatigue at first. This achiness is called delayed onset muscle soreness, or DOMS for short, and it's *not* your typical chronic pain; it's the soreness you get a day (or maybe a day and a half) after you work out. DOMS is a positive sign that your body is building up new tissue. If you exercise one afternoon and feel your usual chronic pain seriously flare up that night, you're not experiencing DOMS—you're getting a signal that you've pushed too hard.

Some people actually like the sensation of muscle fatigue. "It reassures me that my body is working," one woman told me. But if you want to reduce post-exercise soreness, try some of these measures:

- Take a warm bath.
- Apply heat to the affected muscles.
- Massage the muscle—or get a professional to do it for you.
- Take an over-the-counter pain reliever such as Advil or Motrin. (Just don't use these drugs before exercise to *prevent* pain, as you could interfere with the training response that builds muscle tissue. Don't reach for these pills until *after* soreness has set in.)

For some people, DOMS is not the only kind of pain associated with exercise. Take my patient Heather, who developed a wicked case of tendinitis in her shoulder from lifting heavy boxes of files at the office. Heather hadn't exercised in years and was willing to start bicycling and walking—and she accepted that she'd feel a little achy after these activities at first.

But if she wanted to recondition her shoulder, Heather would also need to perform specific exercises designed to stretch her shoulder muscles and open them up, taking some of the pressure off the joint structures. And I was frank with her: She *was* going to feel some pain as she began to work this neglected, overprotected region of her body.

"Out of the question," she said flatly. "No way. I won't risk injuring myself again." But I promised Heather that the exercises I gave her wouldn't damage her shoulder; over time, they would cut down on the chronic pain *and* allow her to use the shoulder again. I sent her to a physical therapist who would show her how to perform the exercises safely. I also offered other therapies, listed here, that would make it easier for her to move the shoulder through the exercises:

- Meditation
- Breathing techniques
- Heat and cold therapy
- Electrical stimulation

- Massage
- Injections of local anesthetic into the painful muscle

We decided to inject the shoulder before Heather went off to physical therapy, which allowed her to exercise without much pain. After working her shoulder, the therapist applied an ice pack to keep any post-workout aches under control. And within weeks, Heather was back at her job with a stronger, more flexible shoulder.

DON'T NEGLECT CARDIOVASCULAR ACTIVITIES

Research shows that if you want to get the benefits of cardiovascular exercise, an occasional workout doesn't help much—you need to get your heart pumping for thirty minutes at a time, three or four times a week. But consistent exercise should not hurt or exhaust you; even if you're in your eighties or have suffered for years, you *can* find an exercise program that makes you feel good.

If you're elderly or in a lot of pain, go lightly at first. You want to feel yourself breathing harder but not gasping for breath, and definitely *not* really hurting. You may also find that certain activities simply feel better than others. It may take some experimentation to discover that, say, swimming makes you very sore and drained but walking loosens you up. Try several methods until you find a few that you like. And be sure to check with your doctor before beginning your program.

Below are some activities that my patients have consistently found doable and helpful:

- *Warm-water walking tanks* are one of my favorite therapies. They're deeply relaxing and allow you a greater range of mobility. If you're in disabling pain, very overweight, or if you simply hate to exercise, these tanks are a good choice. They can be found in many physical therapy clinics. Ask your doctor if he'll write a recommendation for you.

(continued)

- *Brisk walking* is an ideal exercise if you are over sixty-five or out of shape. You'll need to walk at a pace that has you breathing hard—for some people, that's a saunter around the block, but others will need a more challenging uphill hike. If you can, find a route that keeps things interesting for you. Walk in a nature preserve or in an attractive section of town.

- *Tai chi* is another very gentle form of exercise. I consider it primarily an energy therapy, because it purports to affect the flow of life force, but it can provide a decent cardiovascular workout for those who are very frail or deconditioned, including the elderly. (Everyone else can use tai chi for energetic and relaxation benefits but will need a more intense activity to get their heart really beating.)

- *Swimming* allows you to work out without putting stress on your joints.

- *Cycling* is another activity that's easy on the joints as well as on the upper back and shoulders. I always think it's best to get out in nature for exercise if you can, but stationary bikes will also do the trick. If you have back pain and sitting straight up on a regular bike makes you feel worse, try switching to a recumbent bike.

- *Cross-country skiing* or *stationary ski machines* give you a symmetrical workout. They can also make a nice change of pace from walking or cycling.

- *Yoga* can benefit almost everyone. If you want to do yoga for cardiovascular benefits, you'll need to seek out a class in astanga yoga, also called "power" yoga. Astanga yoga requires stamina and strength, so it's not for people who haven't worked out in a while.

HEAT AND COLD THERAPIES

Cold packs and hot baths aren't exactly glamorous, but they *work.* With a bare minimum of expense and effort, they control flare-ups, relax muscles, reduce inflammation, and change your mood. And just as salt enhances the flavors of a meal, heat and cold therapies improve the effectiveness of almost any other treatment you pair them with. Their safety and low cost make them perfect for the elderly, children, or anyone who's looking for a gentler way to manage their pain. (And no, I'm not receiving kickbacks from the hot-water-bottle industry!)

One reason heat and cold therapies work so well is that sensory nerves are highly susceptible to temperature. When their temperature goes down by even a few degrees, their conduction velocity—the speed at which the pain message travels—will change. If you were to secure an electrode to a nerve at the back of a healthy person's hand and then connect it to an EMG machine, you would see waves on the monitor indicating normal nerve conduction. But if you took an ice cube and rubbed it over the back of the person's hand, the machine might give you nothing but a flat line or, after a short delay, a smaller wave. That's because the nerve is no longer able to carry sensory information very well. When the message your nerves are carrying is one of pain, you can see how you'd want to reduce their ability to transmit. (Heat therapies, however, do *not* increase pain—the body's normal temperature is very close to the "speed limit" on pain signals.)

Heat and cold also work on other levels of your body to reduce pain. They provide sensory stimulation that closes the spinal cord's pain gate, at least temporarily; they relax muscle spasms and increase range of motion; and cold tightens up blood vessels and reduces inflammation. Finally, they work at the psychological level. We all know how warmth can comfort and soothe, and that cold can be invigorating.

For the most part, choosing between heat and cold can be based on your personal preference. Heat feels more nurturing to some people; for others, cold instinctively feels more therapeutic. There are some instances, though, in which an application matches up quite nicely with a certain need.

HEAT

One of the best reasons to use heat is that it makes connective tissue more pliable. You can employ any of the therapies below before or after exercise to reduce pain and increase your mobility. They also make a good complement to massage, acupressure, and biofeedback.

APPLICATION	SUGGESTED LENGTH OF TREATMENT	MOST USEFUL FOR . . .	CONTRAINDICATIONS
Hot-water bottle, heating pad, or hydrocollator pack (available in physical therapy). Wrap the unit in a thin towel before applying to your skin. Most people prefer the bottle or pack, because the moistness conducts heat more effectively and tends to feel more soothing.	10–15 minutes every hour as desired. Some people like to apply heat for a short time every day when they get home from work, as way of resting and detensing muscles.	•Reducing muscle spasm as well as stiffness and pain in joints. •Comforting you when pain is especially distressing. •Softening trigger points before or after massage.	•Do not use intense heat on actively inflamed joints. Try a cooler therapy instead. •Do not use heat if you have diabetes, MS, peripheral neuropathies, Raynaud's phenomenon or disease, or anything else that prevents you from feeling temperature normally.
Hot bath or sauna.	If you're in a sauna or extremely hot bath, stay in for no more than 15–20 minutes.	•Whenever you feel achy all over. •Relieving spasm and stiffness. •Reducing stress. •Preventing soreness and pain after exercise, stretching, or physical therapy.	•Don't take saunas or very hot baths if you have a heart problem, high blood pressure, diabetes, or a blood-vessel condition. •Diabetes, MS, peripheral neuropathies, Raynaud's phenomenon or disease.
Paraffin dip. Lower your hand or foot several times into gently heated wax and then seal in the heat with a mitt or towel. You can try this technique at a physical therapist's office or a spa. If it works, you might want to invest in a home unit.	About 10 minutes.	•Osteoarthritis and inflammatory arthritis.	•Do not use on actively inflamed joints, skin lesions, joint infections, or an area with a tumor. •Diabetes, MS, peripheral neuropathies, Raynaud's phenomenon or disease.

(continued)

APPLICATION	SUGGESTED LENGTH OF TREATMENT	MOST USEFUL FOR . . .	CONTRAINDICATIONS
Ultrasound. It heats connective tissues through the use of high-frequency waves, which are not detectable by humans. Unlike other heat therapies, it penetrates the top layer of muscle. Once the deeper structures are heated and loosened, you should exercise and stretch them to restore lost range of motion.	•The session itself will last around 5–15 minutes, depending on the size of the area being treated. You might not see results right away, so you'll need more patience here than with other heat therapies. Plan to try five or six sessions before you decide whether ultrasound works for you.	•Chronic sprains and strains. •Myofascial pain syndrome. •Any condition in which pain has created tightness in the joint or tendon—arthritis, failed surgeries, and neurological disease can all lead to this problem.	•Pregnancy, acute infectious disease, vascular insufficiency, or a tumor. •Do not use near metallic implants, cemented joints, or pacemakers.

COLD

Cold is always the better choice immediately after an acute injury, such as a pulled muscle or a back that's gone out. Unlike heat, it has a strong anti-inflammatory effect, which is useful for rheumatoid arthritis, lupus, and other inflammatory conditions—as long as the area has fully intact nerves. A good rule of thumb here: If it feels hot, cool it.

APPLICATION	SUGGESTED LENGTH OF TREATMENT	MOST USEFUL FOR . . .	CONTRAINDICATIONS
Ice pack. I like a plastic bag filled with ice cubes and wrapped in a thin towel; many therapists say that a bag of frozen peas is their ice pack of choice. You can also dip	10–15 minutes every hour as desired. As with hot packs, some people like to apply ice on a regular, daily basis, especially after coming home from work.	•Acute pain. •Preventing an inflammatory reaction to exercise. If working out tends to bring on a flare-up, use an ice pack immediately after exercise to chill the muscles.	•Diabetes, MS, peripheral neuropathies, Raynaud's phenomenon or disease—anything that reduces sensation in your nerves.

(continued)

APPLICATION	SUGGESTED LENGTH OF TREATMENT	MOST USEFUL FOR . . .	CONTRAINDICATIONS
a washcloth into ice water and wring it out, but you will need to repeat the dip as the cloth takes on the heat from your skin. There's no need to buy commercial ice packs, which don't work as well as the home versions.		•Reducing soreness after an injection. •Fibromyalgia and myofascial pain syndrome. Apply the pack to whatever area feels particularly tender at a given moment. •Neck and back pain. I've found that people with these conditions seem to respond to ice more often than heat, but as always, this is a personal choice.	
Ice massage. You can perform one at home by filling a Styrofoam cup with water, freezing it, and tearing the lip off the top. Hold the cup by the bottom and rub the ice directly onto your skin.	5–15 minutes every hour as desired. Stop when you feel numb.	•Relieving spasms. The massage component of this treatment increases blood flow and helps mobilize the tissue. For this reason, ice massage is often a better way to relieve spasms than a plain ice pack.	•See above.
Spray-and-stretch. This is a technique performed by a physical therapist, in which a vapocoolant spray is applied to a painful area. The therapist then stretches you. In some cases, the therapist may give you some coolant and teach you how to perform the stretches at home.	About 5 minutes (it's usually combined with other treatments). You should give this therapy three or four tries before determining whether it works for you.	•Myofascial trigger points. Injections tend to be more potent, but spray-and-stretch can be a good complement to treatment, or a substitute if you can't use or don't like injections.	•See above.

THE FELDENKRAIS METHOD

Like the Alexander Technique, the Feldenkrais Method is a series of instructions meant to change improper body alignment and posture. Its founder, Moshe Feldenkrais, was a nuclear physicist who developed exercises that freed him from crippling leg pain. Although it can be used by anyone who wants to move more easily and with less tension, Feldenkrais is a particular favorite of people who have suffered serious physical trauma, either recently or long ago. People with spinal cord injury, MS, or stroke say that Feldenkrais helps them maximize their ability to move, and to make those movements with less pain.

Feldenkrais differs from the Alexander Technique in that it involves relearning primitive movements, such as crawling, in an attempt to retrain your nervous system. Perhaps for this reason, Feldenkrais also tends to work well for people who feel that they are still in the grip of abnormal patterns of movement that were set up in childhood. If you had a car accident or a serious fall when you were younger and haven't moved normally since, Feldenkrais might help you break restrictive and pain-causing habits.

Feldenkrais instruction takes two forms. The first is one-on-one training, in which the teacher guides you through basic movements, gently directing your body. She will also look for areas of tension that require special attention. This kind of class is called Functional Integration. The second form, known as Awareness Through Movement, is a group class that teaches correct alignment through a series of slow movements. In both kinds of classes, you learn how to bring focus to your motions so that you perform more naturally and easily.

Try five or six lessons to get a sense of how well this therapy works for you. Your practitioner should be certified by the Feldenkrais Guild; you can find contact information for the guild in Appendix E.

MASSAGE

Massage is as close as you can get to a universal treatment for chronic pain. Almost everyone in pain suffers from muscle tension, either as their primary symptom or as a natural defensive reaction to pain's ongoing alarm bells. By unclenching muscles and other tight spots, massage brings you much closer to that "easy in the harness" feeling.

But massage does much more than loosen your tissues. In the last decade or so, massage has been the subject of many well-conducted studies, and we've learned that it has multiple effects throughout the very place where pain resides—the nervous system. At the level of the spinal cord, the rubbing sensation blocks pain impulses from traveling up to the brain. Massage apparently also depletes substance P, a neurotransmitter that helps communicate the pain sensation, and it increases endorphins. At the highest level of the nervous system—the brain—massage seems to have profound effects as well. It improves cognitive function, reduces stress, and helps you sleep.

In one particularly fascinating study, Dr. Tiffany Field of the University of Miami Medical School asked volunteers to give regular infant massage to premature babies, who would ordinarily spend the first weeks of their lives encapsulated in sterile incubators. Dr. Field discovered that the massaged babies gained much more weight than babies who did not receive massage, and were able to go home in half the time. In a separate study, Dr. Field asked elderly people to give massage to small children on a regular basis. This time, she focused on the massage *givers,* who reported less depression and anxiety—and less pain. It's hard to explain these results except in very general terms: Apparently, giving and receiving caring touch is a basic human need. Without it, we're just not healthy.

Massage is now so widely available that the array of choices can be confusing. Here's a guide to the techniques that are best for pain relief, along with the kinds of conditions they are most likely to help. Any licensed therapist should have a basic familiarity with each of these techniques (with the exception of tui na), but you may want to seek out a therapist who specializes either in your disorder or in the technique that most interests you.

► *Swedish massage.* This is the most commonly available massage in the West, and its primary goals are relaxing muscles and improving circulation. Swedish massage focuses on manipulating the top layers of tissue. You'll receive long, gliding strokes as well as some kneading, vibration, friction, and percussion. Most people will feel better after a Swedish treatment; it's especially good for those with fibromyalgia. If you have deep-tissue pain, however, you may prefer a technique that's a little more aggressive.

► *Myofascial release.* In this deeper, more specialized treatment, the therapist works the fascia—the tissue that surrounds each of your internal structures—in order to reduce pain and make it easier for you to move. Obviously, this technique is especially helpful for anyone with myofascial pain, but it's also good for headaches and other disorders.

▶ *Russian.* Russian technique involves rapid, oscillating movements, especially around trigger points and the joints. Some people just love this feeling, and I'm one of them.

▶ *Tui na.* Tui na is a Chinese technique that's often practiced at the end of an acupuncture or acupressure session. It consists of both long strokes and quicker movements, which are often applied to the points that have just been treated. It has a strong reputation for easing pain, and it does seem to bolster the effects of acupuncture or acupressure.

▶ *Trigger point work.* Trigger points are hard, muscular knots that feel tender when pressed and that also send pain radiating outward into nearby tissues. They're at the root of a lot of muscular pain syndromes, and they're very hard to get rid of. One good technique is trigger point work, which may also be called myotherapy, or Bonnie Prudden Myotherapy, named after a pioneer in this area. In trigger point work, a therapist will locate your trigger points and then apply very firm pressure with her fingers or even elbows for several minutes. Getting your trigger points pressed can be very uncomfortable, but most people identify it as a "good hurt." You may need several treatments before you see results. If trigger points are a serious problem for you, consider combining massage treatments with injections of local anesthetic or spray-and-stretch therapy (see "Heat and Cold Therapies" in this chapter).

▶ *Acupressure* and its Japanese cousin, *shiatsu,* are also good hands-on methods for reducing pain. These techniques, which work in slightly different ways from usual massage, are considered in Chapter 10, "Distracting Your Nervous System from Pain."

No matter which technique you use, your therapist should have the proper licensure. If your state requires certification, then obviously your therapist should be able to produce it for you. If your state doesn't have a certification requirement, she should have passed the national exam for massage therapists, given by the National Certification Board for Therapeutic Massage and Bodywork (contact information for this board and other massage therapy organizations is listed in Appendix E).

Beyond those basic requirements, it's important to hire someone with whom you feel comfortable. You're putting your body into this person's hands, literally, so you'll want someone you can talk to about what feels most useful and what doesn't.

THE MOST MASSAGE FOR YOUR MONEY

I advise that you try weekly massage if your schedule and budget allow. It's often less expensive if you go to a private practitioner instead of a spa. If you live in a large city, consider visiting a suburban therapist, who may have lower rates. The effects of massage seem to build on themselves, so it's best to get one regularly.

In the real world, though, a lot of people just can't afford massage every week. If that's your case, there are a couple of options:

- Try a massage every *other* week. I know several people—fibromyalgia patients especially—who have found this a happy medium. Over the course of a year, they pay half the cost they would for weekly treatments, but they still feel significant relief.
- Schedule massages whenever you have an especially difficult task approaching. If you have to confront your exacting father-in-law or give a presentation at work, get a massage the morning of or even the day before. You'll be more relaxed and less likely to flare up before, after, or during the event.
- Limit massage for treatment of breakthrough pain—that is, severe pain that "breaks through" your regular means of pain management. Have a therapist's number on hand, and when the pain gets bad, go in for a treatment. You may be able to minimize the flare-up and avoid taking extra medication.
- Ask a loved one to give you a massage. Although an untrained person isn't likely to break up muscle tension as efficiently as a therapist, you can definitely receive all the subtler benefits from home treatment. See Appendix B for home massage techniques.

At the beginning of your appointment, a therapist should ask you the reason for your visit and discuss any medical problems, sensitive areas, and so on. This is a good time to speak up. If your shoulders hurt too much to bear direct touch, but you know that massage of your hips will make your shoulders feel better, say so. Don't be shy about stating your needs during the massage, either. Most therapists expect, and even prefer, to receive some direction from their clients. And you shouldn't fear that your modesty will be compromised. When you arrive for your appointment, you'll be left alone to disrobe and cover yourself with a large towel or sheet. The therapist will uncover only the part of the body that she's working on and will cover it back up as she moves on.

Contraindications: Don't use massage if you have a tumor or infectious disease, as the massage might cause it to spread. You'll also want to avoid massage if you have a skin condition that could be irritated by massage (or transmitted to the therapist), or if you have an injury, such as a broken bone, that could be made worse by friction.

PILATES

The Pilates Method is a conditioning technique that's great for opening up and elongating your muscles while building their strength. I especially like that its teachers show you how to bring greater awareness to your movements. Like many of the other therapies in this chapter, Pilates makes the connection between pain and posture, but it stands out for its extra attention to physical strength. This is a good choice for people who've begun to feel a little crimped as a result of constant pain. I also recommend it for osteoarthritis patients, because it allows them to strengthen muscles gradually and carefully, without disturbing their joints.

Pilates was once considered an esoteric technique and was used primarily by dancers who wanted to get stronger without bulking up. Now Pilates classes can be found in gyms and private studios in most cities. The ideal Pilates situation is a one-on-one training session that employs an expensive piece of equipment called the Reformer. The teacher will take you through a series of controlled exercises and ask you to focus on the ways you're using your muscles. He'll also show you how to use those muscles with the greatest precision and power.

If you can't find or afford private training, you can try group lessons. Most often these do not involve the specialized equipment; instead, you'll do all the work on a floor mat. Your treatment won't encompass all the dimensions that a private session might, but you'll definitely get stronger and learn more effective use of your body. Because both kinds of lessons demand sustained mental focus, you may also find that they have a meditative, stress-relieving effect.

Give Pilates at least six sessions before you decide whether it's working for you. After that, you can use your judgment regarding how often you should go. Lots of people go on a weekly or biweekly basis; others find that they can maintain their results—as long as they perform some other kind of regular exercise—with less frequent visits.

Contraindications: Do not try Pilates if you have unstable joints, very severe arthritis, or severe cardiac or pulmonary disease.

ROLFING AND HELLERWORK

Rolfing, also known as Structural Integration, is an intense, deep-tissue therapy that is closely related to massage. It's named after its founder, Ida B. Rolf, a biochemist who felt that the body functions more effectively when aligned with the field of gravity. According to her theory, you can move with minimal effort when all the parts of your body are in proper vertical alignment. Rolfers claim that their technique can improve almost any health problem. I'm dubious of that assertion, but I do think that Rolfing may well reverse underlying postural problems and tension that lead to pain.

Central to the Rolfer's idea of alignment is fascia, the long sheet of connective tissue that wraps around each of your internal structures, including nerves and muscles. Fascia can tighten up or stick together, and when it does, you may feel pain in that location—or that tightness may pull on other, more distant areas, making them hurt. Rolfers believe that the fascia gets stuck or tightened in predictable patterns, and that it can be loosened by very firm, deep rubbing, and some stretching, that penetrates to the fascia and loosens it. When this is accomplished, your posture and ability to move will improve.

Rolfing has a reputation as a painful therapy. When I tried it, I found the massage pretty uncomfortable, but not unbearable. I definitely felt more relaxed and looser afterward, and I know many people who say it's reduced their pain. I can't say for sure that Rolfing stretches out the fascia. When I've cut through fascia during surgery, it's seemed awfully tough, perhaps too tough to stretch out via massage, even one that's specialized and very deep. But that doesn't mean that Rolfing doesn't work. The massage expert and researcher Tiffany Field has found that firm massage has a more profound effect than lighter treatments, so perhaps Rolfing is simply an excellent kind of deep massage. If you have muscle or myofascial pain that feels widespread and out of reach of normal massage, or if you feel that your pain is related to body stiffness and misalignment, Rolfing may be a good option for you. You'll need to go for ten sessions that proceed in a standardized order—you won't get to direct the therapist very much, but you will get treatment that thoroughly works the entire body. Therapists should be certified by the Rolf Institute (contact information is listed in Appendix E); it's nice, although not strictly necessary, if they also have a massage license if your state offers certification.

Contraindications: Don't use Rolfing if you have extremely fragile skin that might tear easily (this is often true of the very elderly), or if you have any of the conditions listed as contraindications for massage (tumors, infections, acute injuries).

In the 1970s, an aerospace engineer named Joseph Heller decided that Rolfing didn't go far enough. Although he felt that the intense, hands-on work was essential, he thought it wouldn't automatically lead people to better movement and posture. In response, he developed his own system of deep-tissue work combined with movement reeducation. Like the Alexander Technique and the Feldenkrais Method, Hellerwork teaches you how to perform basic movement with less stress and greater efficiency. Its practitioners devote special attention to any emotional problems that may be connected to how you hold your body—stress, for example, could affect your breathing or the position of your shoulders. This integration of education and hands-on treatment is well suited for people who want something more intense than other massage or postural therapies can offer by themselves.

A course of Hellerwork consists of eleven sessions, each lasting somewhere between an hour and ninety minutes. You'll get about an hour of tissue work, with the rest of the time spent correcting your patterns of movement. Practitioners must complete a 1,250-hour training course and be certified by Hellerwork International. (Contact information is listed in Appendix E.)

Contraindications: The same as for Rolfing, above.

TRACTION

Traction for neck pain is effective and gentle and feels plain marvelous. In traction, you lie down on a table, where you are fitted with pads under the base of your skull and the back of your head, as well as a strap across your forehead. You relax as a machine pulls directly and slowly out on the pads and strap, stretching your neck and opening up the space between the vertebrae there. By creating more space, traction lifts pressure off the nerves and joints and relaxes muscle spasms. It also helps deliver more nutrients and fluids into the joints and discs, increasing their suppleness and strength.

Traction is a treatment of choice for neck pain caused by pressure on a nerve. It is also quite helpful for neck pain caused by arthritis, disc problems, pinched nerves, or muscle tension. Some people swear by it for headaches, but I find that its usefulness here is limited to cervicogenic headaches, that is, head pain that originates in the shoulders or neck.

You can get traction from a physical therapist and most chiropractors. (Your insurance is more likely to offer complete coverage when you get it from a physical therapist, but check your policy. Of course, you'll almost always need a referral from your doctor, too.) Expect to go for four or five treatments of fifteen minutes each. While you're there, you may want to try some therapies that complement traction's opening effects, such as stretches, massage, or trigger point work.

Contraindications and cautions: Traction is not appropriate for people who have a rheumatoid disorder or any other disease that causes instability or weakens the connective tissue in the neck. If you don't have a contraindication and decide to receive traction, make sure that the therapist doesn't use a jaw strap. This can lead to facial disorders such as temporomandibular joint syndrome (TMJ). I am also leery of lumbar traction, which is traction for the lower back. There isn't any good research to support its use, and I've never seen it significantly help anyone.

8.

MIND-BODY MEDICINE

BIOFEEDBACK / BREATHING TECHNIQUES / COGNITIVE-BEHAVIORAL THERAPY / GUIDED IMAGERY / HYPNOSIS / MEDITATION / PRAYER / YOGA

Doctors aren't supposed to have favorite patients, but I must confess to some hero worship of Captain Stan Wyzynski, a genuine World War II flying ace. Name a major battle in the Pacific theater, and he had been in the thick of it: Iwo Jima, Guam, Guadalcanal . . . not to mention Midway, where he'd been part of the team that sank four Japanese aircraft carriers and turned the tide of the war. I figured that anyone who'd flown those rickety 1940s planes, laden with tons of incendiary bombs, off the deck of a ship and then landed them again might know a thing or two about stress management.

The captain came to my office after a bout of cancer in his upper lung. The tumor was gone, but the surgery on his neck and lung had damaged the nerves leading down his left arm. The arm was swollen and quite painful; in addition, his shoulder had frozen up. As you might imagine, the captain's style was rather tight-lipped and his language a little spicy: "Just cut the damned thing off!" he barked, with the barest hint of a grin. "Hell, I'm right-handed! I could still drive!"

I assured the captain that we could bring the pain down to a manageable level without resorting to amputation. "Stick a needle in me, then!" he said. We could do that, I said, but a better course would be physical therapy to strengthen his arm and return motion to his shoulder. Unless he could perform some exercises, he'd never feel better.

But the therapy hurt too much, even for one of the toughest people I'd ever met, someone who'd survived war and an ugly cancer. Perhaps, I thought, his character and experience might light a path out of his current disability. I suggested that the next time he went to physical therapy, he should try to breathe through the pain. The captain gave me one of his steely looks. "What the hell is that?" he roared.

"Remember when you were flying off the deck of those carriers?" I asked. "How did you breathe then?"

Captain Wyzynski actually laughed. "We breathed like hell! We were about to die! I've never breathed so much in my entire life!"

In war, this pilot had used breathing to control his anxiety, although he never would have described it in those terms. Now I asked him to use breathing in a slightly different way, to control his pain. He'd heard about breathing techniques during his time in Asia, so he was ready to give them a shot. I taught him some ways to focus his attention on his breath, which would relax his muscles and put some distance between him and his pain.

A few weeks later, I saw Captain Wyzynski for a follow-up exam, and he told me that breathing had made the difference for him. It tapped into his immense reserves of courage and focus, making them more available as he brought his damaged arm back to life. Since he was so pleased with the results, I also taught him how to meditate. When I saw him next, he reported that he was meditating every morning. He enjoyed it immensely—and so did his wife, who thanked me over and over for teaching him meditation, adding, "He is *so* much easier to get along with now!"

People who routinely face down death—flying aces, rescue teams, mountaineers, and so on—know that survival is a mind game. By cultivating an intense focus, distraction and fear are set aside and the self is freed to perform the task at hand.

Pain is a mind game, too. When you hurt, nerves conduct messages that push your brain's hot buttons. Those buttons—located mainly in the limbic system and the thalamus, which are discussed in Chapter 3—can trigger panic, anger, and fear. But you can learn to uncouple the sensation of pain from those overwhelming feelings.

A few people are born with the focus of a chess master; they instinctively draw on it to outwit their pain. The rest of us have to practice. Luckily, most civilizations have recognized the importance of this skill and have developed tools for its cultivation. Eastern cultures have brought us meditation and yoga, both Eastern and Western religions have made prayer into a meditative discipline, and Western science has added biofeedback to the list. Each of these methods helps you use your mind to control the body, including aspects of physiology that were once thought involuntary. Now we know that the mind can reduce many of pain's secondary effects: It can ease muscle tension, lower blood pressure, soothe digestive woes, and quiet headaches. You can also use mental techniques to change your internal chemistry, so that you're producing less of the substances that increase pain and more of those that scramble its signals. You can learn to hush nerves that have become hypersensitive or that fire spontaneously. You can reduce anxiety and depression, and even send yourself off to sleep.

Just as I believe everyone in pain needs some exercise, I also think everyone in pain needs at least one mind-body technique to rely on. Most of them are cheap, even free, and once you're comfortable with them, you can use them anywhere, even on the bus or in the middle of a business meeting. Throughout the chapter, I've listed specific exercises that you can try right now.

In Chapter 3, I mentioned Reynolds Price, the novelist whose spinal cord was partially scraped away by surgery for a tumor. He spent three years in a shocking amount of pain before he discovered mind-body medicine. In his book *A Whole New Life,* he describes the results:

> Within that limited stretch of biofeedback and hypnosis, no more than eight weeks, I'd grown essentially free from pain. Not free from its constant presence in my body—it roars on still, round the clock every day, in my back and legs and across my shoulders—but free from any real notice of it or concern for its presence. . . . I can honestly say that now still, six years after approaching my mind for the help it could give, in an average sixteen-hour day, I'm conscious of being disturbed by pain for maybe a total of a quarter hour—in scattered minutes, here and there, at this job or that . . . when I notice the pain, I see it on the far horizon of consciousness like the mute demonstration of a force from which I'm as safe as I generally am from the distant sun.

BIOFEEDBACK

Biofeedback translates information about your body into visual or audio cues. In this modality, you're connected—usually by electrodes taped to your skin but sometimes by handheld thermometers or other painless devices—to computers and monitors that allow you to "see" muscle tension as a pattern on a screen or "hear" your temperature as a series of beeps. Over time, you learn how to control these body functions by paying attention to the feedback and experimenting with ways to manipulate it. After you've figured out how to relax your muscles or raise your body temperature or change some other aspect of your physiology in the practitioner's office, you can duplicate the effect on your own.

One of the most popular kinds of biofeedback, called EMG biofeedback, teaches you to control muscle spasms. EMG is important for pain sufferers, because even if your disorder is not caused by spasms, they may make an indirect contribution to your pain. In a painful bladder condition called interstitial cystitis (IC), patients often clench their pelvic floor muscles in response to the initial pain, making the area tighter and more uncomfortable. EMG biofeedback for the pelvic floor teaches these people how to release their muscles. This form of biofeedback is also good for any part of the body that you feel you're habitually clenching—head muscles, back, jaw—but can't seem to let go of.

Those who want to manage the stress component of pain may prefer a different mode of biofeedback. One kind is based on our knowledge that skin temperature in the extremities often drops in response to stress. (That's because the limbic system, sensing a threat, is directing blood away from these areas and toward your vital organs.) Whereas a normal hand reading might be around 92 or 93 degrees, a reading for someone under stress might go down to 75. Biofeedback can monitor the warmth of your hands; when you learn to raise their temperature, you also learn how to calm your limbic system's response and reduce stress. Another stress-reducing technique, called electrodermal biofeedback (EDR), works by teaching you to lower the salt content of your palms—in other words, it literally helps you to stop sweating over stress.

Biofeedback has been proven to reduce headaches, chronic muscle tension, anxiety, TMJ, and insomnia. There are so many excellent studies behind this mind-body technique that many doctors consider it a conventional therapy, not an alternative one. However, it's not recommended to patients as often as it ought to be. Many health professionals just aren't all that familiar with it; they also know from experience that most patients would rather take a pill than put in the effort biofeedback requires. If you're interested in integrative medicine but are worried about broaching the subject with your doctor, biofeedback might be a good place to start. Although you may have to initiate the conversation, your doctor will likely respond with interest and even enthusiasm.

Unlike most of the other therapies in this chapter, biofeedback can get pricey. However, it may also be covered by your insurance when recommended by your doctor, so check your policy. You'll need to summon up your patience, too. It usually takes eight to ten sessions, lasting thirty minutes to an hour apiece, before you can figure out how to control your physiological responses without the aid of equipment. And some people are never able to do it.

Your doctor or psychologist should be able to recommend a good biofeedback practitioner to you. (There are some home units available, but I don't know anyone who has been able to get consistent results from them. You're better off spending your money on an office treatment.) Make sure the practitioner is licensed by the Biofeedback Certification Institute of America (you can find contact information for this organization in Appendix E); in addition, try to find someone who has experience with your particular problem. It's nice, but not necessary, if your practitioner has a psychology background, too. Biofeedback is painless and has no known side effects—the electricity from the machine rarely enters your body, and even when it does, the amount is minimal.

BREATHING TECHNIQUES

Like good food, good breaths are nourishing; they feed you the essence of life. For millions of people in China, Japan, India, and elsewhere, daily health maintenance and spiritual practice involve some form of systematic, focused breathing. That's not such a difficult concept for most of us to understand. Consider how strong and vital you feel after drawing fresh air deep into your lungs, or think about your mother's admonition to take ten slow breaths whenever you are tempted to act in anger.

But pain can literally take your breath away. Over time, many chronic pain sufferers develop a pattern of shallow inhalations that are the breath equivalent of junk food. When you aren't breathing deeply, you may experience muscle tension or have trouble sleeping. By bringing greater awareness to your breathing, you can induce a state of relaxation at will.

Good breathing comes from your diaphragm, not from the top of your chest. Lie down in a comfortable spot and breathe in your usual manner. Do you heave your shoulders and upper rib cage? If so, your breaths are probably too shallow. To learn how to breathe more deeply, place your hand on your abdomen. Breathe from the base of your rib cage so that your abdomen rises and falls slowly; this movement indicates that your diaphragm is fully engaged. Drink the air down into the very base of your lungs, and then fill your lungs to the absolute brim. Now it's time for a slow, controlled exhalation. Empty the tops of your lungs first, moving down toward their middle, and finally use your abdominal muscles to push the final dregs of air out from the bottom. Continue in this manner for a total of at least ten breaths. Throughout the rest of your day, take time every now and then to notice your breaths. After a week or so, you will fix the habit of deep, diaphragmatic breathing in your body, so that you will hardly need to think about it.

You can also manipulate your breath to control pain and relieve stress. The techniques listed below ask you to become unusually aware of your breathing for a limited amount of time. They give you the benefits of deep breaths, but in focusing your attention on such a simple act, they also help coax your mind away from its usual worries and ramblings. They are most calming when you can spend several minutes in a quiet, comfortable place, but I've also used them while waiting for the elevator or even as I walk from one examining room to the next, when I need to replenish my stores of energy quickly.

YOUR BEST BREATHS FOR PAIN CONTROL

▶ *Foursquare breathing.* In this exercise, you make a kind of square with your breath. Inhale for a count of four, hold for a count of four, exhale for four, and hold again for four. Repeat this for a total of ten full breath cycles.

▶ *Zen breathing for insomnia.* As you're lying in bed, give one count to each inhalation and one count to each exhalation. When you reach ten, start again at one. Don't keep track of how many series of ten you've done; simply use the numbers as a means of

(continued)

focus rather than as a means of marking time. This technique will often send seasoned insomniacs off to sleep. And even if you can't get to sleep, you'll feel much more relaxed and rested than if you spent the night sweating over ever-higher sheep counts. I also use this exercise outside of bed, sometimes when I'm gearing up for a difficult project. It helps me focus on the task ahead.

▶ *The purifying breath.* Imagine that your body is surrounded by a white light. As you inhale, imagine that you're drawing that pure light down into your lungs and throughout the rest of your body—see your bones, muscles, fingers, toes, neck, and head all glowing with the whiteness. As you exhale, visualize that something darker or impure is being expelled from your body, perhaps your pain or sorrow or anger. This is a wonderful technique to use at the end of the workday, when most of us tend to cramp up with tension.

▶ *The flare-control breath.* This technique is specifically for controlling flare-ups. It is harder to do on the fly; instead, find a quiet place where you won't be disturbed for a few moments. Sit or lie down in a comfortable position and take several deep breaths. Notice the breath filling your lungs; it is bringing you vitality. Then imagine that your breath is flowing to the area of your pain. Feel the breath opening up that area and expanding into the area completely. Tell yourself that you're bringing the renewing cycle of breath to your pain, that you're bringing energy, light, and strength to this part of your body. As you exhale, imagine the breath flowing out from the pain. Breathe it out of your body; release it; let it go. Repeat for several cycles.

Deep breathing and breath exercises are useful for almost everyone. For many people with nerve pain, breathing and other mind-body techniques are an especially important source of relief. If you'd like to explore this area further, you might like to try yoga. Yoga teachers are the breath experts in most communities; the more serious they are about yoga as a mind-body practice (as opposed to a purely physical exercise), the more likely they are to know about breath techniques. You can call yoga studios to find out which teacher has a special interest in breath (called *pranayama* in yoga terms).

COGNITIVE-BEHAVIORAL THERAPY

Cognitive-behavioral therapy (CBT) is a form of psychotherapeutic treatment. It works on the principle that we are not bothered so much by events themselves as by our interpretations of these events. If I make plans to meet a friend for dinner and that friend cancels at the last minute, I could interpret the event in a number of ways. I might wonder if my friend has stopped liking me, which would make me sad and possibly anxious. I might feel angry that I've lost my opportunity to go out that night, and so I'd indulge in a good sulk. Or I might chalk up the experience to bad luck and spend a pleasant evening reading a good novel instead. CBT reminds us that it isn't the event—the cancellation of dinner—that's most important. What controls my feelings and my actions is the meaning I decide to give to that event.

This idea can be extended to pain, since our beliefs about it can be more controlling and destructive than the pain itself. When a person responds to pain with thoughts that are excessively, irrationally negative ("I've woken up with another headache. My whole life is a catastrophe"), CBT can help by challenging those thoughts and then replacing them with rational, more realistic ones. Whenever the excessively negative thought comes up, the person replaces it, until she has attained a more productive and realistic response to her pain.

When we hurt, even the best of us have a difficult time responding in a consistently rational, realistic way. And when pain is chronic, it's all too easy to develop thought patterns that actually enlarge pain's role in your life. That's why CBT has become a standard treatment in pain clinics, endorsed by even the most conservative physicians. Even people who hate the idea of psychotherapy tend to find this brand of it very helpful. Instead of talking about your childhood or traumatic experiences, you focus on the problems you need to solve and on finding practical solutions to them. And you don't need to spend a year on the couch to do it. The goal of CBT is to improve your functioning right away. Most people need only a few sessions (although sometimes it takes longer).

How do you know if you could benefit from this therapy? If in your pain diary you found yourself consistently ranking your pain at a 9 or 10, then you may find that cognitive restructuring dramatically changes your life. I also recommend it if you suffer from a progressive disorder such as inflammatory arthritis, if pain has made you feel defective or

REDUCING SUFFERING THROUGH SELF-TALK

Self-talk is the name cognitive-behavioral therapists use for the phrases we say to ourselves. When this talk is needlessly defeating, exaggerated, or unrealistic, it's called a *cognitive distortion*. A key strategy used in cognitive-behavioral therapy is identifying any cognitive distortions and replacing them with more appropriate phrases. Here are some examples:

COGNITIVE DISTORTION	REALISTIC REPLACEMENT
I don't deserve to have this pain taken away. I ought to suffer because I was a bad parent/child/spouse/person.	Feeling physical pain now is not going to undo any wrongs I might have committed in the past. I can't change what's happened, so I am going to do whatever I can to be a fully alive human being today.
I should not have to go through all this effort just to feel like a normal person.	I have pain, like it or not. I'll decide how much time I want to spend managing it, and then I'll devote the rest of my life to other things.
The pain is keeping me from going to the party tonight. I'm going to lose all my friends.	If they're really my friends, they'll understand why I can't go. I'll write the host a nice note and schedule a low-key event with a few people later this weekend.
How can anyone expect me to be nice? I'm in pain!	Behaving poorly isn't going to make me feel better. I'll take deep breaths until I have this bad mood under control.

(continued)

COGNITIVE DISTORTION	REALISTIC REPLACEMENT
Because I'm in pain, people should take care of me.	I will ask for help when I really need it and work on developing as much independence as possible.
I'm having a bad pain day. This must mean that all the progress I was making has been wiped out.	Bad days will happen, even though I'm generally feeling better. Today I'll take it easy and book a massage.
The pain keeps me from lifting my son when he cries, so I'm a bad father. My son will grow up to be damaged.	I can't lift my son, but I can sit on the couch and have him climb onto my lap. By keeping myself calm through pain, I can teach my son how to handle life's difficulties.
The pain prevents me from keeping house the way I used to. Now I'm a failure at the one thing I used to be good at.	No one will die if the house isn't perfect. If I break the work down into baby steps and take breaks in between, I can get a lot done.
I feel better today, but I'm just going to be disappointed when the pain comes back.	I am just going to enjoy today for what it is. If I'm going to live with pain, I need to adjust to its ups and downs.
The doctors can't tell me exactly where the pain is coming from, so it must be untreatable. I'll never get better.	Lots of people with chronic pain never get a diagnosis, but they do improve with time. I'll do what I can to ease the pain.
I can't stand the pain one minute longer. I'll go crazy.	I've lived through pain before, I can do it again. I will try to relax or meditate and separate myself from the pain I'm feeling.

damaged, if you feel helpless much of the time, or if you find yourself blaming others for your suffering.

Every psychotherapist has some training in CBT—there's no official subspecialty—but you should find someone who has experience using this therapy specifically for pain. Try calling a pain clinic or the department of psychology or psychiatry at a local university for suggestions. Cognitive-behavioral therapy is reimbursed under many health plans, especially those that include behavioral or mental health benefits.

GUIDED IMAGERY

Close your eyes for a moment and think of biscuits fresh from the oven, lightly browned and smelling of buttery warmth. Imagine taking one of the biscuits from the pan and breaking it open. It is fluffy and white, and steam rises up from the inside as you reach for the honey. . . .

If your mouth is watering, then you've just experienced successful guided imagery, in which the imagination is used to produce bodily changes. Most people can easily stimulate saliva and stomach secretions by thinking about the aroma of certain foods. I'm sure that if you tried hard enough, you could raise your blood pressure by imagining yourself arguing with someone who really gets under your skin.

To use guided imagery for relaxation, you think of a safe, peaceful place and try to take yourself there in your mind. You might imagine yourself in a favorite vacation spot, lying atop a raft, drifting along a lake, listening to the waves hit the breakfront, feeling the sun warm your bones, and smelling the slightly brackish water. The more details you can conjure up in your mind, the more effective the imagery will be. Writing about the biscuits and the lake has already made me more relaxed (and hungry) than I was just a few minutes ago. If you can take five or ten minutes out of your day for these mini-vacations, you'll probably notice that your stress is under greater control. You may become so proficient that you can leave your pain behind for a while, even when you're having a flare-up.

But guided imagery offers benefits beyond relaxation. By imagining your muscles melting or heating up, you can soften a spasm. If you have a hot kind of pain, then thinking of cold water or ice may cool you down. I also like techniques that convince your mind it doesn't feel pain. Some people accomplish this by imagining that they have a bucket of liquid anesthetic, the kind that deadens pain on contact.

They imagine that they're dipping their hand into the bucket and then bringing that hand to the area that hurts, "painting" it with the anesthetic until it feels cool and numb.

A VISUALIZATION FOR PAIN RELIEF

Find a quiet, comfortable spot where you won't be interrupted. Close your eyes and breathe quietly for a few moments. Once you're feeling relaxed, direct your attention to your pain. Note the location of the sensation, its intensity, and its precise qualities. Now, describe the pain to yourself in terms of color. Is it purple? Black? Green with yellow spots? Stay with that image for a moment, and imagine the area of your pain suffused with that color.

Now find a different color, one that has the power to dissolve or melt the color of your pain. White or silver may be a good choice. Visualize that color pouring into the painful area, dissolving the pain. You have an unlimited supply of the second color, so use however much you need. Dump buckets of it onto your pain; fill fire hoses with it. Let rivers of that color flood over your pain, washing it away.

Try to spend at least five minutes with this visualization.

You can easily perform guided imagery at home (or anywhere you like), either using the suggestions here or by coming up with your own. Don't worry that your imagination isn't good enough or that you don't have the proper attention. Just set aside some quiet time, breathe deeply, and enjoy yourself. If you mind wanders, there's no need to scold yourself. Very few people can summon up immediate focus on any topic. Just gently bring your attention back to your image whenever it wanders.

Some people find that they can relax more deeply when a professional helps them develop an image and takes them through it. Many psychotherapists are skilled in this technique, and your doctor may know of some good ones near you. Hiring a professional hangs a price tag on this otherwise free therapy, but with a doctor's referral it's possible—although not probable—that your insurance will cover some of the sessions. If you want to strike a middle ground, consider buying an audiotape of a professional talking you through a series of images. New-age bookstores and some health-food stores carry these tapes; another source is the Academy for Guided Imagery's Web site at www.interactiveimagery.com. You might also read one of the following excellent self-help books on the subject: *Rituals of Healing,* by Jeanne Achterberg, Barbara Dossey, and Leslie Kolkmeier; *Guided Imagery for Self-Healing: An Essential Resource for Anyone Seeking Wellness,* by Martin Rossman; and *Healing Visualizations: Creating Health Through Imagery,* by Gerald Epstein. (See Appendix F for full details.)

HYPNOSIS

Hypnosis has been an accepted medical treatment in the United States since 1958, when the American Medical Association gave it a seal of approval. More recently, hypnosis as a therapy for chronic pain has been the subject of rigorous clinical trials; over and over, it has shown itself a remarkably useful tool. By slipping into a trancelike, highly suggestible state, patients can learn to control body functions that are usually involuntary. They can reduce their blood pressure, heart rate, and level of stress hormones, and possibly even change how the brain activates during a pain sensation.

When you're under hypnosis, your mind is in a state of deep concentration and is receptive to suggestion. A therapist can use this mental state to offer you alternative, relaxing responses to pain. For example, she may suggest that upon feeling pain, you lower your blood pressure instead of raise it; or she may use imagery instead, suggesting that you imagine that your pain is controlled by a dial that you can turn down at will.

Who can benefit from hypnosis? Almost everyone who tries hypnosis will feel more relaxed, at least temporarily. It seems, though, that some people are more "hypnotizable" than others. For these lucky individuals, hypnosis can have an effect lasting far longer than that of the trance itself, one that is more powerful than biofeedback, general relaxation, or other mind-body therapies. If you can easily lose yourself in your work or in activities such as reading or watching movies, you may be hypnotizable—and hypnosis may be one of your best bets in controlling pain. Headaches, irritable bowel syndrome, and TMJ are among the conditions that have responded well to hypnosis in clinical trials.

A hypnotherapy session works rather simply. Contrary to all those sitcoms in which people are accidentally hypnotized and cluck like chickens for weeks on end, you cannot be hypnotized without agreeing to the procedure and consciously placing trust in the therapist, nor can you be made to do anything you don't wish to do. Once the session begins, the therapist will go over the procedure with you and answer any questions you have. Then she'll go through a routine meant to induce relaxation, perhaps asking you to feel your limbs growing heavy one at a time. In this stage, you're trying to get the conscious mind to settle down and let new ideas have access to the deeper levels of the subconscious. When you're in a hypnotic state, you're fully aware of what's going on—including the fact that you're being hypnotized—but you feel very relaxed and a little bit apart from the world. At this point, the therapist will make suggestions (such as "You're going to sleep soundly tonight") based on your needs. You may receive a tape at the end of the session so that you can play it at home, or your therapist may give you some advice for reproducing the hypnotic state on your own. (If you're interested in home techniques, you could also try the guided imagery suggestions in this chapter. Guided imagery is not hypnosis, but the two have much in common.)

Many doctors, nurses, dentists, psychiatrists, and psychotherapists are trained in hypnosis; ask around to find someone in your area with good experience. Hypnosis is much like biofeedback and even acupuncture in that many health professionals find it interesting, but very few will actually suggest it without prompting. Don't be afraid to ask. And as always, nurses are a good source for references.

Your therapist should be certified by either the National Board for Certified Clinical Hypnotherapists or the American Council of Hypnotist Examiners (contact information for both is listed in Appendix E). It's also a good idea to hire someone who is a licensed health care professional, since you're more likely to get reimbursement from your insurance provider. Hypnosis is safe, with no side effects, although people with serious mental disorders should check with their doctor or therapist before using this technique.

MEDITATION

"I can't meditate."

Most people who come to me know that meditation is good for them. They've heard that it reduces stress along with the risk of heart disease and hypertension. They may also know that it has been clinically proven to reduce chronic pain, and that it stimulates production of endorphins and certain pain-relieving neurotransmitters. They're curious about it and may even have tried it. But still, they tell me, they can't do it.

People who say they can't meditate have usually been misled about the nature of meditation. They believe that a good meditator sits down, assumes the lotus position, and immediately blocks out the rest of the world. After maintaining this perfect focus for a while, he slips effortlessly into a higher mental state. The meditator's attention does not wander, nor does he fidget, or get an itch, or wish that he were out riding his bike.

I say that's a bucket of hallucinogenic hogwash. And I know a lot of Tibetan monks who would agree with me. Before I explain why, let me tell you a little bit more about this therapy.

We're all pretty good at thinking (although cognitive-behavioral therapy can improve those skills). The problem is that most of us are unable to stop. You know the feeling—your mind plays one particular worry or thought over and over, in an obsessively running loop. Or maybe it chatters away at you about a thousand different things.

Meditation is a way of quieting that chatter. By bringing your focus to your breath, a mantra, or the like, you give your mind something simple to hold on to as you gradually let go of the world. By controlling your attention, you're accomplishing something deeply therapeutic. You begin to feel more relaxed, more at peace with yourself. This feeling usually lasts far beyond the meditation itself, so that when stress comes flying your way, you have the psychic resources to deflect it.

But even the most experienced of meditators knows that the mind resists being focused and controlled. The chatter has a way of getting louder and more demanding just as you're trying to shut it off. You're trying to meditate, and your brain is playing the kazoo and banging on pots and pans. This experience is disappointing for some people and leads them to believe that they've failed. It helps to know that it's absolutely natural for your mind to wander and even for you to feel antsy, especially in the opening portion of your meditation session. When this happens, just gently bring your mind back to your object of focus. No need to reprimand yourself. Continue to escort your attention back to the meditation as often as necessary. Even if you spend an entire session doing nothing but bringing your mind back from wandering, you'll receive some benefit. And you may find that after a few sessions, it gets easier.

If you give meditation a try and it *still* doesn't seem to work for you, consider a therapy such as yoga or tai chi, which are essentially forms of moving meditation. Many people discover that it's easier to empty their minds when their bodies are in motion.

I recommend meditation for anyone who's in chronic pain, no matter what their particular disorder. For people with nerve-related pain in particular, meditation is often more effective than any other therapy at turning down that nerve noise and letting you get on with your life.

Meditation is a technique that requires no religious beliefs, even though some form of meditation is common to most of the world's religious traditions. It's free and easy to do in your home or office, as long as you have a quiet place to yourself for a few minutes a day. You can try the meditation suggested here to get you started. For further information, I recommend Jon Kabat-Zinn's book *Full-Catastrophe Living: Using the Wisdom of Your Body and Mind to Face Stress, Pain, and Illness.* (For more information, see Appendix F.) The book outlines Dr. Kabat-Zinn's remarkable meditation program at the University of Massachusetts Medical Center, a program clinically proven to reduce pain in patients when all other efforts had failed. For those who prefer more personal instruction, most yoga studios and Buddhist centers offer classes in meditation.

A MINDFULNESS MEDITATION

Mindfulness meditation is a good choice for beginners; I believe it's one of the best forms of meditation for pain control, no matter what the skill level of the practitioner.

Take a few moments to create a quiet space for yourself. Sit or lie down in a comfortable position, using pillows or other props so that your body is at ease.

Start to bring your awareness to your breath. I don't mean that you think about the mechanics of your breathing, just that you observe the breath as it moves through your body. You might notice the temperature change as your breath enters or exits the tip of your nose, or feel your lungs filling and deflating. The breath will remain your object of focus for the entire meditation. A friend of mine, Joseph Loizzo, M.D., likens the object of meditation to a stake in the ground. Whenever your mind wanders from the breath—and you can be sure that it will—you simply note what you have been thinking

(continued)

or feeling in a nonjudgmental way and then return to your stake. If you begin to worry about your taxes, just let the thought move across your mind as you observe it. "Huh," you might say, "I'm thinking about my taxes. I do that a lot." And then return to the breath. If you start to feel pain, do the same thing. Observe the pain; experience it in the here and now, without judging it or your reaction to it. Just let it pass over you like a cloud floating across the sky. Don't push the pain away; don't pull it toward you; don't try to judge it. Just be there with it, and then return to the breath again when you are ready.

You can continue this meditation for as long as you like. It's best to allow enough time for your mind to settle down. For most people, twenty minutes is a practical amount of time, although of course you can tailor it to your needs.

PRAYER

Are science and religion diametrically opposed? That's certainly what I was taught in school. It's difficult to reconcile religious doctrines about the world's creation with the versions that science presents us. After all, it was the Church that silenced Galileo's theory that the earth revolved around the sun, and today there are some Christian groups that oppose teaching evolution.

Yet religion and medicine have a long history of cooperation. Religious organizations have traditionally sponsored hospitals, for example, and it wasn't long ago that many religious leaders doubled as healers in their communities. Westerners are once again turning to religion as a source of healing, and scientists and doctors are among that number. Many scholarly papers cite connections between the strength of someone's religious beliefs and that person's ability to get well. Harvard Medical School currently offers a class called Spirituality and Healing.

Sorting through the evidence of religion and healing is quite a task, since it's nearly impossible to isolate faith from the things that tend to come along with it. We do know that people who regularly attend religious services (it doesn't matter what kind) are healthier, and that they recover from illness more quickly. Maybe that's because they tend to take better care of themselves and to have more support from their community. Maybe people who believe that there is an order to the world are simply more relaxed. But it is not possible to rule out less earthly reasons for this correlation.

So should you put on your good clothes and go to church next Sunday? Whatever the reason for religion's power, it's unlikely that you can receive its health benefits if your practice isn't heartfelt. But if you have been away from religion for a while and have lately been drawn toward it, perhaps it's wise to heed those feelings.

Thus far I've spoken about having faith in God or a higher power, as opposed to prayer specifically. Many religious people think of prayer as a time of deep reflection; it gives them a feeling of peace and renewal. In this respect it seems that prayer is a kind of meditation—that is, it focuses your attention on one thing to the exclusion of all else, whether that thing is a mantra or your breath or the rosary. Like other forms of meditation, prayer lowers heart rate and blood pressure. Again, if you like to pray, you may want to make a special effort to set aside time for it daily.

But the effects of prayer on health can be most easily measured when another person is praying for you to get better. A famous study of patients in coronary wards separated the patients into two groups: those who were prayed for and those who weren't. Neither group of patients knew about the prayers, nor did any of the patients have any personal connection to those who were doing the praying. Yet those who were prayed for consistently recovered more fully and more quickly. How do doctors and scientists account for this? The most appropriate response may be a deepened respect for all the things we still don't know and may never fully understand.

YOGA

In the 1980s, Arthur C. Klein, a writer and marketing consultant, and Dava Sobel, a medical writer (now famous for her best-selling books *Longitude* and *Galileo's Daughter*), conducted an extensive survey of people with back pain. Four hundred and ninety-two people from all walks of life responded to their questions, and of those who had tried yoga for their pain, a startling 96 percent reported moderate to dramatic long-term help, and the other four percent said their pain had been helped on a temporary basis.

What makes yoga so powerful for back and other kinds of pain? Well, as you know by now, I like therapies that work on several levels, and that's exactly what yoga does. Even its name points toward its multifaceted nature. The word *yoga* means "to yoke" in Sanskrit; when you practice yoga, you use physical exercises, breathing and relaxation techniques, and meditation to help you integrate these different aspects of your being. Such integration has a strengthening effect on your whole self, and fortifies your resistance to pain.

Some of the therapies in this book distract you from your pain so that you temporarily forget it's there. Yoga takes the opposite approach. Instead, it asks you to bring your awareness to your body, *especially* to the parts that are in pain or that just don't feel right. This is especially beneficial for people who feel divorced from their bodies or angry at the part that hurts. Yoga helps you become more accepting of your body and of your pain, less judgmental and reactive. With time, you'll also become an expert on your body; you'll know what makes it feel worse and how to coax it into balance.

Yoga is also an effective way to manage stress. Herbert Benson, a Harvard professor and author of *The Relaxation Response,* has found that yoga lowers your heart rate, promotes deeper breathing, and induces brain wave patterns that are associated with relaxation and optimism. These effects are much like those of meditation, and it's appropriate to think of yoga as a kind of meditation on your body. As you move through the poses, your attention is gently directed to what your arms, legs, trunk, neck, and head are doing at any given moment. In other words, it's hard to worry about the office when you're trying to balance on one foot.

Finally, the poses themselves can ease your pain. They make you stronger and more flexible, improve the circulation to your joints and muscles, and stimulate your brain to produce painkilling chemicals.

Yoga is an adaptable therapy that can be used by almost anyone, but if you have deteriorated joints or any other kind of serious problem, check with your doctor first. You may get her approval to do yoga, with the caveat that you stay away from certain exercises. I suggest that you find a class for beginners, one that's very gentle and that emphasizes stress reduction. Don't worry that you'll be forced into a human pretzel. Beginning yoga classes are extremely easygoing and tend not to stray beyond light stretching and strengthening poses. Most of them are developed with middle-aged adults in mind. For information, you can contact the American Yoga Association; its address, phone number, and Web site are listed in Appendix E.

Yoga classes are fairly easy to find these days, even if you live in a small town. Check yoga studios as well as local hospitals and health clubs. Word of mouth is the best recommendation, but you can also ask a massage therapist, chiropractor, or physical therapist for advice.

9.

THE PAIN-CONTROL DIET: PLUS, THE TOP TWENTY SUPPLEMENTS FOR PAIN RELIEF

Did you know that:

- Fast food can bring on a flare-up of arthritis, PMS, or nerve pain?
- An extra ten pounds around the middle can increase the pain in your knees?
- Walnuts and deep-water fish can help reduce inflammation?
- Berries may strengthen your immune system?
- Spinach salad contains nutrients that can soothe nerve pain and insomnia?

Diet is a basic means of pain control, one that should be an essential element of everyone's plan. Good food choices can subdue pain and pain's side effects: listlessness, fatigue, insomnia, weight gain, and digestive problems. Unhealthful eating, on the other hand, will increase your suffering and need for medication.

It is one of life's great pleasures to eat fresh food that has been prepared with love and care. Compare eating a stew with ingredients you've selected at the grocer's, cleaned and cut by hand, and simmered on the stove with the dismal mess you get from the heat-'n'-eat variety at the convenience store. I think you'll agree there *is* no comparison, and that principle forms the foundation of my diet recommendations: Eat fresh, wholesome food whenever possible.

THE PAIN-CONTROL DIET

In the following pages, I'll show you how food choices can control the inflammatory process, strengthen your resistance to pain, and tame the side effects of pain medications. Even if you do not have the time or ability to prepare homemade meals, you can still improve your diet—and your pain level—by making small changes targeted to your needs. Do you want to control arthritis flare-ups? Swap hamburger for fish a few nights a week. Do you suffer from digestive problems? Introduce a few more servings of fresh fruits and vegetables into your daily routine, and substitute a whole-grain cereal for the morning danish. Is nerve noise driving you crazy? Consider adding two servings of green vegetables to your plate every day. As your palate adjusts and you begin to feel better, you may find it easier to make even more positive changes.

This pain-control diet is simple to follow; I certainly don't recommend spending all your time thinking about what you eat. You don't need a perfect diet to feel better, and an occasional beef Wellington is hardly going to make you ill. Simply by cultivating an awareness about your food and your body's response to it, you will be stronger and more resistant to disease and stress—and you will feel less pain.

EAT FIVE TO SIX SERVINGS OF FRESH FRUITS AND VEGETABLES EVERY DAY

One of the most appealing sights in the world is a farmer's market, with the owners and their employees standing proudly behind their wares, row after row of produce in deep, gorgeous hues—frilly lettuces, carrots that smell like earth and sunshine, the bright primary colors of berries, and, later in the year, the autumnal shades of pumpkin and eggplant and squash. If you think I'm crazy to wax poetic about produce, then you might try attending a farmer's market yourself, or even viewing the displays of fruits and vegetables at your local supermarket with appreciative eyes.

It's no accident that nature has made fruits and vegetables such a sensual pleasure. As a species, we *need* to find them appealing because they are necessary for our good health. If your body is worn down by pain—if you suffer from frequent illness, fatigue, or weakness—fruits and vegetables can act as tonics, strengthening your body with an array of nutrients. Your body will especially appreciate the benefits of *phytochemicals,* plant substances that bolster the immune system, helping you resist cancer, heart disease, and other illnesses. For the most phytochemicals, eat a mix of produce that is richly colored, such as berries, red grapes, leafy greens, carrots, pumpkins, tomatoes, and peaches. By eating these fruits and vegetables, you could even affect pain on the cellular level: Certain substances in deeply colored produce appear to stabilize the cell membranes, making them less likely to produce substance P and other pain-promoting compounds.

Thanks to their high fiber content, fresh fruits and vegetables also improve the digestive problems that are often pain's companions. Fiber, the indigestible component of food, helps regulate your digestive system and encourages peristalsis, the intestinal contractions that allow waste to pass through the body. If you suffer from constipation, irritable bowel syndrome, or Crohn's syndrome, fruits and vegetables ought to be your first line of treatment.

My guess is that science will continue to isolate other compounds in fruits and vegetables with additional health-protective effects. But you don't need to wait for the research to know this basic fact: *If you don't feed your body well, it will not heal well.* Rebuild your bone and muscle tissue with the nutritional offerings of produce, or they will continue to degenerate and inflame. Feed your nervous system with fruits and vegetables, or it may be so weak and unstable that it sends out intensified messages of pain.

In the phrase "fresh fruits and vegetables," the word *fresh* is crucial: You should get most of your fruits and vegetables from the produce department, not from a can or a box. If you must eat processed vegetables, choose frozen over canned, since freezing allows more nutrients to stay intact. When vegetables are deep-fried, as in french fries or sweet-potato fritters, the inflammatory effects of the added fat outweigh the vegetable's nutritional benefits—and some of those benefits may be destroyed by the high heat of the deep-frying process. When you do eat enough fresh produce, you'll feel less sluggish, with more energy to do the things you want to do.

One of the best things about eating the recommended number of servings of fruits and vegetables is that it helps the rest of your diet fall into place. When fresh produce is a priority, you'll be less likely to visit fast-food restaurants, nor will you have room on your luncheon plate for chips or onion rings. Better still, you'll soon develop a taste for cleaner, more robust food—making your pain-control diet that much more enjoyable to follow.

FOR PAIN RELIEF, THINK GREEN

Green, leafy vegetables such as kale, broccoli, spinach, and chard are an abundant source of B-complex vitamins, a deficiency of which is implicated in pain caused by damaged or misfiring nerves. They contain magnesium, which helps relax smooth muscles and possibly reduce stress. They also contain chemicals that encourage the production of serotonin, the neurotransmitter important for sleep and regulation of mood states. I suggest eating two servings of green leafy vegetables every day. This is not as hard as it sounds. You could have a small spinach salad or some broccoli with lunch, and some sautéed kale alongside dinner. If you dislike green leafies, you may want to take a look at how you've been eating them. Too often these vegetables are cooked to within an inch of their life, leaving them dull and even noxious. When they're prepared with a lighter hand, perhaps steamed or sautéed gently, or even served raw with dip, they have a fresh, clean taste that most adults find pleasing. Try buying a different green vegetable every time you go to the grocery store and experiment until you find the kinds you like best.

EAT THE RIGHT FATS

Do your joints feel hot and tender? Is your chronic pain characterized by a burning quality? Do you suffer from PMS pain? If you've answered yes to any of these questions, the kinds of fats you eat can make the difference between a flare-up and significant relief. That's because some fats increase inflammation, while others cool it down.

Normally, inflammation is your body's response to an injury. When you get a cut or sprain, your body floods the damaged area with extra blood and immune cells. The beefed-up circulation and immune activity get the work of healing under way, and they also cause the injured part to become swollen and tender to the touch, telling you to avoid it until the damage has been repaired.

But sometimes inflammation develops in the absence of an injury. That's when it becomes a problem—a chronically painful one. This happens in arthritis, when joints feel hot and tender, or in nervous system disorders such as postherpetic neuralgia, when inflamed nerves transmit a burning sensation. A large degree of PMS pain is caused by inflammation that's set in motion by estrogen.

Inflammation pain is a sign that certain hormones in your body, called prostaglandins, are out of balance. Prostaglandins come in two types: One encourages inflammation, while the other inhibits it. Since both kinds are constructed from fatty acids, the kind of prostaglandins that predominate in your body depends to a large extent on the kinds of fats you eat.

Fatty acids are chains of carbon atoms to which hydrogen atoms are linked. Saturated fats are those formed by fatty acids in which many of the carbon's bonds are occupied by hydrogen atoms; these are the animal fats that are linked to heart disease and other serious illnesses. You've probably also heard about partially hydrogenated oils, in which the carbon atoms of vegetable or seed oils are saturated with hydrogen and then exposed to high heat, converting the oil into a solid, such as

RIGHT FATS, WRONG FATS

Here's a short list of the fats that cool the inflammatory fires, along with those that stoke the flames.

ANTI-INFLAMMATORY FATS	PRO-INFLAMMATORY FATS
Eggs fortified with omega-3 fatty acids	Butter
Flaxseed and flaxseed oil	Corn oil
Herring	Full-fat dairy products, such as whole milk and ice cream
Pumpkin seeds	Margarine
Mackerel	Safflower oil
Olive oil	Sesame oil
Salmon	Sunflower oil
Sardines	Tropical oils (such as coconut, palm, and palm kernel oil)
Walnuts	Vegetable shortening

vegetable shortening, or into a soft, spreadable substance, such as margarine.

Most people know that saturated fats and partially hydrogenated oils can raise your "bad" cholesterol, or LDL (partially hydrogenated oils also lower the "good" cholesterol, HDL). But if you haven't already reduced or eliminated your intake of these substances for the health of your heart, here's another reason: These fats increase the production of pro-inflammation prostaglandins. That's right—they can lead to pain. I can't tell you how many patients of mine have reduced inflammation just by replacing their regular lunch of fast-food burgers and fries with more healthful alternatives. And when they skip the golden arches, they tend to lose weight, too, which means there's less stress on creaky joints.

But the pain-control diet isn't just about *avoiding* food. Other fats are derived from omega-3 fatty acids, highly unsaturated chains of carbon atoms from which anti-inflammation prostaglandins are derived. Omega-3 oils are found in deep-water fish, walnuts, and flaxseed, among other sources. An anti-inflammatory diet that includes these foods (and limits saturated and partially hydrogenated fats) may also inhibit the production of neurotransmitters such as substance P and bradykinins, which increase pain and inflammation.

One way to make a significant improvement in your diet is to eat oily fish such as salmon, tuna, sardines, mackerel, and herring instead of red meat twice a week. If you choose to eat salmon, try to eat the kind that is caught in the wild, since farm-raised salmon does not feed on the plant substances that give the fish's flesh its high levels of omega-3s. However, wild salmon can be a budget-buster, so use canned salmon if you must, and try to eat the wild fish as a treat. (Catfish, the most popular fish in the United States, unfortunately contains none of the omega-3s.) Flaxseed, which must be eaten raw, adds a nice texture to salads or cold cereals. Walnuts, of course, can be eaten out of hand, in salads, or in nutritious baked goods.

If you just can't handle the flavor of fish oil or flaxseed, you can take fish oil capsules (see "The Top Twenty Supplements for Pain Relief," later in this chapter). But it's always better to get your nutrients from food than from a pill.

TONY'S STORY: FROM BURGERS TO BLACK BEANS AND RICE

Tony's knees were so stiff and painful that he hesitated to put weight down on them. When he came into my office, he looked as if he were walking on glass.

Tony had worked in construction all his life, first as a laborer, then as a foreman, and now as the chief officer of the company. Tony blamed his degenerative arthritis on the decades of heavy labor and routine trauma to his knees—a correct assumption. But in a way, Tony's successful ascent to a desk job had added to his pain. While working on construction sites, he'd grown used to eating big fast-food meals and then working them off. Now, he got little exercise but had kept the double-chili-cheeseburger habit. When I first saw him, he weighed nearly three hundred pounds.

I surprised Tony by telling him that his knees weren't really in such bad shape. He had some wear and tear for sure, but he definitely didn't need surgery. I explained that much of the pain was caused by the heavy load he was asking his knees to bear; the extra pounds were stressing his already-weakened joints. And his diet was high in the fats that encourage inflammation.

Tony sighed. He was game for physical therapy and exercise, and willing to try some new medications. "But look," he said, "I've always been a certain kind of guy: I eat like a hog, I work all day, and I drink like a fish at night. That's who I am. End of story."

Tony was right: Foods *are* part of our identities. A good pain diet respects that. So I dug around a little bit.

"You grew up outside of Miami, right? Was your mom a good cook?" Tony nodded, grinning. "And I bet she didn't feed you fast food." Another nod. "So what did she make for you?"

It turned out that Tony's favorite meal as a child had been black beans and rice with chorizo, a spicy kind of sausage. Now, I prefer patients to eat brown rice if they can, but black beans and white rice is *much* more nutritious than chili cheeseburgers and fries. The chorizo, however—well, that's a source of animal fat that increases

(continued)

the pro-inflammatory prostaglandins. "What did you like most about the chorizo?" I asked.

"The spices, doc! It's not black beans and rice without spices!"

We were both having a pretty good time at this point—I think my mouth was watering as much as his was. "Okay, Tony, here's what I want you to do: Go to the Spanish restaurant where you and your wife like to get take-out dinners, and get them to make you some black beans and rice—with just a little chorizo for flavoring. Not much, just enough to make it taste good. And tell them to put in lots of hot sauce and spices, as spicy as you like it. And take *that* in to work for lunch."

Tony agreed. Not only did he drop the fast-food habit, he cut back on the drinks at night (alcohol is highly caloric) and started swimming in the mornings. Physical therapy and a new pain medication formed the rest of his chronic-pain plan. When I saw him for a checkup six months later, the transformation was extraordinary. He'd lost sixty-five pounds. In came a good-looking fifty-year-old man, big-boned but trim—who walked normally, without wincing. Sure, Tony had been resistant to improving his diet as first. He thought it would change a fundamental aspect of who he was. But now, he was more like his old self than he'd been in years.

SUBSTITUTE WHOLE GRAINS FOR WHITE BREAD AND RICE

Once, almost all the breads and rice eaten across the world were whole grains. Most people ate brown bread or brown rice with their meals—and in lean times, they often ate nothing but these products. Only the wealthiest members of a population could afford grains that were refined, meaning that that their fibrous sheath was removed to give them a white color. Slowly, refined grains became a sign of prosperity and good living, to the extent that most of us grew up eating several helpings of white breads or rice a day, along with sweet baked goods that are made with refined flour.

But when the sheath around the grains is discarded, so is much of the grain's food value. Whole grains are a source of many nutrients important for a vital immune system and for pain control, including the B-complex vitamins. They are also high in magnesium, which relaxes cramped muscles, and in fiber, which reduces constipation from irritable bowel syndrome or pain medications.

By contrast, refined products—especially sweet baked goods—cause terrible flare-ups in some of my patients. I most often see this link in people whose nervous systems are wound up and misfiring. Avoiding refined grains may stabilize your nerves and keep them from firing extra or intensified messages of pain. Remember that pain lives in the central nervous system—so the extent to which you can keep it on an even keel is the extent to which you'll feel better.

It's not hard to switch from white bread and rice to whole grains. Many great chefs prefer whole grains, as they have a sweet, nutlike flavor. Whole-wheat and oat breads especially have come into their own in the last few years; look around your health-food store or bakery for fresh products if possible. If you have the time and enjoy the task, you could even bake them on your own—I know one woman in her seventies who takes her mind off her migraines by baking bread. You might also consider eating oatmeal or oat cereal for breakfast. You should be able to find brown rice without much difficulty in your supermarket. It takes no more effort to prepare than the white stuff, although you do need to leave more time for it to cook on the stovetop. It's not necessary to buy whole-wheat pasta, since the ordinary varieties are actually made from whole grains. I suggest, however, that you avoiding overcooking your pasta—let it retain just a little firmness for the best flavor and food value.

MALCOLM'S STORY: PREEMPTING HUNGER

Malcolm, who suffered from back pain, was employed by a prestigious investment bank, the kind where everyone works eighteen hours a day, no grousing allowed. When he was younger and in school, Malcolm discovered arugula salads and marinated tofu—healthful foods that he loved and ate regularly. But now he was an executive in his forties, always running from a meeting to the telephone and back again. Like most of his co-workers, he didn't have time for a normal sit-down breakfast or lunch and often made do with the platters of pastries and sweets that were stacked on the conference tables.

(continued)

Malcolm had long wanted to make changes to his diet, but he hadn't had a compelling reason to do so—until I told him that the extra weight in his belly was putting pressure on the delicate structures of his spine. I also suspected his high-fat meals were leading to some inflammation, and although the sugar provided him with short bursts of energy, the subsequent crashes added to his overall discomfort and moodiness.

Malcolm's hunger drove him to eat foods he didn't even enjoy, so we decided that one goal for him would be to preempt those gnawing feelings. He found a health-food restaurant near his subway stop and began a new morning routine: He'd swing by on the way to work, picking up two meals: first, a breakfast of oatmeal with skim milk and raisins, and then some containers of his old favorites—tofu, salads, curry, and the like. He'd eat the oatmeal at his first meeting of the day. In the afternoon, when everyone else broke for coffee and the now-cold pastries, he'd eat from his stash.

Not only did his back pain improve as he lost weight, Malcolm reported that he even had extra energy and increased mental acuity, giving him an edge in negotiations: "In the afternoon, it's like I'm at eighty-five percent capacity and everyone else is at forty-five percent."

I see a lot of people who were in great shape in their twenties or thirties but then developed bad eating habits as the pressures of business and family took over. Changing just a few of these habits can make a difference in your pain level. You don't need to eat tofu, either (although it's surprisingly good when well seasoned). I know mothers who carry bags of carrots to eat when they'll be running errands for hours, and I've seen truck drivers who avoid greasy spoons by packing chicken sandwiches with cut-up vegetables and dip or containers of black-eyed peas with spinach, cooked with just a little ham for richer flavor.

DO YOU NEED MORE SEROTONIN IN YOUR DIET?

There's been a lot of fuss in recent years over foods that encourage the production of serotonin. Serotonin is a neurotransmitter, a deficiency of which is thought to play a role in depression, insomnia, and increased pain. By eating foods that contain L-tryptophan, a chemical the body needs to produce serotonin, you can theoretically sleep better, feel happier, and have less pain. But how focused do you need to be on these foods?

The truth is that most people with well-rounded diets of fresh food get plenty of L-tryptophan. If you're following the recommendations here and still suffer from depression, insomnia, and pain, you may need to look to exercise, massage, or medication as additional ways to increase serotonin. But if you're getting most of your meals out of the freezer or handed to you from a drive-through window, then there is indeed a good chance that you're deficient in foods with L-tryptophan. Try adding green, leafy vegetables; turkey; or fresh, low-fat dairy foods to your diet. Some people like a small snack of turkey on whole-grain crackers with a glass of warm milk a few hours before bedtime.

THE PAIN-CONTROL DIET AT A GLANCE

FOODS THAT MAKE YOU FEEL BETTER	FOODS THAT MAKE YOU FEEL WORSE
Fresh, homemade food	Fast food and processed food
Fresh fruits and vegetables	French fries
Whole grains	White bread, white rice, and baked goods made with refined flour
Oily fish and eggs fortified with omega-3 fatty acids	Red meat and whole-fat dairy products
Walnuts and flaxseed	Butter, margarine, and vegetable shortening
	Anything that gives you a flare-up

CAN FOOD ALLERGIES CAUSE PAIN?

In a word: yes. In more than a word: yes, but not as often as many alternative health gurus would have you believe.

There are many nutrition experts who will tell you that almost every chronic condition has its roots in food allergies and who immediately saddle every new client with a rigorous elimination diet that forbids almost every kind of food item you can think of, in the hopes of discovering possible allergies or bad reactions. This approach, although well-meaning, has the unfortunate result of making people afraid of food—not to mention that it's so hard to follow that many people simply give up. At the other extreme are many conventional physicians, who mock even the most timid suggestion that foods might contribute to painful disorders.

Although genuine food allergies are quite rare, it seems likely that a small but significant portion of the population experiences a low-grade negative reaction to certain foods. This reaction may contribute to inflammation, stiffness, and irritable bowel. If you suffer from any of these problems, you may want to examine your bodily reaction to some common culprits: wheat, dairy, corn, soy, eggs, and citrus. Try eliminating one of these items from your diet for a week at a time; if you experience no changes in your symptoms, reintroduce that item and eliminate the next. If you do notice a reduction in symptoms, it may be worth your while to avoid that food altogether.

Since body reactions are highly individual and complex, it's also smart to cultivate a higher degree of awareness about how you feel after consuming other foods as well. There's no need to become obsessed, but you may well find that processed, fatty, oily, or other foods tend to give you flare-ups. By avoiding them, you can keep your pain on a more even, manageable level.

THE TOP TWENTY SUPPLEMENTS FOR PAIN CONTROL

Herbs and natural supplements appeal to the romantic streak in us: They make us feel that by gathering flowers, leaves, or berries (or taking a powdered form of them), we can find wellness in our own backyards. I am particularly enamored of the idea that herbs may be easier on the body than many of our present pharmaceuticals. I strongly support those researchers who are reviving the herbalist tradition while bringing it up to date with the latest in scientific testing. Several herbs and supplements show promise in reducing pain, and those that seem most likely to be both effective and safe are listed in the chart on pages 137–147.

"Do I really have to eat vegetables and exercise? Can't I just take a supplement or something?" Lots of patients ask me these questions, and I can't blame them for wanting hassle-free relief. But supplements—like any other treatment in this book—can't do all the work on their own. If you want a truly gentle and holistic approach to pain management, you'll need to combine them with other therapies, starting with exercise, a good diet, and mind-body work.

Talk to your doctor before taking any supplements. You'll need to have her review your medical condition, along with the medications or other supplements you're currently taking. Your doctor doesn't need to love herbs; she just needs to make sure they're not going to hurt you.

GUIDELINES FOR BUYING SUPPLEMENTS

Currently supplements are not regulated by the U.S. government, which means that products may not contain ingredients in the amounts specified on the label. A survey by the American Botanical Council found that of the ginseng products on the shelf, one-third contained *no ginseng at all.* Another third had less than the amount advertised on the package. Products may also be adulterated with undesirable ingredients—the allergen ragweed, for example, is often found in commercial echinacea preparations. Here are some suggestions for navigating the health-food store aisles:

- Look for products that bear the U.S. Pharmacopoeia stamp, which assures you that the product meets a basic set of manufacturing standards. Drugstore brands are actually more likely than small boutique brands to earn this approval, which is pretty good news, since they are usually far more affordable.

- Brands made in Germany, France, and the United Kingdom are often good bets, as these countries have a long history of using herbs and correspondingly high manufacturing standards (which must be met by products that are exported to the United States).

- Buy a product from a large, well-known company, one that has a lot to lose if a product doesn't measure up.

TWENTY SUPPLEMENTS FOR PAIN RELIEF

Always consult your doctor before taking a supplement, especially if you are taking prescription medications, are pregnant or breastfeeding, are taking blood-thinning medications, have special or severe medical conditions (including but not limited to heart, kidney, or liver disease; high blood pressure; stomach disorders; ulcers; blood clotting abnormalities; or depression). Do not give herbs to children without consulting a doctor first.

MULTIVITAMIN	
Benefits	An insurance policy to protect you from deficiencies that can weaken your body and lead to painful syndromes.
Best for . . .	Everyone
Dose	Follow the instructions on the label.
Comments	Don't use a multivitamin as a replacement for a good diet.

B-COMPLEX VITAMINS	
Benefits	Promote proper functioning of the nervous system.
Best for . . .	Peripheral neuropathy
Dose	Take a product containing 50 milligrams of several B-complex vitamins, including B_2 (riboflavin), B_6, and B_{12}.
Comments	You should also eat plenty of green, leafy vegetables and whole grains.

BROMELAIN	
Benefits	Appears to have an anti-inflammatory effect and to encourage healing of repetitive strain injuries.

(continued)

BROMELAIN *(continued)*	
Best for . . .	Chronic sprains and strains
Dose	Take between 1,500 milligrams and 2 grams of bromelain daily. You can also try Wobenzyme, a commercial product containing a mix of bromelain and other enzymes. Take Wobenzyme according to the package label.
Comments	Give bromelain a couple of weeks before deciding if it works for you.

CALCIUM	
Benefits	Relaxes smooth muscle tissue and supports the nerves' ability to fire normally.
Best for . . .	•Headaches •Nerve pain •Pelvic pain, including PMS
Dose	1,000–1,200 milligrams daily.
Comments	Best when used in conjunction with magnesium.

CAPSAICIN OR CAPSICUM (CHILI PEPPER OIL) (TOPICAL)	
Benefits	May reduce substance P, a neurotransmitter that facilitates the pain message. The burning sensation blocks the pain signal from traveling up the spinal cord.
Best for . . .	•Any pain on the body's periphery—hands, arms, shoulders, feet, or legs •Joint pain •Nerve pain, especially peripheral neuropathy and post-mastectomy pain

(continued)

CAPSAICIN OR CAPSICUM *(continued)*	
Dose	Rub a commercially prepared cream onto the painful area three times a day. (If you apply it less often, you won't get the cumulative effect that reduces substance P.) Avoid getting the cream into your eyes or mouth.
Comments	Expect a slight stinging sensation from the cream. Some people find it pleasant; others can't stand it. It should work within three or four days.
DEVIL'S CLAW	
Benefits	Used in southern Africa for centuries to relieve pain and inflammation.
Best for . . .	According to the most recent studies: •Osteoarthritis •Inflammatory arthritis •Tendinitis
Dose	Take 4,500 mg of dried tuber or an equivalent extract every day.
Comments	Give devil's claw a month to work.
FEVERFEW	
Benefits	A couple of good studies have demonstrated a reduction in number and severity of migraines, along with the vomiting that often accompanies migraine pain.
Best for . . .	Migraines

(continued)

FEVER FEW *(continued)*	
Dose	Follow the directions on the product label. Don't try to grow your own leaves and chew them; you could develop mouth problems such as ulcers, swelling, and inability to taste. If you wish to combine feverfew and B_2, try a product called Migraleve.
Comments	Feverfew is a prophylactic—it does not break an existing migraine. You may need to take it for up to a month before you see results.

FISH OIL	
Benefits	Reduces inflammation.
Best for . . .	•Any painful condition •Inflammatory disorders
Dose	10–12 grams of fish oil concentrate daily, or 15–20 milliliters of cod liver oil daily. If the oil repeats on you, try an enteric-coated pill called Fisol, 10–12 grams daily. If you're a confirmed vegetarian, try Neuromins DHA (docosahexaenoic acid), which is derived from plankton and algae. Start with 100 milligrams per day, going up to 300 milligrams daily as tolerated.

(continued)

GAMMA-LINOLENIC ACID (GLA)	
Benefits	GLA appears to have anti-inflammatory properties. One study showed that in people with rheumatoid arthritis, six months of treatment with evening primrose oil (a form of GLA) reduced swelling, tenderness, and pain; another study showed that after a year of taking evening primrose oil, rheumatoid arthritis patients were able to cut back on painkillers or stop using them entirely.
Best for . . .	•Inflammatory arthritis •Pelvic pain •Any inflammatory condition
Dose	There are several forms of GLA available on the market, including borage oil, evening primrose oil, and pure gamma-linolenic acid. Theoretically, they all accomplish the same thing. In practice, however, some people respond to one form of GLA but not to another. I usually start patients with borage oil, which is the least expensive of the three. Try to find an enteric-coated product, which will keep the oil from breaking down in your stomach and repeating on you. Borage oil: Start with 1 gram per day and increase as tolerated, for a total of no more than 6 grams daily. Evening primrose oil: 4–6 grams per day. Gamma-linolenic acid: 1–4 grams daily.

(continued)

GAMMA-LINOLENIC ACID (GLA) *(continued)*	
Comments	No matter which form of GLA you're using, try it for no less than two weeks and maybe even a couple of months before deciding if it works for you. In addition to GLA, make sure to eat oily fish, walnuts, and flaxseed and reduce consumption of saturated fats and partially hydrogenated oils. You may experience some queasiness or diarrhea with these products. People with gastrointestinal reflex disease should take an enteric-coated supplement, not one that will break down in the upper digestive tract.

GINGER	
Benefits	Reduces inflammation and nausea.
Best for . . .	•Inflammatory arthritis •Nausea from pain medications
Dose	For nausea, drink ginger tea (made by steeping peeled and finely chopped gingerroot in a cup of hot water). To relieve inflammation, take 1,000 milligrams of ginger powder daily or 5 grams of fresh gingerroot.

GLUCOSAMINE AND CHONDROITIN	
Benefits	Glucosamine appears to promote growth of new cartilage between arthritic joints; chondroitin seems to keep existing cartilage elastic and supple, possibly preventing further degeneration.
Best for . . .	Osteoarthritis

(continued)

GLUCOSAMINE AND CHONDROITIN *(continued)*	
Dose	1,500 milligrams of glucosamine hydrochloride, glucosamine sulfate, or N-acetyl glucosamine and 500–600 milligrams chondroitin daily.
Comments	You're building up new tissue, so allow one or two months for the supplements to work. I recommend glucosamine and chondroitin to almost all of my patients with osteoarthritis.
KAVA	
Benefits	Used in the South Sea islands as a sedative.
Best for . . .	Occasional relief of: •Anxiety •Insomnia •Muscle tension
Dose	Take 60–120 milligrams of an extract containing kavalactones, kava's active ingredient. A good product is Kavatrol; take according to the package directions.
Comments	Don't use if you have a liver condition or for prolonged periods. Do not mix with alcohol or other sedatives. If used regularly, have your doctor perform liver function tests.
MAGNESIUM	
Benefits	Proven to relax the smooth muscles of the body. A low-grade deficiency of magnesium may make nerves less stable and more irritable.

(continued)

MAGNESIUM *(continued)*	
Best for ...	•Headaches •Chronic muscle spasm •Leg cramps •Peripheral neuropathies •Any nerve-related pain
Dose	400 milligrams of magnesium gluconate daily. About half of long, bad migraines can be broken with intravenously delivered magnesium.
Comments	Fruits, vegetables, and whole grains are even better sources of magnesium than supplements. Magnesium is best taken with calcium.

NIACINAMIDE	
Benefits	Eases pain and stiffness.
Best for ...	Osteoarthritis
Dose	500 milligrams three times daily, or 1,000 milligrams of a sustained-release product two times a day.
Comments	It may take six to eight weeks before you see results. You doctor will need to monitor your liver enzymes.

QUERCETIN	
Benefits	Suppresses inflammatory prostaglandins.
Best for ...	Arthritis
Dose	400 milligrams two or three times a day.

(continued)

ST. JOHN'S WORT	
Benefits	Antidepressant.
Best for . . .	Mild to moderate depression; especially helpful for people who haven't responded to prescription antidepressants
Dose	300–900 milligrams per day of a standardized extract.
Comments	Do not try to treat depression by yourself. Talk to a doctor or therapist. Be especially careful with this herb, as it's known to interfere with several medications. Don't take it without checking with your doctor.
TURMERIC	
Benefits	Anti-inflammatory.
Best for . . .	•Inflammatory arthritis •Other inflammatory conditions
Dose	To make a tea, pour a cup of hot water over 1.5 to 3 grams of the powder and let steep. Drink the tea two or three times daily after meals. Or use 10–15 drops of straight turmeric tincture two or three times daily.
VALERIAN	
Benefits	Mild sedative and muscle relaxant.
Best for . . .	Insomnia, especially from muscle pain.

(continued)

VALERIAN *(continued)*	
Dose	Use a tincture according to the package directions. Since this herb is a bit smelly, mix it with pineapple juice or another drink with an assertive flavor.
Comments	Don't take with other medications or alcohol. Valerian can exacerbate certain physical conditions, especially plant allergies.
VITAMIN B_2	
Benefits	Several papers in medical journals have suggested B_2 reduces migraine pain.
Best for ...	Migraines
Dose	100 milligrams daily; you can also take the product Migraleve, which combines B_2 and feverfew.
Comments	If you don't get results after two weeks of taking B_2 or Migraleve, discontinue use.
WHITE WILLOW	
Benefits	Appears to relieve inflammation and pain.
Best for ...	Early tests tell us that white willow may relieve low back pain.
Dose	240 milligrams per day.
Comments	Don't take if you have had bad results with NSAIDs. Can be taken with acetaminophen; talk to your doctor before taking in conjunction with NSAIDs.

10.

DISTRACTING YOUR NERVOUS SYSTEM FROM PAIN

ACUPRESSURE / ACUPUNCTURE / AROMATHERAPY / ELECTRICAL STIMULATION / HIGHER THERAPIES / TENS

Most people wouldn't think of acupressure and Beethoven in the same category. Nevertheless, you'll find both of them in this chapter. What all the therapies here have in common is a certain effect on the nervous system. They give it other things to focus on, literally distracting its attention away from pain so that you don't feel it as much. Sometimes they go to work on the spinal cord, sending out messages that conflict with the pain signal and prevent it from traveling to the brain. Sometimes they work at a higher level, keeping your brain itself focused on another task or sensation, so that you forget the pain. Many of them have additional benefits, too, such as releasing endorphins, relaxing muscles, improving energy flow, and reducing stress.

Too often these therapies are considered last resorts, things to try when drugs and injections and surgeries have failed. To my mind, this is a backward way of thinking. A last resort ought to be a treatment that's dangerous, one that's as likely to hurt as it is to harm. By contrast, distraction therapies are almost universally safe. Why not try them first, *before* you expose yourself to harsh or invasive treatments?

A friend of mine, an excellent conventional physician with an enthusiasm for acupuncture, likes to tell a story about one of his patients, also a doctor. Like many doctors in these days of punishing schedules and lower pay, he suffered from back pain. He scheduled surgery for himself and was resting at home when my friend sent an acupuncturist over for a house call. After the first treatment, the doctor's condition improved so much that he canceled the surgery and booked a series of acupuncture treatments instead. As my friend says, "If you need surgery later, you can always get it. The surgeons are not going to go out of business. In the meantime, why not use something else if it works?"

ACUPRESSURE

When I was nineteen, I had a friend, Clark, a student of Chinese language and culture. He told me that he'd learned about a traditional Chinese healing technique called acupressure. I had a lot of pain and tension in my neck and back, thanks to a minor bone-growth disorder, so I agreed to let him practice on me. Clark performed what I would later be able to identify as a Jin Shin Do release on my shoulders. I expected it to feel like a static massage, but the spots Clark found on my shoulders were strangely reactive. When he pressed on them, pain began to radiate through my body in odd ways. It seemed to flow from my shoulders up to my head, and then from the center of my head to my forehead, and from the back of my head toward the front of my head. When he was done, the pain ceased. Moreover, my shoulder and back pain was gone. I felt *great,* very loose and refreshed. The next week, I walked into the best acupressure school I could find—I lived in Los Angeles, where there's one on practically every corner—and registered for classes.

Acupressure employs firm, sustained fingertip pressure against certain sensitive points in the anatomy. It's based on the principles of traditional Chinese medicine (TCM), which hold that energy (or *chi*) flows through the body along invisible channels. If this energy gets stuck or is otherwise unbalanced, the result is sickness and pain. According to TCM, you can release blocked energy by pressing on certain points that exist along these channels. Most acupressurists are taught to look for other spots, too, ones that are especially tender. Some of these points are trigger points, the hard knots of muscle that cause pain both at their location and in areas that radiate out from it. In this way, acupressure is also a little like trigger point work, in that it relies on pressure to dissolve these points. A good practitioner will use both Chinese medicine and massage principles to reduce your pain while making you feel more relaxed and balanced.

When I was nineteen, I would have told you that acupressure works by manipulating the energy flow in your body and by releasing muscle tension. I still say both of these things to anyone who will listen. Now, though, Western science has made an important contribution to our ideas about acupressure, and I'd say that a major—but not the only—reason acupressure works so well for pain is that it distracts the nervous system. The nerve impulses that carry the message for firm touch travel faster than those that carry pain messages, blocking them out at the spinal cord. Since the pain messages can't travel up the cord, they never register in your brain. And that "pain gate" at your spinal cord doesn't just pop back open when the acupressure stops; this therapy appears to have longer-term neurochemical effects that can last well past the time of treatment. Acupressure also seems to have some effect on the thalamus. This part of the brain needs a lot of stimulation from every part of the body to keep up normal nerve activity to and from that part. Without that stimulation, the thalamus can produce pain on its own; this is the spontaneous firing I talked about in Chapter 3. In my opinion, acupressure provides the perfect barrage of sensation to keep the thalamus regulated. Finally, acupressure is deeply relaxing and seems to hush the limbic system's emotional alarm bells.

Acupressure, like massage, is one of those therapies that works well for most disorders. I consider it a first-line treatment for myofascial pain, headaches, arthritis, and pain that lingers from an accident or trauma. I've seen it improve range of motion and mobility, too. It's very useful for anyone who has pain that seems out of proportion to their condition or injury, because this kind of intensified pain is usually the result of a malfunctioning nervous system.

Acupressure usually has some kind of stress- or pain-relieving effect on everybody. The real question for you is whether you'll get a significant effect from professional treatment, one that lasts after the session is over. You should be able to determine this fairly quickly; I'd give it anywhere between one and three sessions. Look for someone who has a license in massage (acupressure techniques are part of their training) or a certificate of formal training in acupressure in a state for which there is not a massage license. It's nice if you can find someone who's made a specialty of acupressure techniques, but it's not strictly necessary. Expect treatments to last somewhere between thirty and forty-five minutes.

Contraindications: Acupressure is very safe, unless you have a tumor or serious infection (the deep touch can spread either throughout your body). If you have a skin lesion, don't use acupressure on the affected area.

There are several types of acupressure, and the choices (not to mention the names) can be daunting. The ones below are the best for pain relief, and they're also the most commonly used.

Anmo (also called Ammo or An Mo): Anmo therapists use short, circular strokes over acupressure points and will also rock your limbs back and forth. This technique is gentle and relaxing.

Jin Shin Do Bodymind Acupressure: The practitioner will press spots for up to three minutes each. The pressure will be firm (you may feel some soreness afterward), but the slow, steady technique is soothing.

Shiatsu: This is acupressure Japanese style. It uses deep pressure—the practitioner may dig in with her elbows or even her feet—and follows patterns of points across the body. This therapy moves more quickly than Jin Shin Do does.

You can also use acupressure on your own. I like to use it whenever I'm feeling cramped up with tension or when some achy spots in my back start to bother me. A lot of people use it just before bed as a way to reduce pain and relax before sleeping. As a general principle, you can search your body for those reactive points and then use your fingers or knuckles to apply firm pressure to each point for a minute or so. In Part IV I recommend specific acupressure points for certain disorders. To locate these points on your body, consult the map in Appendix C.

AT-HOME ACUPRESSURE

CATWALK FOR HEAD, NECK, AND SHOULDER PAIN

This is a simple technique you can use at the office or before bed. First, sit in an upright position. Feel along the tops of your shoulder for an area that feels tight or even painful. Then use the index, middle, and ring fingers (or last joint of your thumb, if you prefer) of the opposite hand and walk them along that area, in the same way a cat might knead your belly with its paws. Do this fairly quickly, allowing about a half second for each finger. Repeat on the other side. Now take your thumb and dig it into the base of your skull (use the left thumb for the left side of the skull, and right thumb for the right side), and work back and forth across the tight spots there. You'll be moving against the grain of the muscle, so this may hurt a little. Keep this up, alternating sides as necessary, for three or four minutes. If you

(continued)

like, you can finish up by placing a hot water bottle, heating pad, or ice pack against your neck and shoulders.

QUICK RELIEF FOR LOW BACK PAIN

It's best to lie down on either your stomach or your side for this one. Find a spot in your back that hurts. Take the knuckle of your index finger and twist it into that spot. Keep the twisting motion going in one direction, either clockwise or counterclockwise. You may want to move on to other spots when you're done. If you have time, spend a few minutes afterward with a hot-water bottle or a heating pad on the area. (A variation on this technique is to place tennis balls under your reactive spots. Lie against them and rock gently back and forth.)

ACUPUNCTURE

If your doctor heaves a beleaguered sigh whenever you bring up alternative medicine, ask her what she thinks about acupuncture. I'll bet you get a very different response—maybe not outright enthusiasm, but a piqued scientific interest. Although acupuncture sounds deeply strange to many patients, to doctors it has an element of familiarity—after all, they spent a good part of medical school learning how to stick people with needles. More to the point (that's an acupuncture joke), they've read journal articles that discuss acupuncture's measurable effects on the nervous system. (You can point your doctor toward the May 1997 issue of *Pain* or the National Institutes of Health consensus statement on acupuncture, posted on its Web site at http://odp.od.nih.gov/consensus/cons/107/107_intro.htm.) We know, for example, that people have higher levels of natural painkilling chemicals in their spinal cord after receiving treatment. It also has a counterirritating effect, meaning that the needles produce a sensation that competes with pain and often wins out over it.

That's a Western view of acupuncture, and one that I take very seriously. But you can also take an Eastern approach to this therapy. Acupuncture was developed in ancient China according to beliefs about the way energy flows through the body. The Chinese identified and defined a life force, called *chi*. *Chi* is the force that gets you up in the morning, sustains you throughout the day, and nudges you to sleep again at night. *Chi* moves along invisible channels in the body called meridians, and certain points along those meridians are vital for keeping *chi* flowing properly. Illness or pain is the result of *chi* that's blocked at a certain point or that's moving too quickly or slowly. (This returns us to the concept of balance. In traditional Chinese medicine, *chi* can be thrown off by an unbalanced life.) By inserting needles into the proper points, you can restore the proper flow of *chi*—perhaps by opening up the flow of *chi* in a blocked meridian, among other possibilities—and thus good health.

I feel comfortable with both Western and Eastern theories; that is, I think acupuncture works on our neuroanatomy *and* on our energy. This makes it a dynamic, versatile treatment that's well equipped to handle pain's complexity. Certainly it's a stress reliever. In fact, I've got a second acupuncture joke: You can tell how effective the treatment was by how long it takes the patient to write the check. Acupuncture is so deeply relaxing that some patients seem frankly blotto afterward. Maybe they're just happy that their pain is gone.

The pain-numbing effects of acupuncture can last a long time. One of my patients, Marcia, is on opioids for failed back surgery syndrome. It's an accepted feature of opioids that as your body grows used to them, you need to ratchet up the dosage to maintain their effectiveness. But Marcia also comes in every other week for an acupuncture session. Acupuncture works so well for her that she hasn't needed to increase her opioid dose, even though the textbooks say such an increase ought to be necessary. I can't promise the same will happen for you, but I do have several other patients who've experienced similar results.

Acupuncture has a broad application. I get treatments myself, to relieve stress and to calm down an upset stomach. When it comes to pain, it works for most conditions, especially dental pain, myofascial pain syndrome, arthritis and other joint problems, and painful injuries from accidents or other trauma. It's effective at treating nausea, which is a side effect of many pain medications. Like acupressure, it's also very good when the central nervous system is producing or increasing pain all on its own. Research, however, shows acupuncture is *not* usually effective for people whose pain comes from damaged nerves—this happens in diabetes, alcoholism, toxic nerve injury, kidney failure, and a few other disorders.

Contraindications: There are very few times acupuncture is contraindicated. If you're on blood thinners or if your immune system is compromised in any way, you can still get acupuncture, but your practitioner must be careful with you.

Some people get almost complete pain relief during the course of acupuncture, but when the session is over, the pain immediately returns. If this happens to you, perhaps you're responding solely—and very well—to the counterirritating effect of acupuncture. You should look into TENS, which provides constant, low-grade electrical stimulation and may stop your pain for much longer periods of time. TENS is discussed later in this chapter.

When you go in for a treatment, expect to answer lots of questions about your health, lifestyle, sleep patterns, energy level, and habits. An acupuncturist trained in traditional Chinese medicine may also want to check your pulse and your tongue; Western-style practitioners will probably not. Check around the office; if it doesn't look clean, make a quick exit.

After the consultation, you'll lie down on a table and the practitioner will begin inserting the pins, which are about the size of a coarse human hair. First-time acupuncture patients often say, "Oh, no, I don't want to see the pins, they'll frighten me"—and then, after a treatment that leaves them relaxed and calm, will be surprised when they see the pins once I've taken them out. "Is that all there is?" they'll say, pointing incredulously to the slender pin that's made them feel so much better.

You may feel a little pressure as the needles enter, but you should not feel pain. If you do, tell the practitioner so that he can change the pin's location. An Eastern acupuncturist may rotate the pins by hand; if your energy is activated, you may feel a sensation like warm water flowing through the area, or perhaps a mild ache. Most people will not bleed, either, although you shouldn't be alarmed if every now and then a tiny spot of blood appears at the site of insertion. Someone who follows the Western approach may use a device to deliver a mild electrical stimulation to the points. You'll feel a slight tingle. In either Western or Eastern acupuncture, you may also receive auricular acupuncture, in which pins are placed in the outer ear or taped to it. There's evidence that auricular acupuncture enhances the release of endorphins and gives your treatment a little extra punch. After all the pins are placed, the practitioner will either stay at your side or leave you alone to relax. Many patients fall asleep at this point. Then he'll adjust the pins once more, remove them, and your treatment is done. (It's nice if you can spend a minute or two in further relaxation before you hop off the table.)

Your acupuncturist will probably go easy on you during your first session, gauging your sensitivity. In successive treatments, he should start increasing the number of pins and the time they're left in. You might see results right away, but it's not unusual for people to require five or six sessions before they get maximum relief. If the first couple of treatments don't produce any difference at all, the practitioner might try using electrical stimulators or working another set of points.

Your acupuncturist should be licensed to practice in your city or state, but you should also look for someone who has been certified by the National Certification Commission for Acupuncture and Oriental Medicine (you can find details about professional acupuncture organizations in Appendix E). A small but growing number of acupuncturists have postgraduate degrees in acupuncture; if you can find such a practitioner, all the better. Some insurance companies will pay for treatment, but often the practitioner must be a licensed physician.

Let me close with a word about needles. Almost all acupuncturists use disposable needles, which are what I recommend, and anyone with a license has been thoroughly educated and tested on sanitary needle practice. A recommendation from another professional (good chiropractors often know good acupuncturists) is another way to point you toward someone who's responsible and clean. In my experience, dirty acupuncturists are quite rare. Nevertheless, you should always ask to see the practitioner break open the package of needles in your presence.

AROMATHERAPY

It's fall in the Northeast as I'm working on this chapter, and my house is filled with the smell of fresh apples. Right now I can't think of anything more relaxing than this scent, which reminds me of home and of walks in the country. Aromas are powerful stuff. The olfactory nerve's proximity to the limbic system means that we have a strong reaction to smells; when the brain's emotional center is crackling with distress, scents can calm it down.

Fragrances won't make the pain go away. But essential oils, which are concentrated extracts from scented plants and flowers, can bring you a measure of pleasing distraction. They can also reduce your stress and possibly relax your muscles. A young woman I know who suffers from interstitial cystitis, a pelvic disorder, uses lavender oil in a hot bath whenever the pain is bad. The hot bath soothes the spasm, but the scent soothes her mind. By the time the bath is over, she's not thinking about the pain so much anymore. When my muscles get painful, I like to use oils with a little kick to them, such as eucalyptus or cedar. They clear my head (as well as my sinuses), and it's possible that they have some antispasmodic effect.

Think of a couple of scents that relax or uplift you and try to incorporate them into your life. You can buy vials of oil at most health-food or aromatherapy stores for a few dollars. Add a few drops to unscented lotion or a bath, or use a lightbulb ring to diffuse the scent into your room. You can also scent a handkerchief lightly and inhale it. (Some people develop skin reactions to certain oils, so if you're using a preparation that will touch your skin, test a drop against the back of your wrist first.)

SCENTS TO SUIT YOUR NEEDS

Walk into an aromatherapy store, and you'll find hundreds of oils to choose from. Here are some of the most popular scents, along with the effects they tend to elicit.

ESSENTIAL OIL	SCENT	EFFECTS
Bergamot	Citrus	Soothing
Cedar	Woodsy	Invigorating; may relax muscles; used on the skin, the tingling sensation may block pain signals
Clary sage	Herbal, pungent	Soothing
Eucalyptus	Camphorlike, woodsy	Invigorating, with expectorant qualities; may relax muscles; when applied in a lotion, the tingling sensation may block pain signals
Geranium	Floral	Calming and uplifting
Lavender	Floral	Calming, possibly sedating
Lemon	Citrus	Energizing
Peppermint	Minty	Stimulating; soothes pain that makes you feel sick to your stomach
Rose	Floral	Soothing
Sandalwood	Spicy, woodsy	Soothing

ELECTRICAL STIMULATION

Electrical stimulation sounds like a regimen cooked up by a mad scientist, but in fact it's a standard aspect of physical therapy. During treatment, you rest comfortably as a therapist or chiropractor places electrodes on the part of your body that hurts and then sends a mild electrical current through the skin and muscles. You'll feel a tingling sensation, which beats the pain sensation to the spinal cord and prevents you from feeling it. The stimulation has an additional effect on tight muscles, pulling them into a painless contraction—which ideally results in the muscle becoming so tired that the contraction finally releases.

Electrical stimulation relieves pain temporarily (the effects last anywhere from a couple of hours to two days in most people) so that you're able to perform stretching and strengthening exercises. Without those exercises, you'll soon be right back where you started. Be wary of a therapist who uses stimulation, slaps on a hot pack, and finishes up with a quick massage, neglecting the exercise. Although this can help stop an acute spasm, it's too rushed and superficial to get at the root of chronic pain. Unfortunately, this inadequate combination is so common that it's earned the derisive nickname of "shake and bake." If you want real therapy for chronic pain, look for someone who's willing to spend time with you doing exercises and stretching your muscles.

This therapy is safe, widely available, and almost always covered by insurance with a doctor's recommendation. I suggest it for muscular and joint pain, and especially for arthritis. If you respond well to stimulation, you may also want to consider TENS, which gives you a continuous electrical current and longer relief.

Contraindications: Do not use electrical stimulation if you have a fracture, tumor, or skin lesion in the area.

HIGHER THERAPIES

Bernie was a twenty-something insurance director. She had sickle-cell anemia, a disease that warps the red blood cells and causes tremendous tissue pain. Many people with sickle-cell must yield to long periods of bed rest, but Bernie sailed through her work and social schedule with apparent smoothness. When I asked her how she kept going, she explained that she loved to paint. She set up her easel in front of a window and created delightful abstract works, spending hours mixing colors and applying them to the canvas. "When I'm painting," she said, "I'm in the colors and in the forms. I'm somewhere else." Bernie is still in pain while she sits at her easel. She just ignores it, even forgets about it.

Painting, music, writing in journals, reading, and the like are the ultimate distraction therapies. They so fully engage your brain that, in the words of Carly Simon, it doesn't have time for the pain. (Many of them, especially watching movies and reading books, seem to increase endorphin levels as well.) Consider the German writer Goethe, who suffered from gout—an illness that produces pain so intense that another writer, Sydney Smith, said it felt "as if I was walking on my eyeballs." Goethe found that the only way to lift himself out of his pain was to work for hours in his attic study. Or take the French impressionist painter Renoir. He explained his ability to paint using hands that were gnarled by arthritis in these terms: "The pain passes," he said, "but the beauty remains." I know people who cook, read, or listen to their favorite pop songs for the same effect.

It can be annoying when someone who doesn't have to cope with daily pain gives you the chipper advice to "just take your mind off it." But I will tell you that I have seen people even in the worst situations, people with the lancinating bone pain of terminal cancer or the spastic muscles of MS, draw on higher therapies to reduce their suffering and enrich their lives.

When you hurt, the instinct is to shut down, curl up, and tend to yourself. That's not a bad reaction when you've been injured, but for chronic pain it's not terribly practical. After all, you want to have a life outside this thing, right? Higher therapies—so called because they operate on the mind, the higher level of the nervous system—offer you a temporary respite from pain while calling you back to life. They remind you that you have talents, feelings, memories, connections, and experiences that are all separate from your pain. Some can also help you express your feelings about pain. I hope you'll look into one or more of these strategies. A few of them, such as cooking, require a decent amount of mobility, but others, like listening to music, don't ask anything of you but your attention. Keep them in mind for flare-ups; they may see you through a rough patch without extra medication.

TRANSCUTANEOUS ELECTRICAL NERVE STIMULATION (TENS)

TENS has a reputation as the therapy that works when nothing else has. I certainly agree that it's effective. Many people report total, or near-total, relief while they use it. But I disagree with current medical practice, which is to think of TENS as a last-ditch strategy. TENS is a very safe approach with almost no side effects—so I'd like to see my profession consider it for more patients, and use it earlier in their treatments.

TENS works according to the same principles as regular electrical stimulation. A current passes through electrodes attached to the skin; since the spinal cord gives electrical sensations priority over pain messages, the pain messages are stopped. What's different is that electrical stimulation in a therapist's office usually lasts about fifteen minutes, and you have to lie still to receive it. You might feel great during treatment, but soon you have to get up and leave, and the effects end there. In TENS, however, you are provided with a small, portable unit that you can wear throughout the day or night and that lets you conduct the normal business of your life.

Here's how it works: In the morning, after you shower, you place a couple of disposable, sticky-backed electrode pads onto your skin. Then you attach the wires, which connect at one end to the stimulator, to the pads. You clip the stimulator, which is a little box about the size of a cigarette pack, onto the top of your pants or skirt, and plug the electrode's wires into the side. (Some people prefer to put the stimulator in their pocket.) Then you put on the rest of your clothes. Whenever you like, you turn on the unit, which produces a tingling feeling in the area near the electrodes.

Most people should keep the unit on for a good portion of the day, so that they can work, run errands, exercise, and do other activities, and then turn it off in the evening. (Constant use tends to reduce the effectiveness.) Others, however, turn the stimulator on at night to help them sleep but use it less during the day.

Not everyone responds to TENS, but those who do swear by it. If you get pain relief from acupuncture or regular electrical stimulation in physical therapy, you'll probably like TENS, too. It's best to take advantage of the relief TENS provides by pairing it with exercises that improve your strength and range of motion.

A few words to the wise: You'll probably need to adjust the electrodes and unit settings a couple of times before you find the right location and intensity. Sometimes just a little fiddling can make the difference between total relief and none at all. Make sure that your physical therapist, who will outfit you for the unit, has experience with TENS and is willing to work with you. If he has to pull out the instruction book when you ask a question, it's time to find someone else. Also, prepare yourself to deal with your insurance company. Most will pay for TENS, but some will only do so if your doctor writes a letter explaining that you've already tried everything else. Check under your policy's durable medical equipment (DME) clause to find out. Appendix D at the back of this book offers some advice for talking to your insurance provider.

Contraindications: Don't use TENS for pain near your eye or over any cemented or metallic implants.

11.

ENERGY HEALING

HOMEOPATHY / REIKI / REFLEXOLOGY / TAI CHI / THERAPEUTIC TOUCH

I was lying on a table in someone's living room on the Upper West Side of Manhattan. Six of us—some doctors, some not—had just begun a course in Reiki, a Japanese technique for channeling energy through the healer's body to a patient's. I had convinced a surgeon friend of mine to come along for the ride, and neither of us was entirely sure what we'd encounter. Ben, my friend, was practicing by laying his hands on my lower back and holding them there quietly for several minutes, until he broke the silence.

"I'm feeling more than I should." He sounded puzzled. "I'm feeling something more than I should feel from just having my hands on your back. It feels like a . . . *glow* in my hands." This was from a surgeon, whose hands are his life. I asked him what he thought it was.

"I don't know," he said, "but I'm not going to stop."

I knew what he meant. I'd felt that glow—a kind of heat combined with a mild tingle—when doing acupressure or chiropractic. If someone had a headache, I might put my hands on their right shoulder and feel warmth spread up from their skin through my fingers, hands, and forearms—but feel nothing at all when I moved to the left shoulder. I'd also felt it as a recipient of acupressure and acupuncture, and many of my patients had described the same feeling to me. If you've felt this glow before, you know that it is a rich experience. Like Ben, you don't want it to stop.

This feeling is often described as energy, an animating force that regulates the growth, function, and healing of living things. Each of the therapies in this chapter works to manipulate or shape energy as it moves through our bodies. The philosophy behind all energy healing is that illness is caused by a disturbance in the body's natural state of balance, and that health will return once proper energy flow and balance are restored. These treatments are less about targeting specific illnesses than about making us stronger and more centered. Ben now uses Reiki just before surgery, as the patient is going under anesthesia. He doesn't think that channeling energy is going to cure the patient—otherwise he wouldn't even bother to operate—but he does feel that it helps patients respond well to the ordeal before them.

Of all the therapies in this book, the ones in this chapter are the hardest for us Westerners, especially Americans, to accept. Bioenergy just doesn't fit into our worldview or our vocabulary; at best it seems an amusing relic of hippie culture. We prefer to live firmly grounded in the concrete and the visible. So do our medical scientists, who are captivated by biochemistry—the chemical processes of life—and who believe that all our bodily and mental processes can be explained according to its principles. We have culled so many benefits from this outlook that we cling to it, sometimes forgetting that there are other ways of seeing the world. In China, for example, millions of people wake up early every morning and head for the nearest park to practice tai chi—a sequence of exercises designed to move *chi,* or energy, through their bodies. In India, a doctor may well speak of your illness as a lack of *prana,* or life force. And the nationalized health care systems in Germany and England pay for homeopathy, whose practitioners may explain the healing process in terms of manipulating subtle energies.

It's hard to accept that human creativity, thought, and spirit are nothing more than a series of circularly firing cranial neurons, or that Mozart's music or Michelangelo's art can be explained purely in biochemical terms. As much as biochemistry has enhanced our understanding, energy therapies remain appealing because they suggest that there is another layer to life, one that can't be reduced to a chemical equation. I've devoted an entire chapter of this book to the nervous system's role in pain, and yet I still believe that we can't boil pain down to neurotransmitters and spinal pathways. All my experience tells me that pain just isn't that tidy. How pain is created, and how ordinary humans learn to live in the face of it, remains a compelling and sometimes beautiful mystery.

I can't tell you exactly how energy therapies work. That doesn't mean they're not valid—we don't really know how many pharmaceuticals work, either. But energy therapies are indeed effective, to an extent that seems to go well beyond that of psychology or a placebo. They are also quite safe and often inexpensive. For pain patients, who may be dismissed by doctors precisely because their symptoms do not correspond to biochemical principles, energy therapies offer a deeper and sometimes more sympathetic kind of treatment.

HOMEOPATHY

Homeopathy began in the early 1800s with Samuel Hahnemann, a German physician who was appalled at the crude and invasive medical treatments of his time, which included leeching and bloodletting. He was also curious about quinine. It was known then that this medicine, made from cinchona bark, cured malaria, but the means by which it worked remained mysterious. Hahnemann, using himself as a subject, sampled some cinchona bark and discovered that it gave him the symptoms of malaria, although he did not actually contract the disease. This observation was the basis for his idea that symptoms were really the body's way of *resisting* disease—so that a fever is a strategy to burn up germs, and a cough is a way to propel them outward. He also believed that certain substances such as cinchona could, by stimulating the same symptoms as an illness, encourage the body to successfully resist that illness.

Hahnemann began a lifelong study of thousands of substances, noting carefully what kinds of symptoms they induced. A substance that produced symptoms in healthy people was then used to cure the same symptoms in the sick. Since he was using potent stuff, Hahnemann had to be careful not to accidentally poison his patients. In the interest of a gentler cure, he experimented with smaller and smaller doses—and discovered something rather shocking: the smaller the dose, the more effective the treatment. In fact, the remedies he developed are so dilute that some don't contain even one molecule of the original substance. But the method worked, and to this day millions of people use homeopathy for all kinds of disorders. It's especially popular in Germany and in the United Kingdom, where it is officially included in the national health care systems.

If none of the original substance remains, how could homeopathy work? Most scientists will tell you that homeopathy's effectiveness is nothing but a widespread placebo effect. I find this response inadequate. There are simply too many good studies that demonstrate results above that produced by a placebo; homeopathy has also been shown to work on animals, who presumably are less responsive to the power of suggestion. It seems likely that the substance leaves an energetic imprint on the liquid in which it is diluted (usually water), and that this imprint stimulates the body's own healing force into action. To those who find the idea of an "energetic imprint" laughable, I might point out all the other occasions in scientific history when a ridiculous-seeming idea turned out to be exactly correct. Consider what happened to Ignaz Semmelweis, the first doctor to suggest that his colleagues wash their hands before operating or delivering babies—he was frozen out by the profession. It wasn't until later, when we understood how germs were transmitted, that we all began scrubbing up. Perhaps now we simply lack the technology to see such an energy imprint or to otherwise understand the mechanism by which homeopathy works. Until we know for sure, the evidence suggests that we pay attention.

One of homeopathy's best targets is pain. Homeopathic remedies have been shown to ease (but not cure) the pain of rheumatoid arthritis and fibromyalgia. I've seen several patients improve with homeopathy; it seems to work especially well for people who've tried just about everything else. By this I don't mean that homeopathy should be a last resort, just that certain patients may respond better to its unique (and unknown) means of action than to other treatments. Since homeopathy defines illness by symptoms, and since pain often consists solely of symptoms, with no identifiable underlying illness, there may be a special connection between the two.

If you've been to a health-food store lately, you've probably noticed that homeopathic remedies are available for sale over the counter. Some people try homeopathy on their own by comparing their symptoms to those listed on the container and then buying the one that matches most closely. Although I'm generally an advocate for home care, I don't recommend this approach. Homeopathy usually can't hurt you—at worst, it'll temporarily aggravate your symptoms, which may be rough on those who are already sick—but it's awfully hard to make a good match between your symptoms and the correct remedy. It's another principle of homeopathy that illness is highly individual, and so are the remedies.

A good practitioner will draw on years of training and perhaps a computer database that connects a long series of symptoms and personal traits with a remedy. It's best to visit an experienced practitioner for an initial consultation. You'll spend about an hour talking to the homeopath and answering questions about your disorder, your temperament, and your body's functioning. Afterward, the practitioner will prescribe a remedy for you to try for a short period of time; you'll probably need to go in for at least one follow-up visit to determine whether the remedy is working. It may take several weeks or months before a remedy has an effect, and when it does, your symptoms may intensify at first, as your resistance is stimulated. After this short period of aggravation, which should last no more than a couple of days, you should notice a reduction of symptoms. If you don't, it may be time to switch remedies or to decide that homeopathy just doesn't work for you.

There are no licensing standards for homeopaths in most states, so you'll need to keep your wits about you when searching for a practitioner. Word of mouth can point you in the right direction; I also suggest that you work with someone who has completed a program accredited by the Council on Homeopathic Education. See Appendix E for contact information for homeopathic organizations.

All in all, this therapy is easy on the body. Conventional doctors will tell you that the only side effect of homeopathy is the loss of time and money; others will say that you have to be healthy enough to handle aggravated symptoms.

REIKI

I'll be the first to admit that Reiki rhymes with *flaky* and *fakey* . . . but then I'll also tell you that it works. I think part of being a good doctor is welcoming these paradoxes, of facing things that work despite our beliefs that they shouldn't. (That's not to say you drop-kick science off the roof, just that you keep an open mind.)

The Japanese concept of Reiki is much like the Chinese concept of *chi*. Both hold that there is a life force, or life energy, that moves through the body. Reiki is supposed to radiate beyond the body, so that we are each surrounded by a field of subtle life energy. When Reiki energy is flowing naturally, you feel balanced and well. When it is weakened or stopped up, you'll start developing signs of disease. If this idea sounds too esoteric for you, consider how most of us tend to get sick when we're under emotional stress at work or at home, or under physical stress from winter weather.

Reiki practitioners are trained to be sensitive to Reiki energy, both their own and that of other people. This energy is the mysterious "glow" that I mentioned earlier; Reiki practitioners learn to feel the exchange of energy between bodies and to control that exchange. They believe they can fortify someone who is weak, or smooth out an energy field that feels uneven. I couldn't begin to explain how all this works, but I think many of us know that touch—or simply the company of another person—can have a profound effect. It makes us feel more relaxed, more complete, more welcome in the universe. Reiki may simply be a more focused means of harnessing those benefits.

It's not hard to find practitioners of Reiki; most towns harbor at least a couple. Yoga teachers, massage therapists, and acupuncturists tend to know Reiki practitioners; so do some religious leaders, who tend to be comfortable with the idea of channeling healing energy through touch. (The International Association of Reiki Professionals also offers a directory of practitioners; contact information is available in Appendix E.) You'll know immediately whether you find Reiki relaxing and enjoyable, although it may take two or three sessions before you can judge whether it's helping your pain.

The Reiki treatment is very simple. You'll lie down on a massage table, fully clothed. The practitioner may cover you with a light blanket for your comfort. Some people prefer to work on the energy field that surrounds you, so the healer may or may not actually lay her hands directly on you. The standard Reiki series moves from the top of the head and down along the center of your back or of your chest and belly, but many good practitioners will modify the routine according to how they perceive your needs. They may spend most of the time on the area that hurts, or they may discover a seemingly unrelated area that needs their attention. (This happened to me once as I was practicing Reiki. I was working on a woman with neck pain, but I instinctively felt that something was out of kilter near her lower back. I placed my hands there for a few minutes, and that was that. The treatment didn't seem to have any special effect beyond deep relaxation. The next day, though, the client called to tell me that she'd started her menstrual period that morning, and for the first time in years, she did not feel any attending pain. "I think it had something to do with how you put your hands on my back," she said. Was this another effect of the relaxation, or another kind of purely psychological consequence? Neither of us knew. But for both us, the bottom line was that she felt better.) The treatment lasts somewhere between half an hour and forty-five minutes.

You can use Reiki for any kind of painful condition; it's probably at its best for conditions that include anxiety or depression. It's also possible to practice Reiki on yourself, so if you like the treatment, you could take classes and learn how to channel your own energy.

REFLEXOLOGY

Who doesn't like to have their feet rubbed? A foot rub is one of life's great pleasures, right up there with sunny beaches and ice cream. Even if you don't buy some of its wilder claims, reflexology is a marvelous way to relieve stress and fortify your sense of well-being.

The idea behind reflexology is that every one of your internal organs corresponds to a spot on one of the feet. The brain is connected via biological energy to the big toes, for instance, and the bladder can be mapped to the arch, just above the heel. By pressing on or rubbing the right spots, a reflexologist can theoretically stop a headache or cystitis pain. Is there anything to this theory? Well, I've had reflexology plenty of times, and in most cases I simply had that blissed-out feeling that happens when you completely relax. I've practiced reflexology on patients as a way to calm them down and put them to sleep, and also to reduce headache pain. Beyond these results—which are quite valuable in themselves—I haven't seen much evidence of reflexology's claims.

However, I did have an unusual experience with a highly seasoned Japanese practitioner who teaches at a college of massage and reflexology in Tokyo. He was in Manhattan for a few weeks and came to my office (that's another benefit to energy therapists—some of them still make house calls). It had been a long day, and I was exhausted, but we went together into a treatment room. He began to work on my feet, and I felt the usual effects: My stress was melting, and my tired feet were perking up. But then he pressed on a spot by my little toe and frowned. "You have a problem with your knee?" he asked. I'd banged my knee windsurfing the week before, and indeed, it was still hurting me. Then he moved to another spot. "Stomach not so good today?" Again, he was right.

This experience of mine isn't cold proof that reflexology works in the way its most devoted advocates say it does, but it has certainly piqued my curiosity. I hope that soon we'll see some good studies on reflexology that will give us a better answer than I can currently give you.

Reflexology is probably at its best for headache, insomnia, and stress, but here's the truth: No one who's received reflexology has ever told me that it was a waste of time. It's hard to imagine how a foot massage *wouldn't* make you feel better. (And it's much better for you than that bowl of ice cream.) It's one of those therapies that's great to have around when pain or anxiety flare up; it's also a soothing technique to use in a hospital, nursing home, or other setting in which alternative therapies aren't always welcome. If you can't get to a practitioner, you can always ask your significant other for a foot rub. I don't know if you'll get exactly the same results, but you'll certainly receive the benefit of caring touch.

Many massage therapists have some training in reflexology, but I think it's best to find someone who specializes in the practice. As always, you can ask other alternative practitioners for a recommendation. If you want to try reflexology as a way to heal certain organs (as opposed to relieving stress or temporarily easing pain), I suggest you look for someone with extensive training, like my Japanese therapist. Like most of the therapies in this chapter, reflexology is quite safe. The only people who need to avoid it are those with foot injuries or lesions. You'll know right away if the therapy produces stress-relieving benefits; if you are trying to produce physiological changes to a certain organ, give reflexology two or three sessions before concluding whether it's working.

TAI CHI

If you live in a city, you've probably seen people in the park practicing slow, controlled movements. This is usually tai chi (pronounced "ty chee"), an ancient Chinese exercise that's recently become popular in the West. Tai chi masters say that they can feel energy pumping through their body, pushing against internal obstructions that impede its natural flow. They also say that, with practice, they've learned how to direct this energy flow, giving them the power to maintain their health.

No one has ever been able to prove these claims, but we *do* have documentation of very elderly people in China who demonstrate remarkable strength and health, which they attribute to daily tai chi practice. That alone is enough to inspire many of us to try it. I like tai chi very much, although I can't say that I've ever felt the kind of energy movement that other people talk about (nor do I rule out the possibility that someday I might). For me, and for many other Westerners, the appeal of tai chi is its meditative quality. Professional dancers will tell you that they often feel transported in their work and have a pleasant sense of losing track of time. Tai chi, with its dancelike but easy movements, can have a similar effect. It gives your mind something to focus on, so that it stops its chatter and calms down for a while. This is true whether you practice for an hour or for ten minutes—which makes tai chi a natural for harried professionals, parents of small children, and other people with unpredictable schedules.

Tai chi is also a smart choice for the elderly, because it develops the ability to balance, reducing the chances of a nasty fall, and because it may have some cardiovascular benefits at that age. (There are some claims that tai chi produces aerobic benefits in younger people, but they've yet to be adequately proven. Those of you who are middle-aged or younger should plan to get a workout from some other form of exercise and count on tai chi mainly for its energetic or relaxing benefits.)

Not only is tai chi a flexible therapy, it's also cheap. Although I think it's too difficult to learn it from videotapes, you can sign up for classes, and then, when you've learned the movements, you can continue on your own. You may need five or six classes before you can judge if it's helping you, as it does take some time to get the hang of it.

Like many other energy and stress-reducing therapies, tai chi is good for almost everyone. My suggestion? If you're drawn to it, try it. It could become a meaningful personal practice that wards off anxiety and helps you maintain a cool head when the pain gets bad. And if you're one of the lucky ones, you may also learn to channel your energy in such a way that you reduce pain.

THERAPEUTIC TOUCH

Would you be surprised to learn that there's an energy treatment that's taught at most nursing schools? That treatment, which flies below the radar at these institutions, is Therapeutic Touch, developed by Dolores Krieger, a professor of nursing at New York University. Many nurses I know are enthusiastic about Therapeutic Touch, since it embodies the kind of personal caring that drew them to their profession; frequently they mention their disappointment at not having enough time to use it. The term "Therapeutic Touch" is a little misleading, since often the practitioner doesn't even place her hands on the patient. Instead, she usually holds her hands over the patient, trying to sense the person's energy field and to smooth out any irregularities.

There's a mental aspect, too, which involves the practitioner directing compassion toward the sick person. The treatment usually lasts about fifteen minutes.

You might be thinking that Therapeutic Touch sounds an awful lot like Reiki. They are indeed quite similar; from a patient's point of view, the main difference is that Reiki practitioners take a mystical approach to their work, whereas nurses usually have a more practical attitude. I couldn't say if one is more effective than the other; you should choose the one that makes you feel more comfortable.

There are some good studies on Therapeutic Touch. You may have heard about one that claimed to disprove the treatment, but this study, conducted by a nine-year-old girl and published in the *Journal of the American Medical Association,* did not reproduce the actual conditions of Therapeutic Touch. There are many other studies that prove Therapeutic Touch is an extraordinary tool for reducing anxiety, with results that go beyond that of having someone just talk to you or touch you in a casual manner. There's also a study, with less definite results, that points toward a reduction in pain: People who received Therapeutic Touch required less pain medication after surgery than those who received a sham treatment (a kind of fake Therapeutic Touch). It also seems possible that Therapeutic Touch results in faster healing of wounds. These results aren't conclusive, but since the therapy can't possibly hurt you and will almost certainly reduce your stress, I'd happily recommend it for anyone who wanted to try it. It may be a smart move for people about to go into surgery.

If you're one of these people, ask a nurse if she knows of anyone who practices Therapeutic Touch. Chances are that she will, and even if she doesn't, she'll probably be able to point you in the right general direction. Staff nurses at hospitals and doctors' offices rarely have the luxury of practicing Therapeutic Touch during their working hours, but many can be hired on a private basis.

12.

PAIN PILLS AND OTHER PHARMACEUTICALS

ANTICONVULSANTS / ANTI-INFLAMMATORY MEDICATIONS (STEROIDAL AND NON-STEROIDAL) / MUSCLE RELAXANTS / NMDA ANTAGONISTS / OFFICE INJECTIONS / OPIOIDS / TRICYCLIC ANTIDEPRESSANTS

Conventional painkillers are an important option for most sufferers. They address pain's biochemical element, reacting with nerve cells and body chemicals to stop pain signals from traveling through your nervous system. They can also cool inflammation or relax your muscles.

As a rule, drugs are more aggressive than alternative treatments, and side effects are extremely common. Sometimes those side effects are intolerable; in a few cases, they are fatal. Most of us would prefer to take as few drugs as possible, or none at all. Much of this book is dedicated to that goal. However, the truth remains that pain drugs, *when properly prescribed,* are often necessary for optimal pain relief. By carefully calibrating the class of drug you take, the dosage, or the delivery system, you and your doctor may be able to keep your pharmaceutical intake—and side effects—down to a safe and tolerable level.

The key to pharmaceuticals is the phrase "when properly prescribed." I've said before that pain management occupies a gray area in conventional medicine. Doctors aren't trained in it as a matter of routine. Physicians with patients in pain often have to muddle along as best they can, drawing on their own experience, other areas of expertise, and the bits and pieces of advice picked up from colleagues. Nowhere is this lack of training more evident than in the prescribing of pain-controlling drugs. If you want to get the most appropriate prescription, the one that is most likely to help you and least likely to harm, you'll need to walk into your doctor's office with as much information as possible.

Some of you who have tried medications and abandoned them may be shaking your head. If you're one of them, I hope the material here will convince you to give pharmaceuticals a second look. There have been many developments in recent years, especially in the treatment of pain that seems intractable. It's also possible that you can minimize side effects to an extent that surprises you, especially if prescription drugs have overwhelmed you with their sedating qualities in the past. Of course, drugs aren't right for everyone. Taking medication is a personal decision, and one you should make with your doctor. To help you make that decision, this chapter surveys the many options available today and suggests ways to maximize your chances for success.

AVOIDING PRESCRIPTION DRUG PITFALLS

AUTOMATIC PRESCRIPTIONS

Doctors are taught in medical school to think of most human illnesses as a biochemical riddle, one that can be solved with drugs that change the body's chemistry. When doctors see a patient in pain, they want to help—and, given their training, they will likely turn to pills as a solution. Patients are complicit in this phenomenon, assuming that if they don't leave the office with a prescription, they haven't received good treatment. Prescriptions have become second nature for all of us.

That's unfortunate when so many other treatments are available. I'd like to see pain sufferers try some gentler approaches and lifestyle changes before concluding that a prescription is necessary. If patients do need pharmaceuticals, they should ideally start off with milder drugs first. If those drugs don't work by themselves, it's prudent to add an alternative method or two before going on to a stronger prescription.

I don't mean to lay a guilt trip on those who need heavy drugs for adequate relief. People in crippling pain may well need large doses of a medication just to perform the basic functions of life, and they should not have to apologize for this need any more than a diabetic should apologize for taking insulin. I simply want to challenge the *automatic* nature of prescribing stronger and stronger drugs for everyone in pain.

SIDE EFFECTS

You have some pain, you see a doctor, you take your prescription—and soon you're sick to your stomach and so woozy you can hardly find your way to bed. A day later, you're still sleeping off the effects. Never again, you say. You'd rather have the pain than constant sedation. (Or nausea, constipation, dry mouth, or any other side effect.)

Side effects are a fact of life when it comes to prescription drugs, but there more ways to control them than you might imagine. Here are some strategies for a more comfortable coexistence with pharmaceuticals.

- *Start low and go slow.* Overwhelming side effects may have a simple cause: a dose that's too high for you. Although it's impossible to predict how a certain drug will affect a given individual, you can take steps to reduce the risk of too-high doses by explaining your concerns to your doctor. Tell her you want to "start low and go slow," a phrase most doctors will recognize from their training. Ask if the prescription needs to be adjusted for your age or size or physical condition: If you're elderly, on the small side, or ill, you're more likely to get knocked out by pain medication than the rest of us. Ask your doctor if you should begin with half the prescribed dose, so that you can gauge your response. (But don't tinker with dosages without asking your doctor, since some medications, like long-acting opioids, absolutely must not be broken in half.)

- *Don't give up.* Before you decide that a medicine is ineffective or intolerable, make sure you give your body time to adjust. If after two weeks you're not satisfied, talk to your doctor. He may need to change the dose or prescribe a different kind of drug within the same class. Prescribing pharmaceuticals is not always the exact science we'd like to think it is: It's very hard for your doctor to know how a certain drug is going to act inside your body, and you may have to try several before finding the one that's right for you. Many patients who get sick from one will develop only minimal problems with another. It is also possible that you'll respond better to a combination of drugs than to any of the drugs separately. A careful selection of pharmaceuticals that will work together is known as *rational polypharmacy,* and your doctor should be well acquainted with this term. (Never combine drugs without your doctor's explicit instructions.)

▶ *Make sure you're getting the right kind of opioids.* For extended use, long-acting opioids are more appropriate and result in fewer side effects than the short-acting ones. For more information, see the discussion of opioids later in this chapter.

▶ *Use alternative therapies and home care to control side effects.* Alternatives can help you control pain, but they can also reduce the side effects of pharmaceuticals, including nausea, constipation, dry mouth, and sedation. For your best bets, see the sidebar "Easing the Most Common Side Effects of Prescription Drugs."

EASING THE MOST COMMON SIDE EFFECTS OF PRESCRIPTION DRUGS

CONSTIPATION

Begin the following regimen as soon as you begin taking drugs that can cause constipation.

▶ Drink six to eight glasses of water every day.

▶ Eat five to six servings of fresh fruits and vegetables daily.

▶ Exercise regularly.

▶ Get a massage of the belly or lower back.

▶ Take 100 milligrams of the stool softener Colace (available over the counter) two or three times daily.

▶ You can add Senokot tablets (also available over the counter) in the evening to stimulate bowel contractions.

▶ If you try all of the above and still don't get relief, there are stronger medications that are available by prescription.

NAUSEA

▶ Try acupuncture or acupressure (rub the inside of your wrist for a home treatment).

(continued)

- Drink ginger tea or take ginger supplements.
- Get a massage, especially of the ankles, feet, and front of the hip.

DRY MOUTH

- Keep plenty of water handy.
- Chew gum or suck on sugar-free candies.

SEDATION

- The best way to control this side effect is to reduce your need for sedating medication in the first place. Try appropriate therapies to keep your pain under as much control as possible; I especially recommend breathing techniques, guided imagery, and meditation to help pull you through a flare-up without extra pills.

INADEQUATE RELIEF

You've taken your prescription, but it's like tossing a cup of water on a forest fire. What's going on?

- *You need a higher dose.* It's smart to "start low and go slow," as I mentioned above, but you do need to let your doctor know if you need more relief. An increased dose might do the trick, or perhaps a different kind of drug within the same class will work better for you.

- *You need a different class of medication.* There are several kinds of painkilling drugs out there, and you might have to try a few before you find the one that works best. For pain caused by damaged or sensitized nerves, anticonvulsants or tricyclic antidepressants can help. For pain that's consistently moderate to severe, you might need an opioid in addition to NSAIDs. Check the information in this chapter and in Part IV to find the right medications for your disorder.

- *Your doctor is afraid of opioids.* For many chronically painful conditions, opioids are hands down the best form of pain relief. But opioids are misunderstood drugs, and doctors may prescribe them incorrectly—or not at all—through a misguided fear of causing addiction, or perhaps from a fear they'll be prosecuted by the Drug Enforcement

Administration (DEA). When opioids aren't properly prescribed, they can result in some nasty side effects in exchange for minimal relief. I will discuss each of these issues in more depth on pages 185–195.

ANTICONVULSANTS

Sometimes chronic pain is the result of a nervous system run amok—nerve cells that fire spontaneously or that send out inappropriately loud messages. This is true for outright nerve damage as well as for pain that's inexplicably severe. In these cases, it makes sense to try anticonvulsants (also known as membrane stabilizers), a class of drugs that quiet the nerves and prevent them from misfiring.

Anticonvulsants were first used for epilepsy and seizures, because those disorders also involve overexcited nerve cells; in the late 1980s, as it became more and more obvious that many chronic pain problems originated in the nervous system, doctors began to apply these drugs for pain control. Many patients who have given up on ever finding relief have surprising success with anticonvulsants. Some are able to go off them after a while, because the drugs have given their nervous system a chance to "remember" how it ought to behave. (Nerve pain may also respond to small doses of tricyclic antidepressants, which attenuate pain messages fired by nerves and are discussed later in this chapter. These two medications are often combined for a synergistic effect.)

If you take anticonvulsants, you should know that some side effects are likely. Like many other pain drugs, they can result in sedation, dizziness, fatigue, upset stomach, constipation, nausea, vomiting, and skin rashes. Many of these side effects fade with continued use of the drug. Some kinds of anticonvulsants can also lead to liver and kidney problems or suppress blood cell formation in the bone marrow. These latter problems are obviously very serious, so your doctor should set up a schedule for regular blood and liver tests and a general going-over. If you have a disorder of the kidney, liver, or bone marrow, then anticonvulsants clearly are not a good choice for you, and you may want to try tricyclic antidepressants instead. (By the same token, anticonvulsants are often appropriate for people who can't take tricyclics.)

If you do experience bad side effects, you and your doctor should experiment with the dosage or drug brand to see if you can bring them down to a tolerable level. Many people are able to take a relatively new anticonvulsant called gabapentin (brand name Neurontin) with minimal side effects. Since neuropathic pain also responds very well to mind-body therapies, you could try one or two of them on a regular basis to see if they reduce your need for the drug.

MOST COMMONLY PRESCRIBED ANTICONVULSANTS FOR PAIN

- Depakote (valproic acid)
- Gabitril (tiagabine)
- Klonopin (clonazepam)
- Mexitil (mexiletine, which is actually a heart rhythm stabilizer that acts much like an anticonvulsant)
- Neurontin (gabapentin)
- Tegretol (carbamazepine)
- Topamax (topiramate)
- Trileptal (oxcarbazepine)

ANTI-INFLAMMATORY MEDICATIONS

Anti-inflammatory drugs fall into two broad categories: steroidal and non-steroidal. Although steroid drugs are an extreme measure for pain, the non-steroidal drugs are some of the most frequently used medications in the world.

NON-STEROIDAL ANTI-INFLAMMATORY DRUGS

Non-steroidal anti-inflammatory drugs are known as NSAIDs (pronounced "EN-seds") in medical shorthand. Most of us know them in their over-the-counter incarnations, including aspirin and ibuprofen, although they are also available in stronger doses by prescription. NSAIDs work by preventing the release of certain prostaglandins, hormones that can cause inflammation and have a role in making nerve receptors more sensitive to pain.

For many people, NSAIDs are the first line of treatment for headaches, muscle soreness, arthritis pain, bone pain, and other aches, and with good reason: They work. But people have become so familiar with NSAIDs that sometimes they forget that, despite their easy availability, these pills are still very real medications, with the potential to create significant undesirable consequences.

The most frequent serious problem with NSAIDs is bleeding of the stomach lining. The prostaglandins that most NSAIDs block are also responsible for generating the mucus that protects the stomach lining and platelets from digestive acids. If enough of that mucus is stripped away, the acids can penetrate the lining and cause bleeding. When the penetration occurs near an artery, the bleeding may be unstoppable. Every year, seventy-six thousand people are hospitalized for reactions to NSAIDs, and sixteen thousand of them die. Given that almost all of us take an NSAID now and then, the likelihood that any one person will encounter such a serious problem is relatively low. Yet the danger remains real, and it reminds us that, like any medication, NSAIDs must be taken with reasonable care and good judgment.

In the past couple of years, a new class of NSAID that may be safer has appeared on the market. These drugs are called COX-2 inhibitors, so named because they block prostaglandins on a selective basis, targeting those that increase inflammation and pain but leaving intact those that protect the stomach. At the time of this writing, COX-2 inhibitors are available by prescription only. They do not reduce pain to a greater or lesser extent than other NSAIDs, but they do seem gentler to the body. If you take NSAIDs on a regular basis, you may want to check with your doctor about this option.

You can also use a few commonsense methods to reduce the likelihood of side effects. People with peptic ulcers, kidney disease, or disorders that cause excess bleeding should not take NSAIDs, nor should those who take corticosteroids or drink large quantities of alcohol. People who are taking anticoagulants (blood thinners) should take NSAIDs only if it's absolutely necessary, and they should check in with their doctors regularly. (If you have one of these contraindications, it's possible that you could try the COX-2 inhibitors. You will need to be carefully screened and monitored by your doctor, since it's still possible to develop gastrointestinal and other complications with the new drugs.) When taking an over-the-counter product, do not exceed the dosage listed on the package unless your doctor has specifically advised you to do otherwise. If that dosage doesn't give you enough relief, look into the stronger prescription NSAIDs or perhaps another class of drugs entirely. (Many doctors combine NSAIDs with opioids or anticonvulsants. The effect is synergistic and may keep you from taking higher doses of the opioid or anticonvulsant.) And be alert for the signs of stomach bleeding: pain in the gut, swollen limbs, vomiting of blood, and dark, tarry stools. If you notice any of these symptoms, call your doctor immediately. If those symptoms are severe, call an ambulance.

Of course, one of the best ways to minimize side effects from NSAIDs is to reduce your dependence on them. Alternative therapies offer many ways to accomplish this goal. People who suffer from muscle pain often respond well to physical therapies, including massage, exercise, and postural methods. Those with inflammatory ailments may find that acupuncture or dietary measures can reduce their need for NSAIDs. Mind-body treatments have good track records for managing flare-ups so that you don't have to increase your usual dose. And you may find that Tylenol, a safe but mild painkiller that is not in the NSAID class, can substitute for NSAIDs at times of less intense pain, or you can use it as an adjunct to one of the alternative therapies.

MOST COMMONLY USED NSAIDS

The brand name is presented first, followed by the generic name in parentheses.

- Over-the-counter medications such as Motrin, Advil, Aleve, and aspirin
- Anaprox (naproxen)
- Anaprox DS (naproxen)
- Ansaid (flurbiprofen)
- Arthrotec (diclofenac with misoprostol)
- Celebrex (celecoxib)
- Clinoril (sulindac)
- Daypro (oxaprozin)
- Feldene (piroxicam)
- Mobic (meloxicam)

(continued)

- Naprosyn (naproxen)
- Orudis (ketoprofen)
- Relafen (nabumetone)
- Toradol (ketorolac)
- Vioxx (rofecoxib)
- Voltaren (diclofenac)

STEROIDAL ANTI-INFLAMMATORY DRUGS

Steroidal anti-inflammatory drugs are powerful medications with a set of side effects to match. I won't go into all the side effects here, but suffice it to say that when used for a long period of time they can lead to diabetes, suppression of the immune system, and bone thinning. In her book *Kitchen Table Wisdom,* Rachel Naomi Remen, M.D., who is the co-founder and medical director of the Commonweal Cancer Help Program in California, describes the effects of the steroids that she took for Crohn's disease, a gastrointestinal disorder, as an adolescent. Among other things, they made her bones so weak that they sometimes spontaneously broke underneath her as she stood. An occasional shot of cortisone or a short course of prednisone for major flare-ups is not going to wreck your system, but these drugs are *not* for long-term pain control.

Steroidal anti-inflammatory drugs are mainly used to treat some of the underlying conditions that create pain, such as rheumatoid arthritis and lupus, but in some cases they can also treat pain itself. This approach is usually reserved for serious flare-ups of painful muscles, joints, and discs that press on nerves. When a person is otherwise healthy, I prefer to save these drugs for special situations—such as a horrid flare-up that comes on the eve of the patient's debut concert at Carnegie Hall. In these cases, a short-term dose can allow the show to go on. If you anticipate that you might find yourself in such a dilemma, it's a good idea to talk to your doctor and formulate an emergency plan that will get you through a major speech or performance. Sometimes just having a plan in place can give you peace of mind. Possible side effects of these short-term doses include insomnia, destabilized blood sugar, and a "pepped-up" feeling.

These drugs also make sense for patients who are at the end of their life. Often a combination of a steroidal anti-inflammatory and an opioid can give a person ease and comfort in their final months, when there is no concern for side effects that may not appear for years.

MOST COMMONLY PRESCRIBED STEROIDAL ANTI-INFLAMMATORY DRUGS FOR PAIN

The brand name is presented first, followed by the generic name in parentheses.

- Decadron (dexamethasone)
- Deltasone (prednisone)
- Medrol (methylprednisolone)
- Sterapred (prednisone)
- Sterapred DS (prednisone)

MUSCLE RELAXANTS

Muscle relaxants can be roughly divided into two types: those that relax the muscle tissue itself and those that do so indirectly, by means of sedation. The first type sounds attractive, especially when your muscles are tied up in knots. The list of possible side effects for this type of drug is so long, however, that it's a good idea to use the direct relaxers only in certain circumstances: for short-term relief of spasm (as in a back pain crisis) or for longer use when severe spasms accompany neurological disability. Direct muscle relaxers, which increase GABA, a neurotransmitter that inhibits pain, include benzodiazepines (Valium, Xanax, and the like). Another direct relaxer, baclofen, is the drug of choice for people with MS and spinal injuries, who may experience fierce spasms in limbs that are otherwise motionless. Baclofen may also be used for serious flare-ups of other conditions. Direct muscle relaxers, especially the benzodiazepines, can be highly addictive—despite all the attention the media is currently giving to the supposedly addictive power of certain opioids, Xanax is actually one of the easiest drugs to get hooked on, and one of the hardest drug habits to break—so long-term use should be considered carefully. If you *do* take a regular course of direct relaxants and want to stop, you'll need to be tapered off, as withdrawal (often consisting of agitation, flulike symptoms, panic attacks, or anxiety) or other serious problems could occur.

The sedative muscle relaxants (which include the brand names Flexeril, Robaxin, and Norflex) operate by slowing down your central nervous system, causing you to loosen the tight grip you may have over certain muscles. Of course, they also loosen your grip on the world, and you may find yourself drowsy or asleep after taking a dose. Sometimes this is a blessing: You take a nap and feel better when you wake up. But as a regular means of controlling persistent pain, the downside is obvious. And like the direct relaxers, this type of relaxant can also lead to dependence if taken over the long term. If, however, you find that a sedative every now and then controls your flare-ups, it's reasonable to have a prescription on hand. As with so many other drugs for pain, sometimes the knowledge that you have access to a trustworthy means of relief is a kind of medicine all by itself.

MOST COMMONLY PRESCRIBED MUSCLE RELAXANTS FOR PAIN

The brand name is presented first, followed by the generic name in parentheses.

- Flexeril (cyclobenzaprine)
- Norflex (orphenadrine)
- Robaxin (methocarbamol)
- Valium (diazepam)
- Xanax (alprazolam)
- Zanaflex (tizanidine)

Baclofen, the most commonly prescribed direct muscle relaxant, is a generic drug with no brand-name preparations available.

NMDA ANTAGONISTS

As this book goes to press, NMDA antagonists are still in the research and development phase, but it looks as if they'll reach the market very soon. (Some doctors will now prescribe a currently available drug with NMDA-blocking properties, dextromethorphan, found in many over-the-counter cough medications.) Although the information here is necessarily incomplete, it should alert you to watch for news about these promising drugs.

NMDA is short for N-methyl-D-aspartate, a type of nerve cell receptor. When NMDA receptors are activated, they appear to increase pain sensitivity by allowing greater-than-normal numbers of pain signals to travel along the nerve pathway. If a drug could block those receptors, the thinking goes, we could reduce the signals that get through to the spinal cord and brain. NMDA antagonists seem to accomplish exactly that. It's likely that they will work well with opioids, giving you effective relief while perhaps slowing your body's buildup of tolerance to the opioid. (In fact, one opioid, methadone, actually has some NMDA-blocking properties.) A soon-to-be-released commercial preparation will probably combine the two drugs.

It's not yet completely clear what kinds of side effects NMDA antagonists might have, and of course that's where many drugs in the development stage go sour. You should expect them to have effects similar to opioid drugs, including sedation, nausea, dizziness, constipation, and dry mouth.

OFFICE INJECTIONS

Sometimes a drug works best if it's injected into a painful area. Since the medication arrives directly at its destination without having to take the circuitous route through the digestive system, as pills do, you need a much smaller amount, and you're far less likely to have side effects. Injected drugs also often have immediate results. Because of these attractive elements, injections are a method preferred by many pain specialists, myself among them.

Injections to a structure that's close to the skin can be performed right in the doctor's office—hence the term "office injection," a term most doctors will recognize, although some prefer the phrase "local injection." Office injections are a treatment of choice for myofascial pain, tendinitis, and bursitis, especially cases that involve trigger points, the jumpy balls of muscle that can spread pain outward and through other parts of your body. They can also help joints and ligaments that lie near the body's surface.

(It is also possible to inject medication directly into, or next to, the nerves, spinal cord, or structures that reside deep within the body. Because these injections are more complicated affairs, with greater potential for mistakes and side effects, they are considered invasive procedures and are covered in Chapter 13. However, they can silence a squawking nerve more effectively than many other treatments and are well worth considering after more conservative measures have failed.)

Office injections tend to use two kinds of drugs. The first, local anesthetics, block electrical impulses through the nerves. You can tell from the names—lidocaine, bupivacaine, procaine, and so on—that anesthetics are from the same family as cocaine, which has a notoriously numbing effect on whatever it touches. (When injections for pain were first performed more than a hundred years ago, doctors actually shot pure cocaine into their patients. As you might imagine, that practice has long been discontinued.) Doctors also use corticosteroids for injections, to cool down inflamed muscles, joints, or nerves. Although you should be very wary of taking corticosteroid pills, as they have a thick portfolio of side effects, you need very little in an office injection and are not likely to feel much disturbance. A local anesthetic and a corticosteroid are very often combined into one injection for the most relief.

I've received these injections a few times, on a series of trigger points that pop up in my back, and I won't lie to you. Injections *can* hurt—you feel a pinch, as with a vaccination—but only momentarily, and an ice pack can help ease any soreness that might linger. If the medicine is going to work, it will do so almost immediately. Within minutes, you may be able to move a previously frozen shoulder or turn your stiff neck smoothly from side to side. If you don't feel improvement within a few minutes, your doctor may need to try the injection again from one or two more angles. Patients who still don't feel better after three or four injections should probably move on to something else.

It's hard to predict how long the effects of an injection will last. Recently I injected a trigger point of a surgeon friend. He felt better but needed to return for another injection the next week, and then a month later; after those three treatments, the knots in his shoulder released and the pain disappeared entirely. He may not need to come back again for years, or ever. Most people will get relief of a considerably shorter duration, ranging from hours to weeks. This buys them the opportunity to perform the stretches and exercises that may break the pain cycle, especially in cases of myofascial pain. At the very least, it allows you time to relax and live without pain's alarm bells as a constant background noise. Sometimes that break alone is therapeutic and wards off the return of a spasm.

Possible side effects are the same as for any shot—bleeding, allergic reactions, and infection—and you shouldn't get injections if you're on blood thinners. Since you don't want to be jabbed with needles any more often than you have to, I suggest finding a doctor with a strong history of doing these injections. The more practiced the physician, the more likely you are to experience relief on the first or second try. Just keep in mind that doctors who have specialized in injections may have a certain amount of blindness to other therapies. You may need to ask about physical therapy, exercises, and stretches to perform; otherwise, the topic may not come up at all.

If you are truly too sore to tolerate even light touch on a painful spot, you might be too jumpy to receive a needle. In these cases I advise some loosening-up therapies before attempting an injection—massage, heat therapy, stretching, and mind-body work are all good choices, with massage and heat at the very top.

OPIOIDS

In Chapter 3, I discussed our expanding knowledge of endorphins, the natural painkilling substances produced by the body. Endorphins work like keys that fit certain nerve receptors; when the key turns in the nerve receptor's lock, the receptor's ability to fire off pain signals is partially checked. Endorphins can reduce pain or even stop it altogether; they can also change your mental reaction to the sensation so that it doesn't bother you as much.

Opioids, which belong to the class of drugs known as narcotics, mimic the effects of endorphins. They are very similar in chemical structure, lock into the same nerve receptors, and reduce pain in the same way. The difference is that they're not produced within the body. Instead, they are derived from the opium poppy—it can even be argued that the natural opioids (as opposed to the synthetic products) are a form of herbal medicine.

Because opioids are not natural to the body, they create more side effects than endorphins do. They can make you sedated, nauseated, constipated, euphoric, and sweaty, and they can give you a dry mouth. Even though opioids are not nearly so dangerous as many other drugs, they can certainly be fatal if you take an overdose. There is a very small risk of addiction, which is usually hugely overstated. (See "Won't I Get Addicted?" below.) Opioids are strong drugs, so you don't want to use them for minor complaints. But for moderate to severe pain, they are one of the most effective control measures we have. One especially valuable aspect of opioids is that, unlike other pain drugs, they don't have a ceiling effect—a point at which increased doses no longer result in additional relief. If you and your doctor can find an opioid strategy that results in minimal or tolerable side effects, and if you do not have a history of drug or alcohol abuse, opioids can form the foundation of an intelligent plan for pain relief.

Opioids can be used to treat any moderate to severe pain, but they are not always the *first* drug to turn to. People with nerve-related pain, peripheral neuropathies, spinal cord damage, fibromyalgia, headaches, or pain that's related to insomnia may find better relief with other drugs, most often tricyclic antidepressants or anticonvulsants. People with gastrointestinal disorders will want to be cautious about opioids, since they can relax the smooth muscle of the intestines and cause constipation. If you have a liver or kidney disorder, you'll need to be very careful with opioids, as they are metabolized in these organs; your doctor should start you on low doses and keep a close eye on you.

WHAT YOUR DOCTOR MAY NOT KNOW

If you want to increase the effectiveness of opioids while reducing their side effects, you need to understand the difference between those that are *short-acting* and those that are *long-acting*.

Short-acting opioids, including codeine, hydrocodone, and oxycodone, are a potent way to treat acute pain. If you've ever had a root canal or a serious athletic injury, you've probably received a couple of doses of codeine or hydrocodone, maybe in the form of Tylenol 3, Vicodin, or Percocet. A few pills get you through the worst of the pain, and then their work is done.

But these drugs make less sense for consistent use. Short-acting opioids hit your system quickly. You might feel a powerful wave of euphoria or sedation; whatever response you'll have to this drug, good or bad, you'll get it in a concentrated burst. Then the drug leaves your system as quickly as it came. You might be left with several hours of pain before it's time to take the next dose. With short-acting drugs, you're likely to have fierce side effects, along with an unpleasant feeling of desperation for the next pill. You or your doctor might conclude that you're addicted when that's not really the case at all: You're just looking for pain relief that's more consistent. Too often, this is the end of the line.

These problems can often be alleviated by switching to *long-acting* opioids such as MS Contin (a morphine preparation), OxyContin (made with oxycodone), or methadone. Don't let the names frighten you—for consistent use, these drugs are actually gentler. They release over a long period of time; since your body absorbs them slowly and evenly, you won't feel such a whammy of side effects. You will also receive more consistent pain control from dose to dose. Of course, you'll need to get an appropriate dosage and find the drug that you can best tolerate, but on the whole people are much more satisfied with the results.

Unfortunately, many doctors are reluctant to prescribe long-acting drugs, mainly because they have less experience with them. "Long-acting" somehow translates to them as "big and scary," but that simply isn't true. If your doctor is wary of opioids, see "Talking to Your Doctor About Opioids," below.

WON'T I GET ADDICTED?

I was talking about this book with some friends at a dinner party. Everyone nodded with interest as we talked about alternative therapies, but when the subject of opioids came up, one of the couples protested. It turned out that the husband had been given some codeine after surgery to replace his hip. When the prescription ran out three weeks later, he experienced terrible withdrawal symptoms: shakiness, sweating, and insomnia. He still had severe pain in the other hip, but the thought of taking more opioids visibly upset him. He was terrified he'd become addicted.

"My mother's spine is practically crumbling from osteoporosis, but she won't take morphine," the host weighed in. "She's lived a clean life for eighty years and doesn't want to become an addict now."

"I sure wouldn't want to walk into a pharmacy these days and ask for OxyContin. They'd really think I'd hit the skids."

I'm not one to push drugs on patients, but I hate to see people reject a good source of relief without all the facts. We tend to think that most people, if given the opportunity to become addicted to opioids, will do so. That's just not true. When opioids are given to patients without a history of drug abuse, the rate of addiction is about .01 percent, according to the *Journal of Pain and Symptom Management.* That's one person out of every ten thousand. The risk of addiction is minimal, and any decent physician will monitor you closely to make sure you aren't one of the unlucky few.

Before making a decision about opioids, you need to understand the difference between addiction and tolerance. *Tolerance* occurs when your body adjusts to a substance. This happens all the time. You can get adjusted to spicy food, so that you need more and more Tabasco in your chili before your palate stings. If you take antihistamines for a long time, soon you'll need higher doses before they work on you.

The same thing happens with opioids. Over a period of time, your body will grow accustomed to the drug's presence, and you'll require a higher dose for pain relief. An experienced pain doctor will accept your tolerance and adjust your dose accordingly without any fears that you're an addict.

Addiction is another matter. It is useful to define it primarily as a question of motive. People who take an opioid for its psychological effects—that is, to get high—are considered abusers of the drug; when they can't control their desire to get high, they're addicts. Addicts feel compelled to use a drug even when they are harmed by it; if it begins to wreck their families, careers, and physical health, they still don't want to stop. If your sole motive in taking a drug is pain relief, then you are simply not an addict.

(If you've been addicted to drugs or alcohol before or if you have another compulsive disorder, then obviously you're at a greater risk for addiction than other people. There are some doctors and a few pain centers that will prescribe opioids to former addicts within tightly controlled parameters. You may also prefer to seek out nonopioid methods of pain relief.)

What about withdrawal, such as my friend experienced? Withdrawal is what happens to your body when it's suddenly deprived of a drug it's grown used to. When a body is accustomed to opioids and then stops cold turkey, it will respond with nausea, aching muscles, vomiting, sweating, and other symptoms. You might feel as if you have a really nasty case of the flu. It helps to know that withdrawal is not the special province of opioids. Blood pressure medication and insulin, to name just two, have their own withdrawal symptoms, which are actually much more serious and even deadly.

The key to avoiding withdrawal is for the doctor to taper the patient off the drug, prescribing smaller and smaller doses until the body readjusts to a drug-free state. There should be only minimal symptoms of withdrawal, if any. At that point, the overwhelming majority of people are able to walk away from the opioid without looking back. But the prescribing doctor must know enough about opioids to do the tapering. If my friend's doctor had tapered him off his postsurgical medicine, he would not have felt like he'd been run over by a truck. (It also would have been wiser to give him a long-acting opioid instead of codeine, which is short-acting.) And he would not have spent years rejecting one of his best options for pain relief.

OXYCONTIN: DRUG OF RELIEF—OR DRUG OF ABUSE?

OxyContin, a long-acting opioid, has received a particularly bad rap in the press lately. I get angry when I see media stories implying that OxyContin is highly addictive when taken as prescribed. This kind of sensationalist reporting has turned one of our best pain medications into a drug with a stigma. When patients are too scared to take a drug that can get them out of bed and back into productive lives as teachers, volunteers, grandparents, home builders, and artists, I feel frustrated and outraged.

Yes, OxyContin is abused—but rarely by people in pain who have legitimate prescriptions and who use the drug as directed by their doctors. It's abused mostly by another population: those with addictive personalities, who have deliberately sought out OxyContin as a means of getting high. These are people who buy OxyContin off the street, steal it, or lie to their doctors to obtain it; often they have histories of abusing other substances. In fact, the reason some drugstores have made the highly publicized decision to stop carrying OxyContin is not that their pharmacists are passing medical judgment on the drug, feeling it's especially addictive—they stop carrying OxyContin because criminals in some areas will break into stores to steal it for recreational use. When they are in possession of OxyContin, these abusers don't take it orally, as prescribed. Instead, they break the capsule, destroying the time-release effect that allows the medication to gradually be absorbed into the body over a period of many

(continued)

hours, and snort or inject *all* the medication at once. The effect is similar to that of taking a handful of Percocet or Vicodin.

So yes, if you snort or inject OxyContin, you're in for some big trouble. But if you have not abused drugs or alcohol before, and if you take OxyContin as prescribed, your chances of addiction appear to be the same as for any other opioid medication: one in ten thousand. When I see patients I think will benefit from OxyContin but are wary, I often ask them which choice they want to make: rejecting a drug out of misplaced fear so that they can stay at home, withdrawn and in pain? Or holding their head up high, responsibly using a drug that's been unfairly stigmatized by some people, and resuming their lives?

GWEN'S STORY: METHADONE GOT HER MOVING AGAIN

Gwen is a young woman with a severe bladder condition called interstitial cystitis. In the year or so before she came to see me, she would spend most days curled up on her couch, frozen with pain and unable to do anything but read light novels. She felt like a burden on her husband, began to binge-eat as a means of solace, and grew deeply depressed.

At first, I gave her a fentanyl patch, which slowly delivered opioids into her bloodstream. She felt better, but with time her body developed tolerance to the drug, leaving her with pain between doses. And she was still confined to home for most of the day.

"Gwen," I said, "if you stay on the patch, you'll continue to need higher and higher amounts of the medication to keep the pain from breaking through. I'm beginning to think that you'd do better on another drug. The drug I have in mind is great for tough chronic pain, because it actually prevents tolerance from building up." I paused. "But it's got a terrible social association."

Gwen looked at me as if to say, *Now what?*

"It's methadone," I said.

Gwen practically shrank back into the corner. "Methadone? Isn't that what they give heroin junkies at clinics? I won't take a drug that

(continued)

will make me addicted. I don't care how much pain it takes away, I don't want to end up in the gutter with a needle hanging out of my arm."

She didn't accept methadone at that visit; instead, I renewed her prescription for the patch at a higher dose. But at the next visit, Gwen reported that her pain still wasn't under control and hesitantly brought up the subject of methadone herself.

"Do you really think it would be better than what I'm taking now?" she asked.

"Well, we don't see as much tolerance with methadone as with other opioids, so it's good for big pain like yours." I told her about my other patients on the drug, including an upstanding elderly woman who had come in that morning. Without methadone, this lady spent her days bedridden. But with the methadone, she was able to walk to the senior center to run a sewing circle.

I wrote a methadone prescription for Gwen that day. She felt odd asking for it at the pharmacy, but thinking of my patient who ran the sewing circle gave her some courage. "If a nice elderly lady can take methadone, so can I," she told herself. After Gwen began the drug, her pain settled down enough that she could keep house a little, which made her feel more productive. She was able to begin some exercising and yoga, and went out to meetings of Overeaters Anonymous. These activities brought down her stress level and also released some of the muscular tension in her pelvic area. Even though she was on a very strong narcotic—which might lead you to believe she was always doped up—she actually became much more active. Now she and I are tapering down the methadone as the pain is increasingly controlled by alternative means, including the workouts and yoga but also diet, breathing exercises, biofeedback, and aromatherapy. Notice, though, that most of these alternatives were not possible for Gwen until methadone enabled her to get moving.

THE OPIOID TEST: DOES IT GET YOU UP AND AROUND?

The purpose of opioids is to reduce your suffering while increasing your functionality—that is, allowing you to participate more fully in life. But opioids aren't magic, and they don't always have this uplifting effect. A few months ago I saw a patient named Bill, whose operation for back pain had left him feeling even worse. His previous doctor had prescribed *three* different opioids, a combination that left him so sedated that he was dizzy, and he'd developed constipation that felt as bad as the pain. Obviously, this opioid regimen did not increase his functionality or enjoyment of life. Nor did it allow him the exercise he desperately needed. Slowly we tapered him off the opioids and put him on low doses of anticonvulsants and tricyclic antidepressants, and he began a physical therapy program along with regular massage. He's much more flexible, with a greater range of motion, and he feels much more like himself again. He's still on medication, but he found that opioids were not the answer for him.

Here is the rule of thumb that I share with my patients: Do you have an acceptable level of functioning without opioids? If so, then maybe you don't need them. If not, do opioids increase your functioning? If, after reasonable experimentation, they continue to make you too sick or sleepy to do the things you enjoy, you are probably better off with a different kind of treatment.

HOW WILL THE DRUG GET TO THE PAIN? CHOICES IN DELIVERY SYSTEMS

Pills are convenient and comfortingly familiar. But sometimes pills for opioids are not your best choice. Since pills take the long way to your bloodstream, you need extra medication to account for what's lost in your digestive system. You also risk digestive side effects such as constipation. Here are some other options:

- *The patch.* When medication is delivered via a patch placed over your skin, it enters your bloodstream directly, bypassing your liver, so you need less of it. (The drug used in the patch, fentanyl, is actually a short-acting opioid, but since the patch causes it to leach slowly through the skin and into the bloodstream, it works here like a long-acting drug.)

- *The pump.* When pain is very severe and you require large doses, a pump can be surgically implanted by your spine and filled with morphine or other drugs. It's an extreme option, but it keeps side effects to a bare minimum.

- *The lollipop.* That's right—candy-flavored fentanyl on a stick. About 25 percent of the drug enters directly through the bloodstream. The lollipop is usually reserved for people with unpredictable bouts of pain or who can't swallow pills.

▶ *Suppositories.* Suppositories also bypass the gastrointestinal tract, as the drug flows directly from the wall of the rectum to the bloodstream. They are a good choice for people who suffer digestive problems, especially when nausea and vomiting keep them from holding down their medication.

TALKING TO YOUR DOCTOR ABOUT OPIOIDS

You may find that your doctor is reluctant to prescribe opioids, especially the long-acting varieties that offer the best chance of relief. If this happens, have a frank conversation with your physician. If he is concerned that opioids are addictive (and you are indeed not a current or former drug abuser), refer him to the articles and Web sites listed on the next page, which explain the rarity of addiction. He may also be worried about federal regulations, which, to be fair, can be intimidating. If that's the case, you may want to ask for a referral to a pain specialist. Specialists are accustomed to working within DEA regulations, and federal agents expect them to prescribe opioids in higher-than-usual numbers.

You can help matters along by agreeing to sign an opioids agreement (in which you state that you won't use them for any reason other than your own pain relief and that you will abide by the dosage). Although some general practitioners may not have heard of them, all pain doctors are familiar with these agreements, and most will have their preferred versions on hand in the office. You'll also need to be willing to visit the doctor on a monthly basis, since doctors are not permitted to write prescriptions for more than a month's worth of opioids for a single patient.

FURTHER READING FOR YOU OR YOUR DOCTOR

If you or your doctor would like more information about opioids and addiction, consult the following:

(continued)

- The American Academy of Pain Medicine's Web site, www.painmed.org, which contains its position on the use of opioids for chronic pain. (See also other Web sites listed in Appendix E.)
- J. Porter and H. Jick, "Addiction Rare in Patients Treated with Narcotics," *New England Journal of Medicine,* 1980.
- D. P. Friedman, "Perspectives on the Medical Use of Drugs of Abuse," *Journal of Pain and Symptom Management,* 1990.

MOST COMMONLY PRESCRIBED OPIOIDS

The brand name is presented first, followed by the generic name in parentheses.

SHORT-ACTING OPIOIDS:

- Actiq (fentanyl)
- Darvon (propoxyphene)
- Demerol (meperidine)
- Dilaudid (hydromorphone)
- MSIR (morphine)
- Percocet (oxycodone and acetaminophen)
- Roxicodone (oxycodone)
- Tylenol 3 (codeine and acetaminophen)
- Vicodin (hydrocodone and acetaminophen)

LONG-ACTING OPIOIDS:

- Duragesic (fentanyl transderm)

(continued)

- Dolophine (methadone)
- MS Contin (morphine, slow release)
- Oramorph SR (morphine, slow release)
- OxyContin (oxycodone)

TRICYCLIC ANTIDEPRESSANTS

Dr. Medford is a seventy-four-year-old psychiatrist, a lively man with a dry wit and a set of devoted patients. He also has a punishing case of arthritis that likely involves sensitized nerves. When I first saw him, the pain was making it hard for him to sleep at night, and one day he found himself dozing off in front of a client. The client, luckily, was understanding, but clearly it was time for Dr. Medford to change his pain-control methods. You might not think that someone who thrives despite his pain would need antidepressants, but in fact a low dose has helped him sleep at night, remain alert during the day, and bring his pain under better control.

When it comes to pain, tricyclic antidepressants are usually prescribed *not* for their mood-altering qualities but for their side effect of sedation. They increase available amounts of serotonin and dopamine, which appear to help you sleep. Without adequate quantities of either neurotransmitter, you'll find yourself staying awake at night, and possibly also depressed or anxious. For patients with insomnia that goes hand in hand with their pain, a small dose of a tricyclic antidepressant can give them their first good night's sleep in years. It may also relieve depression and anxiety, although what causes this effect is not clear, since the dose is much lower than would ordinarily be prescribed for psychological disorders. In all likelihood, most people feel happier simply because they have less pain and more sleep; others may be receiving a mood-altering effect from the drug.

It's important to distinguish between tricyclic antidepressants, which are used in pain treatment, and selective serotonin reuptake inhibitors (SSRIs). The SSRIs, which include the brand names Prozac, Zoloft, and Paxil, are excellent for treating depression and anxiety, but they are not usually used for their direct effects on pain. If you need to treat clinical depression in conjunction with pain, it's often best to combine a normal dose of an SSRI with a very small dose of a tricyclic.

When should you consider tricyclics? Clearly, they are a good first choice for pain that involves the nerves. What's not so clear is when nerves have a role in pain and when they don't. Obviously, anyone with outright nerve damage is a candidate for tricyclics. This category includes people with spinal cord injuries, phantom limb pain, multiple sclerosis, postherpetic neuralgia, central pain syndrome, and diabetic neuropathies. A grayer area is pain, stemming from any condition, that's more intense than seems appropriate. This kind of bewildering pain is often helped along by nerves that have gone haywire as a result of an initial pain overload. Dr. Medford, with his arthritis, had so much pain that nerve mischief was probably involved. Tricyclic antidepressants are also used for fibromyalgia, some headaches, and, as mentioned above, anytime insomnia appears as pain's partner.

Common reactions to tricyclics include dry mouth, drowsiness, dizziness, constipation, urinary retention, and a metallic taste in the mouth. If you have heart rhythm disturbances, especially what's known as a heart block, or if you have low blood pressure, you'll need to be monitored regularly by a doctor.

MOST COMMONLY PRESCRIBED TRICYCLIC ANTIDEPRESSANTS FOR PAIN

The brand name is presented first, followed by the generic name in parentheses.

- Elavil (amitriptyline)
- Norpramin (desipramine)
- Pamelor (nortriptyline)
- Sinequan (doxepin)

13.

DEEP INJECTIONS, IMPLANTS, AND SURGERY

DEEP INJECTIONS / NERVE ABLATIONS / PUMP IMPLANTS / SPINAL CORD STIMULATORS / SURGERY

This chapter is devoted to more aggressive pain therapies that tend to act directly on the nervous system. Some of them coat screaming nerves with anesthetic or steroids; others silence those nerves or even kill them. Some stimulate or medicate your spinal cord directly, to block or scramble pain messages. I often consider using them for patients with particular kinds of back and neck pain; pain in the belly, ribs, or chest; or a difficult condition known as complex regional pain syndrome. And if you suffer from severe, intractable pain, these therapies can make the difference between confinement to bed and walking down the street. They also carry more risk—sometimes a little, sometimes a lot—and each of them involves an invasive action into your body, via needle or scalpel.

This aggressive quality does not make these procedures either good or bad. What matters first, obviously, is whether they're appropriate for your condition. Assuming that you *do* have a disorder that might benefit from these therapies, here's the next question to ask yourself: Is this procedure part of a balanced treatment plan?

Consider Lawrence, who has suffered from low back pain for a year. He is about twenty pounds overweight, with most of the excess baggage in his middle. He smokes, and he does not exercise or stretch. He has a low-paying but high-stress job as a restaurant manager. Yet when over-the-counter painkillers fail to give him relief, his primary-care doctor refers him to an anesthesiologist for an injection. A combination of anesthetic and steroids will coat the nerves around his spine.

Lawrence receives the injection. It goes well—none of the possible side effects, which include infection and allergic reaction, occur. After some rest, he goes home, already feeling better. The next day, he goes back to his sedentary job and his diet of cheeseburgers, chips, and Winstons. Every time there's trouble between the wait staff and the kitchen, his heart pounds and his muscles tense. Is it any surprise that soon his pain returns in spades?

I tell Lawrence's story because it's a familiar one. Injections (as well as the other treatments included here) can reduce certain kinds of pain. But they are often used too hastily, before the patient tries out some commonsense measures. And we tend to put too much faith in them, as if they were stand-alone curatives.

Injections, implants, and sometimes even surgery offer a way to get at certain kinds of pain, but they need to be balanced with lifestyle changes. If you and your doctor agree that one of these therapies might help you, great. Just don't forget to follow up your procedure with stretching, exercise, good nutrition, and stress reduction—and anything else that makes sense for your individual needs.

DEEP INJECTIONS

Injections, which offer direct medication of painful body structures, fall into two general categories: office injections and deep injections.

Office injections work for muscles, joints, tendons, and ligaments that reside close to the skin. You can receive such an injection in a matter of minutes, hop off the examining table, and head straight to work or physical therapy. Consult Chapter 12 if you'd like to learn more about these treatments.

Deep injections are more complicated procedures. They target complex structures such as nerves and spinal joints, or tissues that lie far below the skin's surface. Deep injections require a visit to a specialist and a slightly longer time commitment; in a few cases, they produce strong side effects. For these reasons, I suggest that deep injections be considered only after you've already tried more conservative measures. Yet I do not wish to frighten you: Deep injections have a long history of safety and effectiveness. (Consider the thousands of women who are receiving epidurals, a form of deep injection, for labor pain at this very moment.) The doctors in my clinic perform them daily. If you have severe pain with origins in a specific nerve, spinal joint, or deep tissue, deep injections can be lifesavers.

It's beyond the scope of this book to discuss every kind of injection possible, but there are some elements common to most of these procedures. The doctor should meet with you before the injection and take a complete medical history, even if you've been referred by another doctor. Assuming that you're cleared for the injection, you'll go to a procedure room. You'll wear a gown and be connected to machines that measure your blood pressure, pulse, and oxygen levels.

The doctor will sterilize the skin she's about to inject and then give you a shot of local anesthetic, which numbs the skin and tissues below. This shot may be the worst part of the procedure; it feels no worse than the pricking pain of a vaccination. You may also receive a muscle relaxant and pain reliever via an intravenous line.

Once the local anesthetic has taken effect, the doctor will perform the deep injection of medication. In most cases she'll use a combination of anesthetic and anti-inflammatory steroids to coat the joint, nerve, or other structure. Having a needle near your painful nerve or joint may sound like torture, but since the area has already been anesthetized, you should feel no more than a sensation of pressure as the needle goes through.

Usually the procedure will be performed with the assistance of fluoroscopy, an imaging technique that relies on a small amount of radiation, less than you'd get from a day at the beach. The doctor can look at a continuous video of your spine or nervous tissue or joint on a television monitor and use the image to guide the needle to its precise location. Although fluoroscopy helps, it is not strictly necessary, especially for epidurals (again, think of all the women who receive these shots during childbirth without the aid of fluoroscopy).

The injection, including the initial local anesthetic, usually takes somewhere between twenty and forty minutes, longer if you're having more than one area treated. When it's done, you'll probably need a few minutes to rest and recover and then maybe some extra time waiting around the doctor's office, just to be sure you're not having a bad reaction to the procedure. At that point, most patients can go home and take it easy for the rest of the day.

In some cases, you will know immediately whether the injection has worked. Since you'll be awake during the procedure, you can talk to the anesthesiologist about what you're feeling; if the injection fails, she may want to try again from another angle or in a slightly different location. Sometimes, though, you won't feel the results for several hours or days; your doctor should let you know what to expect. Some injections will need to be repeated a few days later.

Some people worry that an injection, especially one to a nerve, will kill sensation to part of their body. Although a widespread numbing effect is the goal for labor pain and for surgical procedures, the injections performed for chronic pain are far more precise. You should feel an absence of your usual pain rather than a total absence of sensation, and you'll be able to move and exercise normally. How long these effects last is a highly individual matter. Some people are pain-free for a few days, others for weeks or months.

The side effects with deep injections are usually minimal. However, anytime you introduce a needle or medication into the body, complications such as infection, bleeding, allergic reaction, and medical error are possible. Steroid injections especially can give you a terrible headache or make you a little nauseated, pepped up, or woozy; still, they do not pose even a fraction of the risk of side effects from steroids taken orally.

If you are considering a spinal injection of any kind, it is important to find a specialist (usually an anesthesiologist, physiatrist, or neurologist) with a strong background in your procedure. You are most likely to find such a doctor in a pain clinic or at a teaching hospital. Keep in mind, though, that in creating a specialty out of spinal injections, a doctor may not have had the time or inclination to explore other methods of pain relief. Such a doctor may not inform you about more conservative options; they may not even occur to her. And she may inculcate expectations that *all* your pain will vanish after a shot, and for good.

Take advantage of injections if they're right for you. But don't forget to try conservative measures—such as physical therapy, dietary changes, and stress reduction—both before you agree to an injection and after you receive one.

MOST COMMON DEEP INJECTIONS FOR CHRONIC PAIN

▶ *Epidural.* This shot is used for back pain, sciatica, and neck pain. It delivers medication to the epidural space, which is the area between the bones at the back of the spine and the dura, the cord's tough covering. This space runs all the way up and down your spine.

(continued)

The specific location of the injection along the length of your spine will be determined by your pain. Shots near your neck are a bit riskier, since the needle and medication come close to the central nervous system.

- *Facet joint injection.* Another treatment for back pain and especially sciatica; in this case, for pain that seems to originate in the facet joints (angular joints that run along the back of the bony spine). Those joints are treated with steroidal anti-inflammatory medication to cool them off and numb them if they're generating pain.
- *Facet nerve block.* Here, the nerves that feed into the facet joints are numbed. Again, this shot is for certain kinds of back pain and sciatica.
- *Selective nerve block.* Nerve blocks are suitable for any pain that seems to come from a specific nerve or nerves. You may receive this shot in the spine or anywhere else on your body, depending on the nerve's location. Selective nerve blocks are especially useful for nerve-related pain in the ribs or viscera and for diagnosing the offending nerve.
- *Sympathetic nerve block.* This block is the first-line treatment for complex regional pain syndrome. The sympathetic nerves, which participate in the involuntary processes of the body, can sometimes go on overdrive and create pain. During a sympathetic nerve block, those nerves are quieted down with anesthesia. The block is initially diagnostic and may allow you and your doctor to confirm the source of your pain. But the anesthetic can also soothe the nerves for a long period of time and even break the pain cycle.

NERVE ABLATIONS

Nerve ablations are a cousin to the deep injections. In this procedure, a pain-generating nerve is destroyed via freezing or heating. It is a more serious affair than an injection, since the nerve is killed rather than just numbed, but it is still relatively noninvasive when compared with surgery. It is usually performed by anesthesiologists in their offices, and patients can go home within hours after the procedure.

During a nerve ablation—some doctors refer to it as a "coagulation"—you'll undergo a routine very similar to that for a deep injection (see the previous entry for more information). You'll get a local anesthetic first, and then the doctor will introduce a very slender wand into the nerve site. That wand will conduct either cold (to freeze the nerve) or radio-frequency heat (to cook it). You may feel a moment of pain as the nerve is destroyed, but the sensation—which is usually no worse than your usual pain—passes quickly. You should feel relief in a matter of seconds and will be able to tell the doctor if the procedure has worked. If not, he may make another attempt. After the injection, you may need to rest in the office for a while. Then you can go home and rest for the remainder of the day.

Nerve ablations don't last forever, but they do relieve pain for a good long time, usually a year or so. The nerves may then grow back and cause you the same old problems; however, since the ablation leaves the nerve's sheath intact, the nerve will regrow into its normal path and will not result in the "angry" nerves that occur with other kinds of nerve destruction, such as limb amputation.

Since nerve ablation is a surgical procedure, albeit a minor one, it does involve certain risks, including infection and surgical error. The closer the ablation is to the spine, the more likely it is that an error will be serious. That's why I always recommend that people try more conservative treatments before undergoing ablation. If the procedure is indeed necessary, make sure to work with an anesthesiologist or other trained physician with a good track record.

IDET: MAKING HEADLINES FOR BACK PAIN

If you suffer from back pain, you'll want to know about a specific kind of ablation called intradiscal electrothermal annuloplasty, or IDET. This new procedure has made some headlines lately, and preliminary studies indicate that it works almost 70 percent of the time for patients with back pain that is a result of a tear within a disc. You can think of IDET as melting the disc from the inside out, so that the disc's covering is sealed, preventing leakage of pain-producing chemicals. You'll need to get a diagnostic procedure, called a discogram, to determine if IDET is right for you. Be sure to work with an anesthesiologist or other trained physician who's experienced in IDET.

PUMP IMPLANTS

In extreme cases of chronic pain, when suffering can be controlled only with high doses of strong medication, it makes sense to deliver that medication directly to the spinal cord. A pump is filled with medication and surgically implanted below the skin of the abdomen; the pump sends a smooth, controlled stream of the drug via a catheter into the spinal fluid, stopping the pain signals from traveling to the brain. Pumps are an invasive means of treatment, and they carry certain risks. But since the direct-delivery method allows you to use much less medication and to bypass many of its side effects, they may actually be kinder to your body than fistfuls of pills.

Before you can receive an implant, you'll go through a screening process. The neurosurgeon or anesthesiologist should make sure that you've exhausted almost all the other avenues, including various pill regimens, physical therapies, and so on. She will also want to make sure that you'll be compliant with the maintenance schedule a pump requires. Once you've passed that screening, the doctor will give you a deep injection of the medication, delivering it straight to the spinal fluid (see "Deep Injections" in this chapter for more information), or she may insert a catheter that sends the medicine directly to your spinal fluid as a trial for a few days. If you get good relief, you and your doctor may agree to surgical implantation of the pump.

As surgeries go, pump implantation is relatively low-key. You will need to go to the hospital for the surgery, but you'll be given a local rather than a general anesthetic; during the procedure, the doctor will ask you questions about whether the pump is working and how it feels. You'll probably stay overnight in the hospital, and the wound area will be sore.

The pump is small—about three inches in diameter and one inch high—and made of lightweight titanium. It contains a reservoir, which holds the medication, and a port, through which your doctor can refill medication via a needle passed through the skin. The catheter is a small hollow tube that's connected to the pump's reservoir at one end and inserted into the space around your spinal cord at the other. Your doctor controls the amount of medication you receive and at the rate at which you receive it; she can also change the dosage and rate by using an external programmer. Most pumps are filled with morphine, but sometimes muscle relaxers or other medications are used.

For people who have made a thorough, intelligent trial of medications and find that they are left unacceptably drowsy or experience other prohibitive side effects, the pump can be gratifying. It makes especially good sense for people with conditions such as multiple sclerosis, spinal cord injury, or pain from cancer or AIDS. Perhaps the best aspect of the pump is that you don't feel like you're on heavy pain medication. Since the drug doesn't pass through your digestive system, you won't feel the same kind of drowsiness, nausea, or constipation that is likely with pills.

Of course, pump implantation does involve a certain amount of life disruption. The surgery aside, there are regular trips to the doctor, a possible feeling of itchiness from the device, and the inevitable alarm bells when you pass through a metal detector (you can carry a medical note to explain your implant). You must also be willing to accept the risks involved. These include infection from the surgical procedure or the implant itself, allergic reaction to anesthesia or to the implant, surgical error, and kinking or breakage of the catheter.

If you and your doctor can prove to your insurance company that you have tried many other therapies and failed to find relief, you are likely to receive coverage for a pump. Check your policy for specific details, and definitely get preapproved, so that you're not stuck with a huge bill.

SPINAL CORD STIMULATORS

In Chapter 10, "Distracting Your Nervous System from Pain," I talked about transcutaneous electrical stimulation (TENS), a noninvasive and underused method of treating pain. A person receiving TENS is fitted with an external device that delivers mild electrical impulses to the painful region. The device works under the gate-control principle: Certain kinds of stimulation—in this case, electricity—travel faster to the spinal cord than pain, thus blocking the pain signal from moving up the cord and into the brain.

Spinal cord stimulators are a more aggressive form of TENS, suitable for those with severe, intractable pain that cannot be adequately relieved by the external stimulator. In these cases, the current generator is surgically buried under the skin along with attached electrodes that lead to the epidural space behind the spinal cord. Most people with this implant (assuming that they are appropriately screened) will see a reduction in pain by half or even more and are able to exercise and perform daily activities.

Before you can receive a spinal cord stimulator, you'll need to undergo a screening process that involves a bit of surgery itself. The anesthesiologist or neurosurgeon will give you a local anesthetic and then, using a needle, will thread an insulated wire under your skin and into the middle of your back. The wire will be attached to a screening device. Since you are awake during the procedure, the nurse or doctor will use the screener to adjust the level of stimulation and ask you how it feels. The doctor may also adjust the placement of the wire and question you about the degree of pain relief. You may then be sent home for a few days with the wire still attached. You'll be given the screener so that you can make adjustments on your own and decide whether you want the surgery. Of course, no matter what you decide, you'll need to return to have the wire removed.

The procedure for implantation itself is quite similar—except, of course, that your body is receiving a larger object: a device about two inches square and an inch thick. You will be under local anesthesia this time as well, so that the doctor can test the device and you can report on the degree of relief. Although you'll likely have this surgery performed on an outpatient basis and will be able to go home within a few hours, you're going to be sore and tired for a day or two.

Be aware you may not be able to use the stimulator twenty-four hours a day, since your nervous system may eventually grow inured to constant electrical stimulation, and the pain-blocking effects will be lost. (However, the pain relief may continue even when the stimulator is turned off.) You will be given a handheld programmer that allows you to turn the stimulation off and on and to adjust its frequency. The stimulation itself usually feels like a tingle, a sensation that most patients far prefer to that of pain. You will need to prepare yourself for this feeling, though the screening surgery will help—as well as for certain inconveniences.

The presence of the stimulator is disturbing to some. The electrodes are placed against the spinal cord, inside the bony spine; if you're slender, you might be able to feel the wires if you press against the skin of your back. The stimulator itself, which is about the size of a cigarette pack, sits at the side of the belly, and you might be able to see a bump at your waist. You may even feel itchy at first, but most people adjust to the sensation.

You must commit to regular doctor's appointments, as your physician needs to monitor the device and check you for possible side effects. Every four or five years or so, the stimulator will wear out and require removal and replacement. It is also possible to receive a stimulator with an external battery that you wear like a beeper. You will avoid needing surgical replacement, but you won't be able to get the battery wet. In addition, no matter whether your stimulator's battery is internal or external, you'll have to deal with the hassle created by theft detectors, security systems, and aircraft communications systems that may interfere with your device or that might be disturbed by it. You cannot receive certain diagnostic or therapeutic treatments, including MRI scans and external defibrillation—used in case of heart attack—with a stimulator in place, nor can you take certain medications.

Any implant, especially one that's close to the central nervous system, comes with a certain number of risks: infection, allergy to the anesthesia or to the materials in the device, mistakes in surgery, and devices that malfunction. Those risks must be weighed against the severity of the pain and the level of disability it causes.

Spinal cord stimulator implants are not given to people who have pacemakers or cardioverter/defibrillator implants. They are also not appropriate for patients, such as those with serious mental illness, who might be upset at having a foreign object in their body, or who cannot maintain the schedule of checkups.

Medicare and many insurance companies will cover the surgery and maintenance of a stimulator implant, provided that your doctor can prove a host of other measures has been tried. Your policy will give you the specific requirements. You may find that getting the all-clear from the insurance provider demands some persistence; it is extremely helpful if your doctor will act as an advocate for you with the insurance company.

SURGERY

Say you suffer from hideous, unrelenting pain. No one can tell you where it comes from or why it torments you; or perhaps the source is known but incurable. But one doctor has a idea: an operation that will cut off the pain messages. It's rarely performed, perhaps experimental. You must agree to surgery on your spinal cord, or even your brain. What do you do?

Sometimes surgery for a painful condition makes obvious sense, as in reconstructing a degenerated arthritic knee. But that kind of surgery doesn't really address the pain itself. It targets the underlying condition that causes the pain. The next section of this book discusses painful conditions, along with any operations that are appropriate for underlying causes.

But there's another breed of operation: surgery solely for pain control. The assumption is that the underlying condition can't be found or can't be healed; the goal of surgery is to stop the pain message. One of the first procedures of this type was amputation. Desperate people, with equally desperate doctors, simply had their painful arms or legs cut off. Often, the result was phantom limb pain, in which nerve pain comes back with vengeance.

This early experience was instructive. It taught us that pain isn't located in one particular area of the body; it's all over your nerves, your brain, and the part that hurts. So surgery to stop pain messages has a pretty poor track record. If you're going to receive a procedure on your nerves, it will more likely be a deep injection or nerve ablation.

Of the pain-control surgeries that are still being performed, the cordotomy is the most common. It's most often used for pain that occurs below the neck. In this operation, the bundles of nerves that carry pain and temperature sensations through the spinal cord to the brain are severed. The procedure is usually performed under local anesthesia, so that you can talk to the doctor about what you're feeling. Often there's no need to cut open the skin—instead, a needle is inserted just below the ear, and the nerves are killed with radiofrequency heat. But make no mistake: This is a major operation. You'll be kept immobilized for a day or two in the intensive care unit and then spend several more days in the general ward. After the nerves are severed, you won't be able to feel pain or temperature below the neck on the affected side of the body; you may even lose total sensation or function where the pain was. In addition to the usual risks of surgery (infection, bleeding, and so on), it's also possible that you may lose coordination, develop mental dysfunction or mood changes, or lose neurological control of your bowels, bladder, or sexual organs. And when you're talking about the spinal cord, a surgical slip could be devastating. You should also know that the success rate of cordotomies varies from surgeon to surgeon, and even when the pain disappears, it often makes a return several months later. These factors make cordotomies most appropriate for people whose pain comes from terminal illness.

Medical scientists are constantly working on new surgeries for pain control, so it's possible you may encounter other surgical options. If a doctor suggests such an operation to you, don't agree before (1) trying all other methods of pain relief and (2) getting all the facts. Ask the doctor to show you journal articles that discuss this procedure, and ask him how often he's performed this procedure, what his success rate is, how many patients feel relief after six months or a year, and how often he turns down patients for this surgery. Be wary of a neurosurgeon who claims a 100 percent or other astronomically high success rate, or one who never turns down patients who request the surgery.

When pain is intractable, surgery can sometimes be a compassionate option, especially at the end of life. But keep in mind that although surgery for pain control has a long history, that history has seen only rare successes.

PART IV

PAINFUL CONDITIONS

HOW TO USE THIS PART

Each of the following twelve chapters focuses on a chronic pain condition. The chapters all follow a similar pattern: (1) a description of the condition, including its symptoms and possible causes, (2) the tests your doctor should run to diagnose the disorder or to rule out other problems, and (3) therapies that either have been scientifically proven to help or have strong anecdotal evidence for your condition.

Therapies highlighted with a ►► should be your first choices. These usually include customized elements of good nutrition, exercise, and relaxation, which are inexpensive and easy on the body. You may also see certain pharmaceuticals or other treatments highlighted as well.

Therapies indicated with a ► also have a good record for the condition, but they may be riskier or appropriate only for a particular set of needs. Or perhaps they are simply excellent runner-up therapies.

Each therapy that is <u>underlined</u> is discussed in detail in Part III, "Therapies." You may also be referred to the Appendices for information about stretching, exercise, and acupressure points. Consult with your doctor as you make choices. And don't forget to listen to your innate wisdom: The therapies that appeal to you are the ones most likely to help. For further assistance in choosing therapies, see Chapter 6.

14.

HEADACHE

TENSION / CERVICOGENIC / MIGRAINE / CLUSTER

Recurring headaches afflict 40 percent of the U.S. population, according to the *Journal of the American Medical Association.* If you're a woman, there's a greater than 17 percent chance you suffer from migraines; if you're a man, that chance drops to a small but still significant 5 percent. For those who like to measure pain by its cost to the workforce, headache vies with back pain as the leading cause of missed days at the office.

Yet about half of headache sufferers don't ask for help. It's common for people to think that their headaches are not important enough for treatment or to assume that nothing can be done. Neither is true. There exists an extraordinary variety of options for headache relief, including effective medications for migraines. Even if your headaches aren't bad enough to keep you from work or socializing, you may find that some simple changes to your health routine will reduce the frequency and intensity of your episodes.

Headache treatment is one area in which the integration of conventional and alternative medicine is already well under way. Almost every physician who specializes in headache is familiar with strategies such as biofeedback, dietary changes, supplement routines, and physical therapies. One reason for this open-mindedness is the unfortunate effect of many headache medications: They may provide initial relief but then rebound the sufferer into daily bouts of head pain. Patients must reduce their reliance on pharmaceutical treatments if their headaches are to get better and then stay at bay. When it comes to headaches, there really isn't an alternative to using alternative medicine.

Headaches fall into four broad categories: tension, cervicogenic, migraine, and cluster.

Tension headaches are the most common type. As their name suggests, they are caused by muscular tension in the head. They tend to feel like a vise clamping down on your skull, are mild to moderate in intensity, and affect both sides of the head equally. Often they are brought on by recognizable triggers: stress, caffeine, alcohol, skipped meals, lack of sleep, atmospheric changes, or exposure to heat, noise, or fumes. Particularly frequent is the "weekend headache," brought on by drinking caffeine at the office and then suddenly withdrawing from it on Saturday and Sunday.

Cervicogenic headaches are a cousin of the tension headache. Although they are caused by muscular tightness as well, their origin is not in the head but in the neck and shoulders. The pain is usually felt either in the back of the head or radiating up from the back of the neck. There may or may not be pain located in the neck itself; often there is simply a sensation of stiffness or tightness. Moving the neck may make cervicogenic headaches worse, and some people will also feel pain upon awakening in the morning. These headaches are often caused by stress or poor posture.

Migraine headaches are moderate to severe; frequently they are disabling. They are usually characterized by a pulsing sensation on one side of the head and are often accompanied by nausea, vomiting, and extreme sensitivity to light, sound, and odors. Some people temporarily lose their vision, which makes migraines especially frightening if they occur while driving or on the street. Migraines last much longer than most tension headaches, usually between twelve and seventy-two hours, although occasionally they go on for days or even weeks. About 10 percent of migraine sufferers experience a visual aura, in which areas of the visual field appear to be sparkling or shining, or develop other odd sensations before the migraine hits.

Despite decades of research, the cause or causes of migraines is still a mystery. You may have been told that migraines are caused by constriction of blood vessels in the head. This is a dramatic oversimplification. Constriction certainly occurs with migraines, but whether it *causes* them remains to be seen. In addition, many scientists believe that a sudden dilation (opening) of blood vessels follows the constriction—but again, no one is sure if this action actually causes the migraine or is merely associated with it. And it's clear that much, much more is going on inside the head of a migraine sufferer. Brain scans show definite changes in the occipital lobe, where vision is processed; these changes are probably linked to the visual aura that many sufferers experience. There are shifts in the levels of certain neurotransmitters, including serotonin (which affects sleep and mood and may have a role in constricting blood vessels) and dopamine (which has many functions; possibly it helps regulate pain). In some people, the trigeminal nerve, which supplies sensation to the face, may be malfunctioning. In addition, there are several factors that can trigger a migraine: Stress, certain foods, caffeine, the menstrual cycle, alcohol, and bright lights are the most common.

In women, estrogen appears to be linked to migraines, although its role remains unclear. Many women experience migraines at about the same time as their menstrual period, when estrogen levels drop rapidly. Other women are first affected by migraines during menopause or the years before its onset, when estrogen levels are falling. Since estrogen is a vasodilator (it widens blood vessels), the prevailing theory is that lower-than-usual levels of estrogen may trigger the constriction of blood vessels and set off a migraine. That women normally afflicted by migraines often do not experience them during pregnancy—when estrogen levels are high—seems to bolster this theory.

Cluster headaches appear far more often in men than in women. They occur in groups (hence the name), usually during the same period every year or at times of heavy emotional or physical stress. They are usually felt on one side of the head, behind one eye; there may be tearing of the eye's mucous membranes and dramatic, even frightening, facial swelling. Cluster headaches don't last nearly as long as migraines—usually between ten minutes and two hours—but what they lack in length they make up for in intensity. One of the most painful and unbalancing disorders I've ever witnessed, cluster headaches sometimes drive their victims to suicide. The cause of cluster headaches is unknown, but if you suffer from them, it's critical to learn how to manage both the pain and your response to it.

TESTING, TESTING

D*o I need a brain scan?* Most people with severe or lengthy headaches worry that their pain is due to a tumor or an aneurysm. Such disorders are extremely rare; even when I was working in a headache clinic, I saw only a handful. If your headaches fit one of the symptom sets above or have followed a stable pattern of their own for some time, it's usually not necessary to be tested for a growth or vascular disturbance. Your doctor can make this judgment. Should you experience an unusual group of symptoms, or if the headaches have just started or deviated from a previous pattern, then it's reasonable to run an MRI or CAT scan to rule out an underlying cause. The vast majority of scans in such cases will come back negative; when this happens, you can relax and focus on treating the chronic headache.

Have you been in an accident or experienced a blow to the upper body? Cervicogenic headache is sometimes a symptom of whiplash. Even migraines and other head pain may stem from injury to the head, neck, or shoulders. If you've been in an accident recently, you should be checked for whiplash and treated accordingly (see Chapter 18). Those with old injuries or who have accidents in their history should report them to their doctor.

RED FLAGS: WHEN A HEADACHE ISN'T JUST A HEADACHE

Chronic headache that's settled into a familiar pattern is rarely cause for grave concern. But everyone—not just headache sufferers—should know that a serious *acute* headache can be a sign of stroke or other disease. If you experience severe head pain that breaks cleanly from the usual routine, you should talk to your doctor. *Get immediate medical attention* if a new headache is intense and is accompanied by neurological symptoms: dizziness; loss of coordination, balance, or motor skills; personality changes; or loss of sensation.

CHRISTINE'S STORY: THE YEARLONG HEADACHE

One of the first things that strikes you about Christine is her air of practical intelligence, a no-nonsense approach to life that's tempered by her smile and warm demeanor. This combination of attributes stands her well as an oncology nurse in one of New York's major hospitals. They also helped her get through an extraordinary health crisis of her own—a headache that lasted for an entire year.

(continued)

The pain began shortly after Christine was hospitalized for an asthma attack. She felt it in the front of her head, just at the back of her right eye—"I felt that if I could just get my hand behind my eye, I could rub the pain out," she says—and the headache was so strong that she was sick to her stomach. As a cancer nurse, Christine immediately thought of the worst-case scenario: a brain tumor or an aneurysm waiting to burst. Repeated brain scans failed to show an anatomical problem, but the apparently inexplicable pain, one that defied all known categories of headache, continued for weeks, then months. Sometimes it would fade a little, only to creep up the side of her head again like a tentacle. She wondered if the scans had missed something: "I was afraid to go out or walk down the street for fear it was a tumor, that I'd pass out and no one would know me."

Not surprisingly, both the pain and fear took their toll. She kept working—she didn't miss a single day at the hospital—but after her shift she went straight home to lie down. Her personal life all but ceased, and Christine became irritable, depressed, and despondent.

What saved Christine was her refusal to be helpless. Her first doctor offered her opioids for the pain, but Christine turned them down, afraid they would interfere with her job. When she came to me, she was taking absolutely no pills for her headache—but she would not accept that the pain was something she'd have to live with. She was willing to try a wide array of techniques for her pain, in the hopes that something would stick. Although acupuncture didn't work (a serious disappointment for Christine and for me as her doctor), regular exercise did. She agreed to try a low dose of Elavil, a tricyclic antidepressant that inhibits pain signals but does not cause drowsiness, and found that this drug helped considerably. She also found a surprising amount of relief from a combination of acupressure and Reiki, which brought a pleasantly warm feeling to her head and, as she describes it, "put a cap" on the pain.

It took a full year for Christine's headache to break completely. Now she may get some pain once or twice a month, but it doesn't disturb her quite so much, since she knows which therapies will help. Her advice for fellow headache sufferers is characteristically hopeful and practical. "There's a tendency to say 'I'm in pain and there's nothing I can do about it.' But I don't believe that's acceptable. There's always something you can do. . . . There were times I came into the doctor's office crying. But I'm not crying now."

THERAPIES

Again and again, successful headache sufferers have proven the adage that simpler is often better. Basic changes in exercise and nutrition, along with the regular use of a mind-body technique, can decrease the number of headaches and soften those that do arrive. Once you have a healthful routine in place, you may well feel that your headaches are under control, especially if they have never been very intense. Keeping a pain diary (see Chapter 4 for details) can help you and your doctor pinpoint possible headache triggers, such as the menstrual cycle, caffeine consumption, or stress.

Some people will need further relief and can choose from a variety of practitioner-centered therapies. I also recommend that anyone who suffers from frequent migraines, cluster headaches, or any other debilitating and chronic head pain see a doctor regarding medication.

PHYSICAL THERAPIES

▸▸ Cardio, cardio, cardio! Thirty minutes of aerobic exercise three or four times a week will address multiple causes of headache: stress, upper body tension, and (possibly) serotonin deficiency. Yoga can also work as a cardiovascular exercise, but only if you take a truly challenging class.

▸▸ In addition to cardio, try the exercises and stretches listed in Appendix A, focusing on those that involve the neck. Perform them daily as directed. This goes for headaches of all kinds.

▸▸ Check your home and office for potential headache-causing setups. Your computer screen should be at eye level, so that you don't need to raise or lower your head. Get a headset if you find yourself cradling the phone receiver between your head and neck. Check your purse, backpack, or briefcase—if it's heavy enough to pull against your shoulder, it could be a source of your pain.

▸▸ Anyone with headache pain can develop muscular knots in their neck, shoulders, and upper back—which will create more headaches and lead to more pain. Massage, especially the deeper techniques such as myofascial release and trigger-point work, can help break these up. If pressing a knot sends pain radiating out to another part of your body (say, pressing on a knot in the shoulder creates pain in your head), consult Chapter 24, "Myofascial Pain Syndrome."

▶ For cervicogenic headaches, there are a few therapies that may go straight to the heart—or the neck—of the problem. The Alexander Technique, the Feldenkrais Method, or Hellerwork can teach you how to perform everyday motions with less stress on your neck and head.

▶ Traction gently creates more space between the joints in the neck and can halt a series of powerful cervicogenic headaches.

▶ Spinal manipulation therapy, a chiropractic technique, can help in a limited number of headache cases. If your neck is stiff, not just tense, or if you have a history of upper back injury, a chiropractor or osteopath may be able to improve your range of motion.

▶ I've also seen several headache patients (not just those with stiff necks) helped by craniosacral therapy, which claims to manipulate the imperceptible motion of sutures that hold the skull together. This technique is practiced by osteopaths, chiropractors, and others.

▶ Patients often ask me about pillows that are promoted as headache aids. It's true that your neck should be in line with the spine as you sleep, not angled forward or propped way up with a fluffy pillow or two. But you don't need specially designed pillows to accomplish this alignment. A relatively flat pillow bought off the department store shelves and positioned by you so that your neck and head are in proper position will do the trick.

NUTRITION AND SUPPLEMENTS

▶▶ Follow the pain-control diet outlined in Chapter 9; be especially sure to eat plenty of green, leafy vegetables, which are high in magnesium (which eases muscle cramping and is necessary for nerve health).

▶▶ Supplement your diet with magnesium and calcium, both of which relax tense muscles and support nerve stability. For recommended doses of these and other supplements, see Chapter 9.

▶▶ Many headaches are triggered by certain foods. Read "Can Food Allergies Cause Pain?" on pages 135–136 and keep an eye on your diet. In addition to the usual pain triggers (wheat, dairy, corn, soy, eggs, and citrus), foods containing tyramine, a substance known to affect blood vessel constriction, can bring on headaches, especially migraines. These foods include aged cheese and red wine, pickled and marinated foods, and anything aged or fermented. Still other foods trigger migraines in some people for unknown reasons: yogurt, bananas, dried fruit, buttermilk, MSG, aspartame, whiskey, and beer. If you can rule out these foods as triggers, however, there's no need to avoid them.

▶▶ Cut out the caffeine. People with headaches often use caffeine, consciously or not, to medicate themselves. Caffeine constricts blood vessels; it also causes changes in the central nervous system, increasing adrenaline-type neurotransmitters that can trigger stress and muscle tension. You may feel temporarily better after drinking coffee, tea, or cola, but caffeine can cause rebound headaches that appear every day. Caffeine can also lead to sleep problems, which in turn can cause headaches or make them worse.

▶ Avoid alcohol during a series of cluster headaches. It often brings on an acute attack.

▶ Moderate daily doses of vitamin B_2 may help ward off migraines. This vitamin is important for nerve cell function and may quiet down irritated nerve pathways (although no one knows for sure why B_2 appears to help migraine sufferers).

▶ Migraine sufferers can also try feverfew, an herb that may reduce the number and intensity of migraines when taken on a regular basis. You may wish to try a product called Migraleve, which contains both feverfew and vitamin B_2. If you use Migraleve, don't take additional supplements of B_2.

▶ If you suffer from insomnia, consider taking valerian at night. If anxiety is a component of your sleeplessness, try kava instead (but don't take kava for long periods).

▶ A *slow* intravenous push of magnesium, delivered at the hospital or in some doctors' offices, can break lengthy, severe migraines in about 50 percent of cases (magnesium that's delivered too quickly can have serious cardiac effects). Ask your headache doctor whether she can provide this option.

MIND-BODY MEDICINE

▶▶ Make it a priority to cultivate a daily relaxation practice, even if you have only ten minutes to spare. Of all the mind-body therapies, hypnosis probably has the most science and testing behind it for headache relief, so your doctor may be willing to write a referral for you—and might even be enthusiastic about it. (If she needs some encouragement, direct her to the Web site www.odp.od.nih.gov/consensus/ta/017/017_statement, where the National Institutes of Health say that the evidence of hypnosis for headache relief is strong.) Biofeedback is another good choice for you.

▶▶ Many headache sufferers have found that daily meditation helps ward off episodes; when a bad headache is active, breathing techniques can help you feel more in control. They may also keep you from tensing your head, neck, and shoulder muscles in response to the pain.

▶▶ If you prefer a more active form of relaxation, try yoga. Not only does it relieve stress, but many poses relax the muscles in your upper body. For cervicogenic headaches, it may be the best mind-body option.

HEALING ENERGY

▶ Consider Reiki. Although the evidence is only anecdotal, this therapy has loosened a headache's grip for several of my patients.

▶ Reflexology is another energy option that can soothe away a headache.

DISTRACTING YOUR NERVOUS SYSTEM FROM PAIN

▶▶ I love acupressure for headache pain. If you want to try some home care, use points B 10, GB 20 and 21, and TH 15. See the acupressure map in Appendix C for the location of these points and instruction in using them. You can also try the Catwalk for Head, Neck, and Shoulder Pain on pages 151–152.

▶ Orthopedic supply houses, back stores, and sporting-goods stores sell sets of small balls that can be inserted into an accompanying platform. You can adjust the balls on the platform to your liking and place the device under the edge of your skull, where it meets your neck. The balls will press against the muscles of your neck and head, resulting in something like a home shiatsu treatment.

▶ Try acupuncture to break a migraine; for a truly bad case, you may need more than one treatment. Acupuncture also works as a maintenance therapy for some headache sufferers.

▶ It may be harder to distract your mind from headache pain than from any other kind, perhaps because mental concentration reminds us of where we hurt. But if you can tolerate sound, listening to music—or playing it—can be deeply soothing.

PAIN PILLS AND OTHER PHARMACEUTICALS

People who frequently dose themselves with medications to stop headaches may get a rebound effect, or even something called a transformed migraine, which—trust me—is no fun at all. This doesn't mean that you can't use pharmaceuticals, only that you should not rely on them exclusively or use them every day. (There is an exception for drugs used to prevent headaches rather than stop them. These drugs must be taken daily and usually do not cause rebound headaches or transformed migraines.)

I've broken the pharmaceutical options down according to category of headache, since the treatments for each can be very different.

IF YOU GET A HEADACHE EVERY DAY . . .

It's a sad cycle: You experience severe, recurring headaches, so you take medication on a daily basis, hoping to stave off any possible pain—and unknowingly push your neurophysiology to a straining point, so that it responds by creating *more* headaches. Soon the headaches appear every day. The more pills you take, the worse the pain gets. Although the exact mechanisms aren't fully understood, daily medication may change the density of nerve receptors at the

(continued)

synapse (the gap between nerve cells where communication takes place) and manipulate neurotransmitters (no one knows which ones) in a way that results in a daily headache.

Unknown to many primary-care physicians, this phenomenon is called a rebound headache or chronic daily headache. When it happens to migraine sufferers, it's called a transformed migraine, because the headache doesn't feel like the usual pain. Typically, rebound headache or transformed migraine feels more like a classic tension headache, with pain on both sides of the head. These headaches are usually less intense than migraines, although they can sometimes be disabling. They often last all day long.

Medications that cause rebound are usually abortive treatments, meant to stop headaches or reduce pain once they've set in. This includes caffeine, a drug people often use as a means of self-medication, whether consciously or not. Prophylactic treatments, which prevent headaches from occurring, do not cause rebound or transformed migraine.

If you suspect that you suffer from a rebound headache or transformed migraine, a headache specialist is best equipped to diagnose the problem and to wean you off the daily doses of pills. When I encounter patients suffering from rebound, they are usually taking four or five medications daily. If they are game, I may ask them to devote a three-day weekend to withdrawing from these drugs. Starting on the first day, they stop *all* their usual headache medication. This really hurts; most people will need to stay in bed the entire weekend and to take a high-dose opioid (a drug that does not contribute to rebound) that I've prescribed. Some will even need to be hospitalized for their pain. By the end of the weekend, the worst is over, although there is usually some lingering pain over the course of the next week, as well as wooziness if the person is still taking the opioid. At that time, the patient and I will work out a simpler regimen of headache drugs that aren't likely to cause rebound. I also encourage patients to cultivate nondrug options for managing the headache. Do *not* attempt to withdraw from headache drugs before consulting with your doctor.

Tension and Cervicogenic Headaches

▶ Be aware of drugs that can trigger headaches. Appetite suppressants, oral contraceptives and other estrogen products, and antihypertensive medications are all possible culprits. *Do not go off blood pressure medication without talking to your doctor first.*

▶ NSAIDs remain the mainstay for tension and cervicogenic headaches. You can also try acetaminophen or an aspirin/caffeine combination, as in Excedrin. (Again, though, be very wary of relying heavily on anything with caffeine in it.)

▶ If you have trigger points (hard but tender knots of muscle that cause pain elsewhere in the body when pressed) in your neck or shoulder, you can have an office injection to calm the pain and perhaps release the spasm. Make sure to follow injections up with stretches of your neck and shoulder. For more information about trigger points, see Chapter 24, "Myofascial Pain Syndrome."

▶ Headaches that don't respond to conservative care may be treated with low doses of tricyclic antidepressants, most often Elavil (amitriptyline), Pamelor (nortriptyline), or Sinequan (doxepin).

▶ Severe, debilitating tension headaches are rather rare, but if you do get them, your doctor might prescribe a short-acting opioid for very occasional use.

▶ Do *not* use tranquilizers to treat headaches. People who do so often become dependent on them, not to mention that tranquilizers only mask tension—they don't resolve the cause.

▶ You may know Botox as a poison that's often used for cosmetic purposes, to smooth out furrowed brows by paralyzing the muscles. But plastic surgeons performing this injection soon noticed that their patients reported fewer headaches as well. Now you can get injections of Botox in small quantities in your temples and forehead. (Those with cervicogenic headaches may need injections in the neck area as well.) The idea is to release chronic tension that doesn't respond to more conservative methods. Side effects include mild aching or malaise, and there's always the risk that the needle will miss its mark and paralyze (temporarily) the wrong muscle. See a neurologist or headache expert who is experienced with these injections. You should know after the first set of injections whether this treatment is working.

Migraines

Medications offer specific, effective help for migraines; most sufferers can't imagine doing without them. If you get more than four or five migraines every month, however, it's wise to break the cycle of gulping down medication each time a headache comes on. Otherwise, you're in danger of getting the rebound effect. Instead, you should try a preventive program of medication.

Abortive (to stop the pain once a migraine has begun)

▶ NSAIDs can help, especially if taken at the first sign of a migraine.

▶ Alka-Seltzer is effective for some people, also when taken as soon as a migraine comes on.

▶ The combination of acetaminophen or aspirin with caffeine (available over the counter as Excedrin) may work when the first two options on this list do not. Remember that caffeine is one of the worst culprits for rebound headaches. Don't become dependent on it.

▶ Triptans, which came on the scene in the mid-1980s, revolutionized the treatment of migraines. Why they work remains controversial, but many scientists believe that these medications mimic serotonin, which may stop blood vessels from constricting; many migraine sufferers think of them as a godsend. Brand names include Imitrex (sumatriptan), Amerge (naratriptan), Zomig (zolmitriptan), and Maxalt (rizatriptan). You'll know right away if triptans are working for you; if your first prescription doesn't work, you and your doctor may wish to try a different brand before giving up. These drugs are inappropriate for people with cardiovascular disease, and side effects can range from itchiness and aching to (rarely) hallucinations and cardiac arrest.

▶ Ergotamines, which are made from a fungus that grows on rye, can be used as a last resort for disabling migraines. Your doctor can prescribe pills (brand names for ergotamine include Ergomar, Wigraine, and Ercaf) or use something called a DHE drip, administered intravenously in the hospital. Typically this drug won't be used unless the migraine has lasted for twenty-four to forty-eight hours and shows no sign of retreat. You'll know immediately if the drug works. Ergotamines are toxic at high doses (doses that are used to break a migraine are not at toxic levels) and when used for long periods of time can result in dependence. More common side effects include nausea, vomiting, dizziness, numbness in the fingers or toes, chest or abdominal pain, and possibly dangerous blood vessel contractions. Like triptans, ergotamines should not be taken by people with cardiovascular conditions.

▶ Another option for last-resort treatment is an IV of a steroidal anti-inflammatory drug. It's not completely clear how steroids affect migraines, but they do stabilize cell membranes and, of course, reduce inflammation. They are also powerful antistress agents; in fact, they were used in World War II on fatigued soldiers who needed to fight one more battle. You will know at once if the steroid is working.

▶ If your doctor suspects that the trigeminal nerve is a source of your pain (a good sign is that the pain appears along the nerve's path in the face), he may wish to apply lidocaine, a form of anesthetic, to the nerve bundle, located at the back of the nose. He can use a special cotton swab to apply the medication.

Prophylactic

Prophylactic drugs prevent migraines from occurring. They are taken on a daily basis; depending on how often you experience migraines, you may need to take them for a few weeks or even months before you can determine if they're working.

▶ NSAIDs are used as prophylactic as well as abortive treatments. The classic NSAID for this purpose is naproxen, found in the over-the-counter medication Aleve.

▶ Tricyclic antidepressants and anticonvulsants are more recent prophylactic treatments for migraines. They appear to work by quieting down the nervous system, perhaps reducing some of the unusual brain activity associated with migraines.

▶ You can try injections of Botox, which appears to reduce many kinds of headaches by temporarily paralyzing certain muscles. (See medications for tension and cervicogenic headaches.)

▶ Two classes of heart drugs, beta blockers and calcium channel blockers, have long been used to prevent migraines. Common brand names include Inderal LA (propranolol), Corgard SR (nadolol), and Calan SR (verapamil), along with the generic verapamil. They appear to work by preventing sensitization of the trigeminal nerve, which is the primary nerve of the face and jaw. However, they may cause dangerous drops in blood pressure, so it's best to try other prophylactic treatments first.

Cluster Headaches

▶ Medications for cluster headaches are generally the same as those used to abort migraines. A cycle of cluster headaches rarely lasts long enough to try prophylactic drugs.

DEEP INJECTIONS, IMPLANTS, AND SURGERY

▶ Most cervicogenic headaches can be eased, if not completely relieved, by a combination of posture changes, exercise, and mind-body therapies, perhaps along with massage and acupressure. When those therapies aren't enough, a deep injection of the occipital nerve at the base of the skull can help matters considerably. Be sure to find an anesthesiologist who is experienced with injections in this location.

15.

BACK PAIN

GENERAL BACK PAIN / DISC PROBLEMS / SCIATICA / PAIN FROM SERIOUS INJURY OR ILLNESS

GENERAL BACK PAIN

Americans now have an 80 percent chance of experiencing back pain at some point in their adult lives. Back pain is one of the most common reasons for emergency room visits, and it competes with headache as the number-one reason for missed work days. And when the back hurts, we really *suffer.* With back pain, it's hard—or even impossible—to stand up, sit down, sleep, drive to work, shovel the sidewalk, stroll through the park.

On a higher level, the pain can feel like a wound to one's essential capacity. The back is a site of great spiritual significance: It represents our humanity and separates us from animals by allowing us to get up on two legs and walk. It is a source of our strength, our ability to stand tall and face the world. When this symbol of confidence and pride starts to hurt or malfunction, many people experience more than just physical pain. They feel they've lost their robustness and vigor. "Guess I'm getting old," they sigh. "Old and weak."

When I hear patients talk like this, I know that my most important job is to offer them hope. Not a falsely chipper pep talk, but the straight truth that most people who walk into an integrative clinic with tough back pain will eventually walk out feeling much better. It may take some time, I warn them. Back pain is notoriously complicated, and it's nearly impossible for me or any other doctor to put a finger on the sole cause of the problem. Even if a friend has relieved his own back pain through chiropractic, say, or abdominal strengthening exercises, there's no guarantee that these same techniques will have a similar effect on them (although both therapies can be great places to start). So, perhaps even more than with other disorders in this book, control of back pain takes persistence. It takes determination and energy to make the necessary lifestyle changes and to experiment with newer therapies such as IDET (a minimally invasive microsurgery for pain that originates in discs), facet joint blocks (to soothe nerves irritated by the bony joints of the spine), or anticonvulsant and tricyclic antidepressant medications (to control pain that's amplified by central nervous system changes).

A note on what constitutes chronic back pain: Technically, back pain isn't chronic until it's hung around for six months or more. Some people definitely experience this kind of long-term, daily pain, and there's no doubt in anyone's mind that they are chronic-pain sufferers. But not everyone in my office has back pain on a regular basis. Instead, their backs "go out" at unpredictable intervals, when they feel an abrupt onset of gripping, knifelike back pain, often when bending over or reaching. Sometimes there is a sensation of the back locking up, so that it's impossible to straighten up or move. This debilitating pain usually passes on its own within a few days, often helped along by medication and/or chiropractic manipulation. But once a person suffers from an acute episode of back pain, the problem is likely to return. It's common to feel fragile or tense between episodes, wondering when the pain will strike next. I put sufferers of this kind of back pain into the category of chronic-pain patients as well.

THE SPINE

There is no single cause of back pain; even within one individual, back pain may be triggered by a variety of factors. This is easier to understand when you know a little about the anatomy of the spine.

The spine is the body's support system, made up of several elements—all of which can be pain generators. Twenty-four vertebrae link together to form the length of the spine. At the rear of these doughnut-shaped bones are several bony protrusions, each of which have interlacing ligaments that anchor the backbone and hold the back's shape. Some of these bony protrusions form the posterior facet joints, which interlock with the facet joints of the vertebra above and below. (Lace your fingers together and you'll get a rough sense of how the facet joints link up, with your palms serving as the vertebrae.) This connecting structure of individual bones and joints is what carries the upper body and allows you to arch, bend, reach, stretch, and twist. Muscles and ligaments that surround the spine offer both support and stability to the vertebrae so that they stay aligned as you move.

The "doughnuts" of the vertebrae are separated by discs, made of a jellylike, springy core that's protected by a tough, fibrous covering. Often called the shock absorbers of the spine, these flexible discs help protect the vertebrae by providing a cushion between bones and compressing whenever you apply pressure by jumping, lifting, twisting, or bending.

Perhaps the spine's most important function is to house the spinal cord, which runs through a canal surrounded by the vertebrae. The spinal cord is the set of nerves that connect the brain with the rest of the body. Branching off the spinal cord are nerve roots, which pass through gaps between the vertebrae on their way to and from other parts of the body.

Any of these anatomical structures can malfunction or experience injury, causing back pain. Below is a look at the most frequent triggers of these malfunctions.

CAUSES OF BACK PAIN: MYTHS AND REALITIES

The intensity and persistence of back pain leads most sufferers to wonder if they have a serious, perhaps life-threatening, disorder. You can probably relax about this: Less than 5 percent of all back pain is caused by serious medical conditions. A good physician should be able to rule out these causes fairly quickly, often in the course of a single exam. Once that's done, you can focus on treating the pain itself. (Signs that you might need special tests such as an MRI or CAT scan to check for serious illness are listed in the "Testing, Testing" section. Back pain that is caused by injuries such as car accidents and illnesses such as advanced osteoporosis is discussed at the end of this chapter.)

A few years ago, it was generally believed that most back pain was caused by the degeneration of one or more of the discs that cushion the vertebrae. Today we know that almost all adults over forty have some disc deterioration; moreover, many of those with degenerated discs don't feel any pain at all. There simply isn't the strong causal link between disc damage and back pain that once was thought to exist.

Another myth is that disabling episodes of back pain—the back "going out"—are caused by a vertebra popping out of place or a disc slipping when you twist. That's absolutely not true. Discs are fully anchored to the spine. They don't slide around like hockey pucks over ice, and making a sudden movement or reaching the wrong way won't make them pop out to the side. Nor does treatment require snapping those discs back into place.

So what causes chronic or recurring back pain, if not a serious illness or the mythical "slipped disc"? Most of the time, a cause simply can't be found. There might have been an initial injury, but that injury is usually insufficient to explain the long-term pain or a person's continued vulnerability to acute back pain episodes. That's frustrating to hear when you're in so much pain you can't make the bed—or even get out of it. But it also helps to know that a doctor who tells you "I just can't find anything" may well be more honest and forthright than one who claims to know exactly where your pain is coming from. I've seen too many back patients who've gone from doctor to doctor to chiropractor to massage therapist, hoping that one professional will hit upon a definitive source of their problem with an equally definitive cure. By the time they come to me, they're understandably angry and disappointed. If I can help these patients accept that the one-symptom/one-cause/one-cure model doesn't work for back pain, that they will have to commit to experimenting with gentle lifestyle changes as well as more aggressive medications or injections, I know they are more likely to heal.

Back-pain patients and their doctors aren't left entirely in the dark, however. There are many known contributors to back pain; you can use this knowledge to embark on a solution to your chronic back pain.

Nerve irritation. Back pain is often caused when structures of the back irritate the nerve roots that pass from the spinal canal through the vertebrae. Although degenerated discs don't have the simple cause-and-effect relationship to back pain once thought to exist, they can definitely contribute to nerve impingement and irritation. When discs degenerate, their protective outer layers of collagen may tear, allowing the highly inflammatory fluid of the jellylike core to leak out and irritate nearby nerves. (This leakage of fluid may be one cause of a back that "goes out.") Facet joints that have deteriorated or are misaligned can impinge on nerves as well. Note that many of the other possible causes of back pain in this list can encourage nerve pressure and irritation.

Poor diet. A diet high in inflammation-promoting foods such as cheeseburgers and pastries can make back pain worse. These foods probably don't affect the structures of the back directly (unless you have arthritis, which is made worse by inflammation), but they do tend to make pain worse by depressing your overall health and the biochemical stability of nerves, joints, and connective tissue. And when people cut back on these foods, they also tend to lose weight, further reducing the pain.

Poor posture. When your posture is good, your body's load is more efficiently distributed across the structures of the back; the muscles can relax because they're well aligned. But when you slouch over your computer keyboard or hunch over housework, you're pulling on the spinal joints, muscles, ligaments, and tendons, and putting more pressure on the discs.

Sensitized nervous system. This is discussed in detail in Chapter 3. One of the secrets of pain medicine is that pain itself can sensitize your nervous system, in essence reprogramming your nerves, neurochemicals, and brain so that they send out messages of pain that are stronger and more alarming than is warranted by any bodily injury present. A lengthy encounter with severe back pain from leaking disc fluid or torn muscles might wear out your body's ability to produce endorphins (natural painkillers), for example, or leave your nerve receptors exquisitely sensitive to normally painless sensations such as the touch of clothing against your skin. Medications and mind-body techniques can soothe a jangled nervous system and help you cope.

Stress. As the foundation of the body, the spine is also a symbol of the foundation of personality, especially of mental and spiritual toughness. It's no wonder that many of us rely on the back to absorb our stress, leaving us with tensed, tight, painful muscles. Stress can also inhibit pain-blocking endorphins, and as I discussed in Chapter 3, it may have the power to reconfigure your nervous system so that it becomes highly sensitive to pain. In his book *Healing Back Pain: The Mind-Body Connection,* John E. Sarno, M.D., theorizes that *all* back pain of unknown origin is an unconscious manifestation of emotional stress. Although I wouldn't make such a strong statement—as you can see from this list, I believe there are multiple factors involved—Dr. Sarno's book has been helpful to many of my patients.

Weakened muscles. Without the soft tissues, including muscles and ligaments that help align the spine, the vertebrae would be nothing more than a collection of loose bones. When abdominal or back muscles weaken, those bones may shift into a painful configuration. In particular, the pelvis may tilt abnormally and the discs may be forced to carry more of the body's weight, increasing the risk of compression. And weak, stiff muscles are more vulnerable to injuries such as sprains and tears, which can cause acute back pain. Strengthening these muscles is an important part of healing back problems.

Weight gain. People who consider their back pain an inevitable, irreversible sign of aging sometimes forget that they've put on a few pounds since the age of twenty. Extra weight around the middle pulls on the delicate structures of the back, requiring them to shoulder more than their already heavy load. The muscles, tendons, and ligaments especially tend to groan, strain, and tighten under the additional burden; worse, the excess pressure can pull the back's structures out of alignment, causing them to impinge on nearby nerves. If you're overweight, exercise and a good diet should form the first steps of your chronic pain solution.

SO WHEN ARE YOU GOING SKIING AGAIN?

When I work with back pain patients who feel disabled, who are sure that big pieces of their life are gone forever, I try to reset their thinking. "You're right, the MRI shows some disc degeneration," I'll say. "So when you are going skiing again?"

At this point, the patient looks me, half hopeful, half incredulous. "Really?" he'll say.

"Sure!" I tell him. "It's starting to get cold outside!"

"I know I'm over the worst of the pain, but . . . really? Won't I wear down my discs? What if I throw my back out again? It still kind of hurts."

"Look, I don't want you going down those treacherous black-diamond runs right away. It's true—if you fall, you could hurt yourself again. But you can still take your family to the mountains and spend some time on the bunny slopes with your kids. As your healing progresses, you may eventually be able to work your way up to the more challenging hills. *But don't let the pain ruin your life.*" I finish up with a reminder to continue with stretching, strengthening, and all the other elements of the patient's pain control solution.

As with most painful disorders, back pain is often met with disbelief and suspicion of fakery. But back pain is unusual in that it also elicits the opposite response. Back pain has come to occupy a special status in our culture: We've built legal, medical, and economic structures that are heavily invested in the notion that back pain is, and always will be, debilitating. Well-meaning friends and family may issue proclamations of doom. Personal injury lawyers, sometimes with less noble motives, may do the same. Your doctor might recommend an operation, with potentially harrowing results: About one-third of patients who undergo back surgery are left in pain that's as bad or even worse than before. (Some of the newer techniques that are performed with scopes or other instruments that are less invasive have better records.)

This grim situation is just one more example of imbalance in pain treatment. Practitioners of traditional Chinese medicine, who believe that balance is the key to health, would say that the Western approach to back pain is too *yang,* meaning too aggressive, too hasty, and too dramatic. I agree—and so, I think, would all those patients who are now truly disabled as a result of failed back surgery. More common than failed surgery, however, is the mentality of disability. In this mentality, sufferers are convinced that their pain equals dysfunction and decrepitude. They withdraw from favorite activities and feel pessimistic and blue—giving themselves a giant push down that slippery spiral of chronic pain.

Much wiser is a gentle, optimistic *yin* stance. With proper exercise, stretching, diet, and mind-body techniques, you can address most of the known contributors to back pain and help yourself heal naturally. Acupuncture, TENS, and other therapies can speed things along. A positive outlook—one that avoids the disability mentality—can keep you engaged with friends, work, and recreation. When the pain is severe, some *yang* is usually called for, in the form of injections and medications that can pull you through a rough patch and get you moving again. In a few cases, surgery is in fact necessary.

If you have back pain, you are not disabled for life. By taking advantage of conservative healing methods—and using the stronger stuff when you need it—you may even feel stronger and more flexible than you did before.

WHAT IF I HAVE A DISC PROBLEM?

Every day I see patients who come in, defeated and depressed, because they've been told that they have a degenerated (or herniated or bulging) disc and are permanently disabled. This makes me depressed, too—because these people have been misled about an issue critical to their well-being. Disc degeneration does *not* have to lead to disability or even to pain. If this statement surprises you, you're not alone.

Discs are often described as the spine's shock absorbers; they are

(continued)

pads with a gel-like inner core that act as cushions between each of the spine's vertebrae. In degenerated discs, the core material has swelled and pushed outward, sometimes putting pressure on surrounding nerves. The disc's outer covering may also tear, so that some of the core material spills out, again irritating the surrounding nerves.

These disc changes may sound violent, but several large studies have shown that disc degeneration isn't the medical crisis it was (and often still is) thought to be. On the contrary, it's a normal part of aging, much like arthritis. Nor is disc degeneration necessarily a cause of pain; lots of people with striking disc changes—to the extent that you'd expect them to be almost paralyzed—report no pain or disability at all, or very little. Multiple studies (beginning with those by Dr. M. C. Jensen and his colleagues) have looked at people who have never suffered any back pain at all—and guess what? Consistently, more than 60 percent of these pain-free people show herniated discs in the low back.

The precise relation of degenerated discs to pain remains cloudy. For now, it appears that a new rupture or bulge causes pain—often quite serious—in some people but not in others. If you have pain *and* a degenerated disc, the pain might come from the disc, *or* it might come from muscle tension *or* lack of exercise *or* any of the other causes discussed in this chapter. Quite possibly it comes from a combination of them. When a degenerated disc causes pain, it's important to know that the disc does eventually heal itself (sometimes by shrinking back to its usual size and sometimes by forming scar tissue that seals a leak or tear), removing the pressure on the nerves. If you're suffering from a degenerated disc that hasn't healed yet, your challenge is to get through this painful period without resorting to surgery and without doing those things—indulging in junk food, getting depressed, stopping exercise—that make the pain worse. The techniques below can help dramatically.

TESTING, TESTING

Do I need an MRI or CAT scan? Probably not. These scans can reveal disc changes, but disc changes often don't correspond to pain. (See "What If I Have a Disc Problem?" above.) And only about 5 percent of all back pain can be traced to a serious illness. A good physical exam and medical history are usually enough to rule these out. The doctor should test your range of motion, perform a neurological exam, and palpate your back to locate the pain. However, if you fall into one of the categories below, a combination of scans, X rays, and nerve conduction studies may be in order. These studies rule out hidden fractures, tumors, and other causes. Consider more tests if:

- You've experienced a trauma or bad blow to your back.
- The pain is severe—on a scale from 1 to 10, your pain rates a 7 or higher—or the pain prevents you from participating in the activities of daily living.
- You've experienced inexplicable weight loss.
- You're over sixty-five.
- You have a history of serious medical illness.
- Your immune system is compromised.
- Your doctor is considering giving you a deep injection or performing a surgical technique. (You'll need tests to help the doctor pinpoint the procedure site.)
- You experience increasing numbness or loss of muscle strength in an arm or leg.

Could the pain originate in the facet joints? If your doctor suspects that your facet joints—those protrusions of the vertebrae that link the spine's bones together—are a factor in your pain, he may perform a facet joint injection. If you feel better after this deep injection of nerve-cooling medication, chances are that you've located the source of the pain. For the most part, you'll need to rely on your doctor's diagnostic skills to determine if this injection is needed, but if your pain is worse when you bend backward, you can ask your doctor if a facet joint injection makes sense in your case.

Could a discogram help? In this procedure, a needle is inserted into the disc to increase the disc's volume. If your typical pain is reproduced, you and your doctor will know that the pain comes from a disc itself and not from any surrounding tissues. Although the procedure can be painful (in that you'll have to steady yourself to feel an intense version of your usual pain), it does point you toward a new therapy, IDET, which so far boasts an impressive record of significantly helping 70 percent of patients whose pain originates in a disc.

THERAPIES

Most pain develops when several burdens such as poor diet or inactivity are heaped upon the back over a period of time. This is true even for pain that involves irritated nerves or a torn ligament. To reverse the pain, you'll need to unload each of these burdens to the extent possible. That means exercising *and* stretching *and* relaxing *and* eating well. Make these conservative therapies the cornerstone of your chronic pain solution.

But if the pain keeps you from the physical activity, sleep, and mental quiet you need, don't hesitate to call on the help of medications and injections. You may wish to add further strategies according to your personal needs and the intensity of your pain.

MIND-BODY MEDICINE

► All of the mind-body therapies in Chapter 8 are good ways to loosen muscular tightness and ease your mind. Choose one or two that most appeal to you and practice them daily. My personal favorite is yoga, which I think is the ideal back pain therapy: It stretches, strengthens, and reduces stress. If your pain is severe, look into rehabilitative yoga classes, offered by many hospitals and private studios.

► If the pain is dictating the terms of your life, look into cognitive-behavioral therapy. This therapy can show you how to break out of the disability mind-set and put the pain into perspective. When the pain is very strong and persistent, it can help you develop mental coping techniques.

PHYSICAL THERAPIES

►► Are you making enough time for cardiovascular activity and stretching? It's all too easy to neglect physical fitness, especially as the demands of adult life take hold. Back pain is your body's way of telling you that it needs more attention. Start with the exercises in Appendix A and perform them daily. In addition, perform thirty minutes of low-impact cardiovascular exercise, such as swimming, cycling (recumbent bikes are good if regular bikes give you pain), and fast walking, three or four times a week.

▶▶ Poor posture contributes to back pain. Check your habits at seated activities. Are your feet flat on the ground? Is your spine straight? When you walk, is your purse, backpack, or briefcase pulling on your back muscles? If you feel you need some help correcting your posture, try the Alexander Technique, Feldenkrais Method, Hellerwork, or Pilates.

▶▶ Heat and cold therapies may both be useful. If your pain is acute or has a "hot" dimension, try a cold pack, especially after exercising or a stressful day. For a low back that feels stiff, heat is a comforting way to loosen up.

▶▶ When low back pain flares up, you need to strike a balance between rest and motion. Don't tax your back with lifting or vigorous exercise, but try to continue your normal activities as best you can. Prolonged bed rest, once the favored treatment for back pain, only weakens your muscles and makes the pain worse.

▶▶ Spinal manipulation therapy, practiced by chiropractors and osteopaths, has been proven to improve acute flare-ups of low back pain. I also like it for pain in the middle back and have used it myself for this problem, with good results. You will always need to combine spinal manipulation therapy with stretching, exercise, and other lifestyle changes.

▶▶ A paper in the *Archives of Internal Medicine* by Daniel C. Cherkin, Ph.D., indicates that massage may have long-term effects even greater than those of conventional techniques or acupuncture. Deep massage, such as myofascial release and trigger point work, is best.

DO YOU HAVE TRIGGER POINTS?

Trigger points are knots or taut bands of muscle that feel tender when pressed; they also produce pain that radiates to another part of your body. They are frequent contributors to back pain. Luckily, there are several treatments that can release trigger points and significantly reduce aches and sleeplessness. For more information about trigger points and their treatment, see Chapter 24, "Myofascial Pain Syndrome."

▸▸ Use safe lifting techniques. First of all, don't lift anything that you know is too heavy for you or too awkward to lift properly. Get someone to help you or to do it for you. When you do decide to lift, keep the object as close to you as possible, planting your feet apart to give yourself a wide base. Bend from the knees, tucking in your pelvis and keeping your abdominal muscles tight. Use your leg muscles, not your back muscles, to carry the load. *Never* twist to one side while lifting. If you lift for a living—and this includes parents who carry small or not-so-small children—you need to train for your job. Strengthen your arm and leg muscles and keep yourself in good cardiovascular shape. A physical therapist can help you get in the best condition possible for repeated daily lifting.

NUTRITION AND SUPPLEMENTS

For recommended doses of supplements, see Chapter 9.

▸▸ Extra pounds around the middle make back pain much worse. So do inflammation-promoting foods such as red meat and anything that's fried or greasy. The pain-control diet in Chapter 9 will help you lose weight and decrease inflammation.

▸ White willow bark is thought to relieve pain generally, but early reports indicate that it also appears to help low back pain specifically. Take it for occasional relief of pain as directed, but not if you have problems tolerating NSAIDs.

▸ If you suffer from insomnia, try valerian before going to bed. When anxiety is the cause of sleeplessness, take kava instead (but don't use kava on an ongoing basis).

DISTRACTING YOUR NERVOUS SYSTEM FROM PAIN

▸▸ Acupuncture is one of the best ways to control a painful flare-up. For some people, regular use will also manage ongoing pain. For tough low back problems, I like electroacupuncture, which blocks pain signals from traveling up the spinal cord, stimulates pain-blocking endorphins, and may defuse a hot-wired nervous system.

▸ Acupressure is another helpful distraction technique. A self-care acupressure technique for low back pain can be found on pages 151–152.

- When pain is consistently severe, TENS can help by blocking the pain signal. If you use TENS, make sure that you take advantage of the pain relief by exercising, stretching, and relaxing.

- If you are lethargic or fatigued, aromatherapy with peppermint, lemon, eucalyptus, or other invigorating essential oils can give you a lift.

CHAIRS, MATTRESSES, AND BRACES: THE BUSINESS OF BACK PAIN

Back pain sufferers beware: There's a huge industry out there waiting to make big bucks off your pain. Therapeutic mattresses, ergonomically designed pillows and chairs, braces that look like old-fashioned corsets . . . manufacturers promise instant back relief with their gizmos and gadgets. Before you succumb, bleary-eyed and aching, to those television ads that come on in the wee hours and promise relief from sleepless, painful nights with their product, give a few lower-cost alternatives a try.

If you think that your *workplace* equipment is causing your pain, talk to other employees in your office. When chairs and desks are uncomfortable and poorly designed (no one was meant to sit in a folding chair for eight hours a day!), chances are that you're not the only one who's suffering. With a group of aching employees standing behind you, ask the boss to hire a professional ergonomics analyst, who can determine if the furniture and equipment may be causing or contributing to your pain. The analyst can tell if your office needs better chairs and tables, if the height of computer screens should be adjusted, and so on. Sometimes an analyst can offer creative solutions to apparently unsolvable problems. I know an architect who hurt from bending over a drafting table all day and considered her pain an unavoidable occupational hazard . . . until a professional suggested a tilted table that could be used from a standing position. That may sound uncomfortable, but she much preferred this arrangement. It took the pressure off her back muscles and distributed her weight more evenly. If your boss is unwilling to hire an ergonomics analyst, be aware that the Occupational Safety and Health Administration

(continued)

(OSHA) sets standards for the workplace and may be willing to play the role of advocate for you.

If, on the other hand, you are tempted to spend thousands of dollars on specialized mattresses and reclining chairs for your *home,* first ask your doctor if he'll write you a prescription for physical therapy. A therapist who understands back pain can evaluate your body—where it's tense and cramped, where it's strong, and where it's weak—and make suggestions for both exercise and equipment. You may find that you don't need to invest in anything more than some comfortable workout clothes to get yourself in shape, or perhaps a reasonably priced firm mattress if yours is soft and sagging.

Should you continue to feel that some special equipment could help you at home, here's a list of the most popular mechanical back aids and my opinions on their usefulness:

- *Mattresses:* If you find that sleeping on the floor makes your back feel better, if your pain is at its worst in the morning and improves throughout the day, or if you find yourself rolling down into the dips and craters of your bed at night, you might need a new mattress. I recommend a firm mattress, one made by a well-known, reputable company. There's no need to pay extra money for special beds or "therapeutic" brands.

- *Pillows:* To help the spine align itself as you sleep, try placing a pillow between your knees. You don't need expensive sculpted pillows, although you can certainly use them if you like the way they feel. But ordinary pillows should do just fine.

- *Chairs:* One size does not fit all when it comes to chairs. If you sit for long periods at a desk, make sure your chair's back, seat height, and armrests are all adjustable. It should have a lumbar support feature, also adjustable. Office furniture supply stores and mail-order catalogs usually feature several models with varying price tags. You don't necessarily need the most fashionable, expensive chair; what you do need is a chair that's comfortable and adjusted to *your* body.

- *Braces:* It's a myth that back braces prevent or improve garden-variety back pain. People who use braces at work to prevent injury experience just as much pain as those who don't—and worse,

(continued)

constant use of a brace weakens the abdominal muscles as well as the extensor muscles in the back, leaving you even more vulnerable to aches and physical stress. I recommend back braces only for occasional use, when a little extra support can get a person through a particularly long and bumpy car trip, or when someone with a seriously injured back needs to get from one place to another.

▶ *Tilt boards, traction tables, and gravity boots:* All of these aids purport to improve back pain by stretching and relaxing muscles, but I haven't found them useful for this purpose at all, nor have many research inquiries. Although traction tables and tilt boards can help some people with neck pain, they don't do much for pain in the low back (probably because the head and neck are lighter structures that are easier to open up than the low back). Gravity boots, also called inversion boots, are not just ineffective for back pain; they can be dangerous if you have high or low blood pressure, cardiac disease, diabetes, weak leg joints, or impaired feeling in your feet, or if you're frail.

▶ *Abdominal strengthening devices:* Strengthening the abdominals is a great way to support your back, but you don't need devices to work them out. You just need to follow some simple exercises, such as those listed in Appendix A. If buying an exercise aid will motivate you to work out, that's fine, but don't waste your money on electrical devices that supposedly work your muscles without any effort from you. If you want a device—and again, I don't think you really need one—I recommend handheld rollers that allow you to roll forward from a kneeling position, using your abdominal muscles to pull your arms and torso back in. These rollers are available at sporting-goods stores for a reasonable price. You don't need the higher-priced versions sold on late-night TV. And remember: *Buying* the device isn't enough—you need to perform the exercises to see results!

PAIN PILLS AND OTHER PHARMACEUTICALS

▶▶ NSAIDS are often the pain pills of choice for low back pain. If ordinary over-the-counter NSAIDs such as Advil or Motrin are not strong enough, ask your doctor about a prescription. The new COX-2 inhibitors, which appear to be gentler on your stomach, may make good sense if you need regular doses for relief. In addition to

NSAIDs, some people need even stronger medications, such as opioids, and those with sensitized nervous systems often benefit from tricyclic antidepressants or anticonvulsants. No matter what kind of NSAIDs you use, try to reduce your need for them with some of the alternative therapies suggested here. A further note on NSAIDs: When a patient is incapacitated by acute back pain, emergency room doctors may sometimes provide injections of ketorolac or indomethacin (also available in oral doses), heavy-duty NSAIDs that can temporarily resolve the pain and get the patient moving again. They can be a smart solution in the ER, but unfortunately, these medications can't be prescribed for routine pain relief. They are two of the most destructive medications of their kind, resulting in an alarming number of digestive bleeding and kidney problems—so they are not prescribed for long-term use.

- When muscle spasms appear to be a significant component of back pain, a short-term course of muscle relaxants can help, especially during acutely painful episodes. Your doctor should be able to diagnose muscle spasm, but you can assist the diagnosis by reporting if your muscles feel hard and rocklike to the touch. Muscle relaxants are sedating (which can be a welcome side effect during painful flare-ups) and can lead to dependence, so they are not good choices for regular use.

- Anticonvulsants or low doses of tricyclic antidepressants may help when the pain keeps you from sleeping or when your doctor suspects that your nervous system's alarm bells are having trouble shutting themselves off.

- If your pain is severe, you may need opioid medications to bring it down to a more tolerable level. No one should make you feel guilty or ashamed for needing this option. Remember that opioids should make you *more* functional, not less—if you're too woozy to exercise while on the medication, you need to talk to your doctor. Another dosage or a different kind of opioid might improve the situation.

- When you're truly debilitated by a disc that's pressing on a nerve and need to get moving quickly, steroidal anti-inflammatory medication can be used on a very limited basis.

DEEP INJECTIONS, IMPLANTS, AND SURGERY

▶ For pain that is moderate to severe, epidural injections of local anesthetic and steroidal anti-inflammatory medication can allow you to start moving (and relaxing) again. Most people receive a series of three injections that are spaced a week or two apart. You will need to follow up the injections with exercise and stretches.

▶ If your doctor suspects that the pain originates in the facet joints, a facet joint injection or a facet nerve block may help relieve the nerve pressure and irritation. (One sign of facet joint problems is pain on bending backward.) If these injections help but you would like further relief, you might try a nerve ablation.

▶ A new procedure called intradiscal electrothermal annuloplasty (IDET) is showing exciting results for pain caused by pressure within a disc. This form of nerve ablation deadens nerves on the disc's surface by heating them up. It also stabilizes the material inside the disc, so it is less likely to irritate nerve fibers. When a discography has confirmed that the pain originates with the disc—admittedly, most patients, even those whose MRIs or X rays show disc degeneration, don't fall into this category—70 percent of patients report significant relief.

▶ In a few instances, surgery on the back is both necessary and appropriate. (See the box "When Surgery Makes Sense" for more details.) A good rule of thumb is to ask your doctor if he'll agree to a waiting period of four to six weeks, during which you can try more-conservative therapies. If the pain fades and any nerve losses do not get worse, you may be able to avoid surgery. If surgery is indeed necessary, I suggest preparing for it by learning some relaxation techniques. Guided imagery can be especially helpful in calming your spirits before surgery. Plan on intensive rehabilitation afterward, lasting several weeks to a couple of months. After that, you'll need to incorporate a program of regular self-care, including appropriate exercise (ask your doctor or physical therapist), diet, and stress management.

WHEN SURGERY MAKES SENSE

Surgery is often needed when the following conditions are present:

- You have clear and progressive neurological losses, such as weakness or a loss of reflexes.
- The pain is strongest in the leg. You may need an operation to remove pressure on the nerve roots leading to the sciatic nerve.
- Spinal joints have become unstable.
- Infection or a tumor is present.
- A fractured bone leaves the area unstable.

In most of the above circumstances, there are several surgical possibilities. In a *discectomy,* a small incision (about six centimeters) is made in the skin of the back. A window of bone is taken from the spine to allow the surgeon to see a disc that's putting pressure on nearby nerves, along with the nerves themselves and any inflammatory material that's leaked from the disc. Using a delicate instrument that looks like a stick with a pincer at its tip, the surgeon removes the offending disc and any leaked material. In the best of circumstances, the surgeon uses an operating microscope to see the structures with greater precision, reducing the risk of damaging spinal nerves. An even less invasive procedure is the *percutaneous discectomy,* in which a tiny catheter outfitted with surgical cameras and instruments is inserted into the back. At the end of the catheter is a device that allows the surgeon to remove the disc's core material. However, the surgeon's view of the inside of the back is limited. He can't see the internal field very well, so this procedure should be done only by surgeons who have experience with it and can be alert to any subtle problems that could be present deep in the back. Both kinds of discectomies may be appropriate when neurological losses or leg pains are present, as they take pressure off nerves that cause these symptoms.

The next surgeries are much more invasive. They require a long incision and surgical penetration of a larger area of muscle and bone.

(continued)

In a *laminectomy,* part of a vertebra is removed from the back of the spine, either to relieve pressure on a nerve or to stabilize the spine. This procedure is usually reserved for spinal infections, tumors, abscesses, or instability. Another surgical option is *instrumentation and fusion,* in which bone is harvested from the hip and laid down on either side of the spine to form a bridge between joints that have become unstable. Metal rods and screws may be inserted for additional stability. In some cases, a laminectomy is performed along with instrumentation and fusion. Instrumentation and fusion is responsible for many cases of failed back surgeries—most often when it is performed on back pain of unknown origin in the hope that a drastic technique will provide dramatic relief. But it can be very useful in cases of fracture or anytime a surgeon identifies a need to stabilize the spine.

HEALING ENERGY

▶ Reflexology is a healthful indulgence for people with low back pain. If you've been exercising, stretching, and eating well, why not reward yourself with this specialized foot massage?

▶ Tai chi has kept millions of Chinese people strong and flexible well into their old age; perhaps it has some effect on the back that remains unknown to us. Certainly it's a great way to relax, especially if seated meditation is too uncomfortable.

SCIATICA

The sciatic nerves run down either side of the body from the base of the spine, through the buttocks, and down into the foot. When a sciatic nerve or a nerve root that feeds into it is compressed or irritated, you feel a crampy, tight, burning pain on one side of the back that radiates down the leg. It is usually worse when bending forward or sitting down, and there may also be some numbness or tingling in the leg or foot in any posture. Like many chronic pains, sciatica often flares up for long periods of time and then withdraws.

If you want to treat sciatica properly, you'll need to uncover the source of nerve irritation. Technically, the word *sciatica* does not name a condition; it merely refers to the symptom of back pain traveling down the leg. Most often, a bulging or herniated disc is behind this symptom, pushing against the nerve or irritating it with leaking fluid. That's not such bad news: The disc will eventually heal itself as a bulging disc shrinks back to its normal size and a herniated disc forms scar tissue over any tears in the cartilage, and the source of nerve irritation will be removed. The danger here is that until this healing occurs—and it may take months—you may withdraw from exercise, stress management, and good eating, sending yourself into a downward pain spiral. So it's important to bring the pain under control so that you can continue (or begin) healthful habits. (For more information about herniated discs, see the sidebar "What If I Have a Disc Problem?" above.)

Herniated discs are not the only causes of painful sciatic nerves. Irritated spinal joints—usually the facet joints that run along the back of the spine—can also be at fault. Irritated joints are treated with an injection of anti-inflammatory medication, along with the other gentle therapies recommended for all back pain. Another cause of sciatic pain, which is less frequent but not rare, is piriformis syndrome, in which the sciatic nerve is entrapped by a muscle of the buttocks. Treatment includes anything that will relax the muscle: stretching, physical therapy, and sometimes injections of local anesthetic. If you have sciatica, it's important that your doctor check you for *all* the possible causes and not simply assume that a herniated disc is to blame.

TESTING, TESTING

Appropriate tests for sciatic pain range from the simple to the highly technical, depending on your symptoms.

▶ *Medical interview.* Your doctor should ask you several questions about your pain, especially the degree to which it radiates down your leg. Your answers will help him determine the cause of your pain. If he has given you a diagnosis of a pinched nerve caused by disc herniation but hasn't questioned you in detail, it's possible that he's failed to consider other possible causes. Ask him if he's ruled out spinal joint irritation and piriformis syndrome.

▶ *Straight-leg-raising test.* The doctor should lift your straight leg to a forty-five-degree angle. If this action causes the pain to radiate down your leg and below the knee, the pain is probably coming from the nerve roots in the spine.

▶ *Neurological exam.* This exam checks for changes in the nervous system. The doctor will check your reflexes, scratch the soles of your feet, and perform other very simple tests.

▶ *MRI and EMG nerve conduction studies.* These advanced tests are usually unnecessary, but occasionally they can help pinpoint the cause of nerve pressure. If you've had disabling sciatic pain for a long time, or if you've had numbness, weakness, or tingling in your leg, either or both tests may be in order. If your doctor is trying to diagnose piriformis syndrome, be aware that the H-reflex (the name given to the shape formed by the electrical impulse sent from the back of the knee to the spinal cord and back again) test is the gold standard. The H-reflex text should be performed in side-lying position, meaning that you're lying on your side with your knee pulled up.

BRIANA'S STORY: BACK IN HER BOOGIE SHOES

Briana was hobbling down the street to work one day when an older gentleman stopped her and gave her his cane. "You need this more than I do," he said. Although Briana was only in her thirties, the pain and numbness of sciatica threatened not just her mobility but her livelihood. She worked for a global marketing firm that was expanding rapidly, and she was afraid that if she missed many more days at the office, she'd be fired.

Briana saw an orthopedic surgeon, who told her that she needed a discectomy to remove the source of pressure on her sciatic nerve. She consulted with me; I told her that although surgery isn't right for most back pain, it would probably help her. However, Briana wanted to seek out other forms of treatment first, and I told her that I'd support her decision. She and I worked out a plan of stretching, combined with Naprosyn (naproxen), an anti-inflammatory medication, and supplements of magnesium to reduce her muscle spasms. Because Briana was familiar with Zen Buddhist meditation, she chose to draw on that technique as well. These four therapies helped her get back to work—and avoid surgery—but I discovered that Briana had another goal: She wanted to go out dancing again in her high heels, and as soon as possible. Was there something that would help her heal even faster?

(continued)

Asking a pain doctor to approve of high heels is like asking a politician to approve his own pay cut. But I *do* heartily approve of dancing. So I asked a colleague, Sekhar Upadhyayula, to step in. Sekhar gave her a series of three epidural injections that reduced the painful pressure on her sciatic nerve and coated it with anesthetic. With the pain level temporarily brought down by the injections, Briana was able to stretch more deeply during her daily routine. She continued the magnesium and meditation, cutting back on the Naprosyn to occasional use only. A couple of weeks after the epidural series ended, Briana was managing a full workload at the marketing firm *and* shopping for a new pair of dancing shoes.

RED FLAGS: POSSIBLE NERVE DAMAGE

In a few cases, sciatic pain is a sign of serious nervous system damage. Call your doctor right away if you experience a loss of feeling in the groin region, if you have difficulty controlling your bowel or bladder, or if you experience any sudden numbness or weakness.

THERAPIES

As with other forms of back pain, you'll need to apply the basics of exercise, stretching, eating well, and managing stress. See the list of therapies starting on page 237 for more specific ideas. In addition to the basics, you may need other treatments that address the particular source of nerve pressure or irritation. These are listed below.

PHYSICAL THERAPIES

▸▸ One of the best reasons to try spinal manipulation therapy is sciatic pain. See a good chiropractor or osteopath, who will prescribe stretches and exercises along with manipulation. You should see results within six or eight weeks; if not, then it's time to try something else.

▸▸ If you have piriformis syndrome, you need physical therapy to stretch out the muscle. The exercises in Appendix A are a good start, but you'll probably need to work with a physical therapist to fine-tune a regimen that suits your individual needs.

▶ I often use osteopathic stretching techniques to relax the piriformis muscle. Before you see an osteopath for this problem, call ahead to ask if he practices this form of manipulation.

PAIN PILLS AND OTHER PHARMACEUTICALS

▶ If the piriformis muscle is very tense, an office injection of the tissue with local anesthetic or Botox can help it relax. Unfortunately, not many physicians practice this technique. Before agreeing to it, make sure your doctor has experience with this injection. Remember that an injection is not a substitute for physical therapy. It simply allows you to stretch and exercise.

DEEP INJECTIONS, IMPLANTS, AND SURGERY

▶ When sciatica is caused by irritated facet joints in the spine, a facet joint injection or a facet nerve block can cool down the pain considerably. This injection is not a cure in itself, but it allows many people to exercise, stretch, and relax when the pain would otherwise be too great.

▶ A series of three epidural injections can ease the pain caused by pressure from a herniated disc. Again, you'll need to use the relatively pain-free window that follows to perform the basic back therapies listed starting on page 237.

BACK PAIN FROM SERIOUS INJURY OR ILLNESS

Unlike many conditions discussed in this book, this pain comes directly from major injury or illness. In this category are spines that are gnarled or crumbling from disease, that have been cut up in surgeries (some of which have been necessary and some not), or that have been smashed in accidents.

If you suffer from spinal pain as a result of serious injury or illness, you need to be under the care of specialists who understand your condition. You also need to build a pain-management team to coordinate treatment with your primary doctor and focus on making you as comfortable, independent, and active as possible. It's quite possible that you'll need a multitude of therapies to keep the pain at a bearable level. Finding the right mixture requires some effort and persistence, but the payoff is worth it.

For an example of someone who has successfully negotiated the trial-and-error process, see Stephanie's story, below. To get you started in your own experiment, I've listed the therapies that have most consistently produced good results in my patients. But you need not feel confined to my suggestions. It's a good idea to review the therapy chapters in Part III so that you can draw upon all your options for pain relief.

STEPHANIE'S STORY: CANCER AND A CAR CRASH

Stephanie was only twenty-nine when she was first referred to me. She had already recovered from breast cancer and Hodgkin's disease, but her incapacitating pain came in the wake of two failed back surgeries following a serious car accident. Formerly an active equestrienne, now she could barely walk. At times, she couldn't even feel her legs, thanks to permanent nerve damage; at other times, every little movement felt as if it were knifing through her spine. She was on extremely high doses of short-acting opioids, which left her woozy, sick, and painfully constipated.

Stephanie discovered the value of experimentation as she cast about for ways to get moving again. We started by changing her prescriptions. Instead of short-acting opioids, which gave her bursts of inadequate relief, she moved to long-acting opioids. She began a course of anticonvulsants and tricyclic antidepressants, which helped her sleep. They also hushed her nervous system, which was firing off extra pain signals as a result of her trauma. On the new drugs, her pain levels went down, but neither of us wanted to stop there. She was game for yoga, but unfortunately even its gentle activity was too much for her. I then tried some acupressure with her, and she responded so well that she agreed to try Rolfing, a deeper form of bodywork. Not only did this approach help Stephanie use her body more efficiently, with less stress on her painful spine, but it also helped

(continued)

her release some of the strong emotions she was holding in about her cancers and accident.

After several more months of trial and error, Stephanie could walk and move about more comfortably, but she couldn't really exercise yet, and she was still anxious and depressed about her pain. At that point, we hit upon something that kept her pain under control for weeks at a time: electroacupuncture, which is just like regular acupuncture, except that tiny electrodes are attached to the needles. We lowered her opioid prescription significantly, and she began a program of gradually increasing exercise. Eventually, she was able to ride her horse again, a testament to her persistence as much as to any pain control therapy.

Since then, I've found that electroacupuncture improves pain in many patients with severe back pain. And Stephanie's work continues. She wears a back brace at times (usually when traveling), receives trigger point injections when her muscles ball up in jumpy knots, and practices relaxation techniques, including the yoga that was off-limits before. Recently, she spent a week at Commonweal, a program for cancer patients, where she found that art therapy lifts her out of her pain for hours at a time.

THERAPIES

MIND-BODY MEDICINE

▶▶ Meditation, breathing techniques, guided imagery, and prayer are all powerful ways to relax your muscles, soothe your soul, and hush any nerves that might have been overstimulated in the aftermath of great pain. Use at least one of them every day.

▶▶ Biofeedback and hypnosis are only slightly more complicated techniques that can help you create distance between you and your pain.

▶▶ Cognitive-behavioral therapy can teach you mental techniques for responding to overwhelming suffering.

▶▶ Yoga can be remarkably effective for even the worst back pain, but you must be extremely careful not to jeopardize any unstable joints in your back. Talk to your doctor before doing any kind of exercise, and seek out yoga classes with an emphasis on rehabilitation.

PAIN PILLS AND OTHER PHARMACEUTICALS

▶▶ Don't be afraid to use opioids to control the pain; most people in your situation need them. You may reduce your need for them, however, by adding gentler therapies to your regimen.

▶▶ A lengthy bout with acute pain (such as you might feel after an accident) can disturb the body's mechanisms for handling pain signals. Anticonvulsants and low doses of tricyclic antidepressants can calm down a nervous system that's producing its own pain. These drugs can also help when the pain keeps you from sleeping.

PHYSICAL THERAPIES

▶▶ Everyone needs some form of exercise, even people who are bedridden or in wheelchairs. Work with a physical therapist to create a routine that's right for you, and make sure to include stretching.

▶▶ People with a significant disability or illness often miss being touched in a caring, compassionate way. If your spine is unstable, you might get a light massage that avoids your back. People with stable joints have their choice of massage techniques. Swedish massage is great for relaxing, but deep forms such as myofascial release and Rolfing can help you let go of muscle tension and difficult emotions you may be holding in. Trigger point work is another good way to get out the kinks.

▶ You may need to relearn how to hold yourself and how to move. Hellerwork incorporates some of the elements of Rolfing and is very good after an accident; for pain that stems from childhood disease or trauma, try the Feldenkrais Method.

▶ Back braces have a poor track record for garden-variety back pain, but in your case, a little extra support may help you get around more comfortably.

DISTRACTING YOUR NERVOUS SYSTEM FROM PAIN

▶▶ Acupuncture is one of the best ways to manage your ongoing pain. If regular acupuncture doesn't do the trick, make sure to try electroacupuncture, also known as Western acupuncture, which incorporates gentle electrical stimulation.

▶ TENS is another effective technique that prevents pain signals from moving up your spinal cord and into your brain.

▶ Acupressure distracts pain signals, releases tension, and gives you compassionate touch. Consider shiatsu, a Japanese acupressure technique that works the muscles deeply.

▶ Paint, draw, read, write in a journal, play music … do whatever engages your mind at its highest level.

NUTRITION AND SUPPLEMENTS

For recommended doses of supplements, see Chapter 9.

▶ Your body is already under deep strain; support it with the pain-control diet in Chapter 9.

▶ Make sure to get sufficient B-complex vitamins, especially if you're older. Your nervous system has been challenged by constant pain, and these vitamins help it function properly.

HEALING ENERGY

▶ Reflexology is deeply relaxing and possibly therapeutic, especially when you can't tolerate massage or are confined to a hospital bed.

16.

JOINT PAIN

OSTEOARTHRITIS / RHEUMATOID ARTHRITIS / LUPUS / SCLERODERMA / ANKYLOSING SPONDYLITIS / OTHER INFLAMMATORY JOINT DISEASES

OSTEOARTHRITIS

Some alternative practitioners believe that ancient humans didn't suffer from joint degeneration and that arthritis is a disease caused by our modern lifestyle. That's a tempting philosophy; if it were true, it would mean that by looking at our ancient ancestors and their habits—how they ate, exercised, and cared for themselves—we could devise means of avoiding the disease.

But I'm afraid that's just wishful thinking. Skeletons of prehistoric humans show clear signs of joint degeneration. This disease has always been with us, no matter how many nutritious plant foods we ate or how much exercise we got while chasing antelope over the savanna. It turns out that osteoarthritis is a bit like gray hair or wrinkles—it's a normal part of aging. Very few people hit forty or fifty without some degeneration in their joints. But that doesn't mean you have to accept disabling pain. It just means that you don't need to feel guilty about living a modern life.

Arthritis is caused by a thinning of cartilage, the spongy material that acts as a cushion and lubricant between bones. Cartilage is constantly dying and being replaced, but as we age, the rate of replacement slows down and is unable to keep up with the need for new tissue. The bones begin to rub against each other, and that familiar sharp, creaking pain sets in.

Any joint in the body can be affected by osteoarthritis, but the common targets are those that perform most of the body's hard work: hips, knees, spine, and hands. (The disease usually strikes one side of the body—say, the right hip but not the left, or in the left wrist only. If you have pain in the same joint on *both* sides of the body, you should see a doctor to rule out inflammatory arthritis, a category of more serious disorders.) People who have sustained repeated blows to a joint—athletes, for example, or construction workers who hold jackhammers—are at increased risk for arthritis, as are obese people, whose excess weight stresses the joints. Anyone in these categories may develop arthritis earlier than the rest of us. No matter what the contributing factors, a majority of elderly people have arthritis, and their condition may be compounded by other problems such as osteoporosis.

Arthritic joints tend to be stiff but not so painful upon awakening. As the day wears on, the stiffness fades and the pain sets in. By late afternoon or evening the pain, possibly accompanied by tenderness or swelling, is in full swing. People with severe arthritis, especially in the hip, spine, or knees, may experience serious nighttime pain that keeps them from sleeping. If the disease progresses, no matter where it occurs, joints can become deformed. They can also become dysfunctional. Every joint has an expected range of motion, the arc that it can travel in various directions—to the side, out to the front, to the back. Some joints, such as the ankle, can move forward, to the right and left, and back. Others are naturally more limited—the elbow, for example, bends up toward the front of the shoulder but not backward. A person with arthritis may experience a range of motion that's more restricted than normal. The hip that could normally flex to an angle of 140 degrees can now flex only to 90 degrees, or the knee that once eased into deep bends can barely move at all. Progression is not inevitable, however, and there are several therapies that may keep arthritic degeneration at bay.

It's natural, upon feeling arthritis pain, to tense the surrounding muscles or to use the joint less. But these reactions stiffen the ligaments and tendons that surround the joint. Connective tissue will shorten unless it is stretched regularly; it must be worked and used to remain pliable. When the early astronauts come back from their missions, during which they were forced to hold a seated position for a long period of time, their joints contracted so severely from lack of use that some of the men were temporarily unable to walk upon returning home. In fact, there's a phenomenon here on earth known as "frozen shoulder," in which a person who has injured a shoulder protects herself from pain by keeping the shoulder still. She stops lifting even light objects and reaching overhead. After three or four weeks, the tissue in the shoulder has shrunk, so that it's now impossible for this person to raise her hand past her waist. She needs physical therapy to regain a normal range of motion.

In people with arthritis, range of motion can be limited by the disease itself, but most doctors, as well as the Arthritis Foundation, believe that *most* loss of mobility—I'd estimate about 90 percent—is caused by decreased use of the joint in response to pain. *If you have osteoarthritis, you must keep the joint in motion.* Otherwise, you will experience additional stiffness and immobility that may feel worse than the degeneration itself.

You may be saying, "Work out on my arthritic knee? Is he *crazy*? I'd rather have my teeth drilled without anesthesia!" It's true: Exercising the joint without some kind of pain relief isn't a very palatable solution to chronic pain. This chapter contains suggestions for reducing arthritis pain so that physical therapy or other appropriate exercise hurts less. With time, as your connective tissue stretches and becomes looser, working out may even become pleasurable.

Inflammation appears to be another element of osteoarthritis, even though osteoarthritis is not a true inflammatory illness. In rheumatoid arthritis, lupus, and other inflammatory joint diseases, the body's immune system turns traitor and attacks its own tissues; many of these illnesses are life-threatening. This process does *not* occur in garden-variety osteoarthritis. However, the wear and tear of normal arthritis does appear to spur on the body's immune response. The immune system reacts to the cartilage damage by arthritis in much the same way it reacts to skin damage from cuts and scrapes: by increasing blood flow to the injured area and sending extra white blood cells to encourage healing. But one theory about arthritis pain is that this inflammation may become *too* exuberant. Just as the central nervous system may become sensitized in the presence of chronic pain, producing stronger and stronger pain signals even after the tissue has healed, it's possible that the immune system goes overboard in response to arthritis, sending such an overload of blood and immune cells to the area that your joints become tender and puffy. You can control inflammation by making proper food choices and taking certain medications.

One source of joint pain that many doctors are unaware of is a sensitized nervous system. When severe arthritis pain hangs around for a while, it doesn't just hurt—it can alter the way your body sends and receives pain signals. You might think that someone in constant pain would eventually grow accustomed to the sensation (if you've lived with serious arthritis, maybe you already know better), but often the exact opposite happens: With time, the pain signals that travel from nerve cell to nerve cell are amplified. If you've been told that you feel more pain than you ought to, given the extent of your joint damage, you may suffer from this phenomenon. (For more information about the nervous system's role in pain, see Chapter 3.) Mind-body therapies and pharmaceuticals such as anticonvulsants and tricyclic antidepressants can settle down this sensitization, or at least prevent you from suffering so much.

So far, I've made arthritis sound like a pretty straightforward kind of illness: We get older, cartilage wears out, pain occurs, end of story. But strangely enough, that's not always the case. Bone rubbing against bone sounds inescapably painful, like breaking a leg—and yet many people whose X rays or MRI scans show severe degeneration report *no pain at all.* Conventional wisdom tells us they should hurt—a lot—but they simply don't. By contrast, other people whose tests reveal little damage feel high levels of pain.

It's hard to know what to make of these findings. Some scientists have postulated that the bone-on-bone element may be less important to pain than some other, still-undiscovered mechanisms. Certainly a nervous system whose pain signals have run amok can lead to a feeling of horrid injury even when the damage to the joint is minor. From what I've seen, lifestyle factors such as appropriate exercise, an anti-inflammatory diet, and stress management make some people more resistant to pain than others. (So perhaps our cave-dwelling ancestors, with their plant-based diet and nearly constant exercise, suffered less from arthritis pain after all, even though they experienced joint degeneration.) What *you* can take from this news is hope: Although arthritis may be inevitable, pain and disability are not.

Although we don't know exactly why some people hurt from arthritis and others don't, we do know many strategies for decreasing the pain and improving function. Medications can help, and yoga, certain supplements, dietary changes, and other methods will improve your condition naturally, without side effects. Many of them are relatively inexpensive and easy to use on your own. If the arthritis should prevent you from getting around and performing basic tasks, then conventional science can step up to the plate with injections or joint replacement surgeries.

TESTING, TESTING

In most cases, your doctor can make a good diagnosis of osteoarthritis from just a physical exam and medical history. However, there are a few instances when further testing is in order:

- You feel significant pain in symmetrical joints (left *and* right wrists, knees, or hips, for example), or you experience general achiness or fatigue. A blood test will rule out inflammatory or collagen-vascular diseases.
- The pain appears in only one joint, which is hot or swollen. You should be checked for infection, gout, and a few other disorders.
- You have risk factors for cancers in the painful area or have sustained a physical trauma around that location. You should have X rays to rule out hidden tumors or fractures in the bone.

Some doctors like to get X rays on all their patients with arthritis. That's fine, but you should know that there's a poor correlation between what appears on the film and the symptoms reported. If you feel only minor pain but X rays show advanced wear and tear, don't let well-meaning people convince you that you're disabled or going downhill. What counts is how you feel and how you function. *You* should be treated, not your X rays.

DO YOU HAVE TRIGGER POINTS?

Trigger points are knots or taut bands of muscle that feel tender when pressed; they also produce pain that radiates to another part of your body. They are frequent contributors to arthritis pain. Luckily, there are several treatments that can release trigger points and significantly reduce aches and sleeplessness. For more information about trigger points and their treatment, see Chapter 24, "Myofascial Pain Syndrome."

THERAPIES

PHYSICAL THERAPIES

Note: If a joint is unstable or excessively mobile, meaning that it moves beyond the joint's normal range, certain exercises may not be safe for you. Talk to your doctor.

▶▶ Much of arthritis pain comes from connective tissues that have constricted, restricting mobility and accelerating the degenerative process. By keeping tendons and ligaments limber and strong, you can greatly reduce your suffering—and maybe ward off the disease's progression. Perhaps the best activity for this purpose is gentle yoga. I usually group yoga with mind-body therapies, but when it comes to arthritis, yoga's physical benefits really shine. Look for a class that emphasizes slow stretches over rapid, energetic movement; most yoga studios and some hospitals offer basic classes with middle-aged and older adults in mind. If you need inspiration, look at photos of old yogis, who can still swivel around on their knees and dip into back bends. (However, back bends and other rigorous poses, such as headstands, may not be advisable for you. Check with your doctor before starting class to see if you need to avoid certain movements, and inform your instructor about your condition.) If you don't like yoga, a physical therapist can show you how to combine stretches with very light weight lifting.

▶▶ Cardiovascular exercise will also prevent you from increasing pain by holding your muscles too tightly. Swimming is a good choice, and so is Pilates (although Pilates should not be used by those with very severe conditions or unstable joints).

▶ Light massage, which helps loosen up tissue, makes a relaxing adjunct to exercise and can reduce pain before or after a workout. Russian massage, which features quick, repetitive motions, works very well around achy joints—consider that this treatment has been a mainstay of Russian Olympic teams for more than a century. I've had Russian massage on my stiff left knee and can happily report increased mobility and decreased pain. Swedish massage, with its long, gliding strokes, may be slightly less therapeutic but is certainly worth trying. Avoid any kind of massage around a joint that is tender and swollen.

▶ Heat and cold therapies won't cure your pain, but they can allow you to handle exercise with less pain when applied before and after working out. Even independent of exercise, they offer comfort and relief of symptoms. A hot paraffin dip is a favorite for people with hand, foot, or elbow pain, but you can use whatever mode you like. One caveat here: Don't use heat on joints that are tender and swollen.

▶ A couple of published papers have indicated that magnets and copper bracelets *may* help with arthritis pain—possibly by increasing circulation or manipulating pain receptors in the nervous system—but most of these studies are on small groups of people and have not been duplicated. Wearing these items is almost certainly harmless, however, and I see plenty of patients who swear by them (although these patients aren't *just* wearing magnets or bracelets—they're also following a multifacted approach to their chronic pain).

THE NIGHTSHADE CONTROVERSY

There's a folk tradition that connects arthritis pain with consumption of foods in the nightshade family—that is, potatoes, bell peppers, tomatoes, and eggplants. (They get their name from the deadly nightshade, which is a member of that plant family but which none of us—I hope—is putting into stews.) However, study after study has failed to find a link between the two. Given the lack of evidence, and since these foods are staples of a good diet, I'm hesitant to suggest that you eliminate them. But if you do notice that you feel worse after eating dishes heavy on the nightshades, then you might find a brief trial (a week or two) of elimination worthwhile. If you don't experience symptom reduction after that time, then by all means reintroduce these foods and eat them without guilt.

NUTRITION AND SUPPLEMENTS

For recommended doses of supplements, see Chapter 9.

▶▶ Your body requires a wide array of nutrients to rebuild joints and cartilage. Follow the pain-control diet in Chapter 9 and take a multivitamin every day. I especially recommend that you eat "good" fats. Your body is likely producing a constant low-grade inflammatory response to the damage caused by arthritis; this inflammatory response contributes to pain and tenderness. By eating deep-water fish, walnuts, flaxseed, and other "good fats"—the ones that contain anti-inflammatory prostaglandins—you can settle down inflammation and reduce some of your aches. But when you eat animal-based fats and partially hydrogenated oils, you're encouraging the production of pro-inflammatory prostaglandins, the kind that make your pain worse.

▶▶ It's rare that I'm so excited about a supplement that I recommend it to *all* my patients. But I do encourage everyone with arthritis to try glucosamine and chondroitin. Glucosamine appears to reduce subacute inflammation; more astonishingly, it may stimulate new cartilage to grow between arthritic joints. One study showed that although ibuprofen brought faster relief to patients, the pain reduction they experienced after taking glucosamine for eight weeks was more significant. Chondroitin's effects are more preventive: This supplement seems to maintain the pliability and suppleness of cartilage that's already present. Try these products for at least a month or two before determining if they're worth continuing.

▶▶ Rub a lotion made with capsaicin (chili pepper oil) onto the painful area three times a day. Its heating sensation travels faster from one nerve cell to the next than pain does, so it beats the pain signal to the spinal cord, thereby "closing the gate" on the pain. Allow the lotion a few days to take effect. It may burn a little (and for some people it burns quite a bit), but most people prefer the burning sensation to that of pain.

▶ Devil's claw may reduce arthritis pain and inflammation.

▶ Try ginger, turmeric, or quercetin to relieve inflammation. Introduce them to your body one at a time so that you'll know which one is working or causing a particular adverse effect. For example, you might try ginger and not feel much improvement; you could then discontinue it in favor of turmeric or quercetin. Remember that more is not always better, especially when it comes to supplements.

▶ If you're over sixty-five, take a B-complex supplement. A deficiency of the B-complex vitamins—frequent in older people—can lead to increased pain.

▶ Try niacinamide to reduce pain and stiffness.

▶ Zinc seems to have a slight effect on arthritis pain, but if you're taking a multivitamin, there's absolutely no need for additional dosing.

WORTH YOUR MONEY?

I often talk to my patients about the potential side effects of therapies. Most people are used to hearing that a pill can cause vomiting or headaches, or that some exercises can hurt you if your joints are unstable. But patients are usually surprised when I warn them of another possible danger: emptying of the pocketbook. They laugh, but I'm serious. Many of the arthritis sufferers I see are on fixed incomes, and I'd hate for them to spend a disproportionate amount of their monthly check on supplements that don't have much scientific or anecdotal weight behind them.

However—and this is a big "however"—I know that arthritis pain eats away at a person's quality of life. If there is a treatment out there that could help, I don't like closing off options. If you have tried the other therapies listed in this chapter *and* if you can afford experimenting with costly supplements that might not work, you might consider giving these items a try. Just remember that there aren't any miracle drugs out there; you'll still need to exercise your joints, eat well, keep stress under control, and use conventional medications when necessary. And you must always check with your doctor before taking any supplement.

Below are some supplements patients often ask me about:

▶ *SAM-e.* SAM-e stands for S-adenosylmethionine, a substance involved in many of the body's biochemical reactions. Proponents say that it repairs cartilage, but the doses you'd have to take for this supposed (and unproven) effect are awfully high. That's not a risk I'd want to take—I'd rather stick with glucosamine and chondroitin myself, since the doses are lower and the effects better understood. Of my patients who have tried SAM-e, many have reported less pain, and some feel very strongly that their pain is significantly reduced. Some experience diarrhea while taking the supplement, and nearly all who try SAM-e complain about its cost.

(continued)

▶ *MSM.* MSM (methyl sulfonyl methane) is a chemical compound, one that supposedly reduces pain by pulling toxins that cause inflammation out of the cells. There isn't much evidence for it, and I haven't seen many patients who feel it's helped. Most of those who've tried MSM have moved on to glucosamine and chondroitin.

▶ *DMSO.* A few years ago, it seemed that everyone was taking DMSO for arthritis—and reeking to high heaven. DMSO is dimethyl sulfoxide, a derivative of the material that bonds the cells of trees, and it causes the skin to give off a garliclike odor. The idea was that a 90 percent solution of DMSO, applied topically, would reduce inflammation and pain. There is still no evidence to back up this claim, although there *is* evidence of short-term side effects such as skin irritation. I saw many patients who'd decided to give DMSO a try, but very few reported relief. As far as I can tell from my personal practice, DMSO use has fallen dramatically.

DISTRACTING YOUR NERVOUS SYSTEM FROM PAIN

▶▶ <u>Acupuncture</u> is one of the best-kept secrets for arthritis pain—for some reason, people who would consider acupuncture for back pain or smoking cessation don't tend to think of it for arthritis. I've used it personally for joint stiffness and felt that it improved mobility in my knee. I've also seen a great many patients improve with regular treatment. One of my colleagues told me of a woman who suffered from extreme hip pain as a result of a youthful diving career; for her, acupuncture was so successful that she used it instead of medication for months as she awaited a double hip replacement. Such anecdotal reports on acupuncture's effects are common.

▶ <u>Acupressure</u> blocks pain signals and can also relax the connective tissue and improve motion. Consider shiatsu (which makes a nice close to a session of acupuncture) or anmo (its quick motions improve circulation).

▶ <u>Electrical stimulation</u> can also help. If you like this therapy, you might want to look into TENS, which is a portable and longer-lasting method of electrical distraction.

► If you hurt constantly and at a moderate to severe level from knee, hip, or spinal pain, TENS can distract your spinal cord and prevent it from processing pain signals. It's less helpful for joints that are out at the periphery, such as fingers and toes.

HEALING ENERGY

►► Tai chi has helped millions of Chinese people stay active and limber well into old age. If you're over sixty-five, it will also improve your balance and reduce the chance that you'll hurt yourself in a fall. People of all ages can benefit from its gentle range-of-motion exercises and meditative quality.

CHERYL'S STORY: "JUST GIVE ME SOME PILLS AND I'LL GO AWAY"

When I first met Cheryl, she was succinct and clear about what she wanted from me: stronger medication for her arthritis pain. She looked tired and a little dejected, I thought, so I asked her to tell me more about herself. Cheryl was in her late thirties, with a government job that provided a decent income but not much excitement. It was the practice of aikido, one of the martial arts, that had added juice to her life. She held a second-degree black belt; practicing at the dojo (a studio where martial arts instruction takes place) was her favorite source of relaxation, exercise, and social activity. Teaching classes to children brought her particular enjoyment—that clear, straightforward demeanor I'd just witnessed made her a gifted instructor, and, as I was to learn later, she had a wide smile and open countenance when she wasn't in pain.

Over the past year, Cheryl had developed wicked, stabbing pains in her elbow. She brought in her X rays, which showed signs of massive degeneration; there was even a hook at the edge of the joint, where the bones had rubbed together. "Aikido did it," she told me. Her doctor told her she'd have to quit the martial arts and wrote her a prescription for naproxen, an NSAID. The naproxen helped some, but not enough. She came to me looking for something stronger.

(continued)

That's when she said what I've heard from so many demoralized arthritis sufferers, worn down by the sense that a part of their life has been shut closed: "Just give me some pills and I'll go away."

I still held the X rays in my hand. "You know," I said, "these look pretty bad. I'll give you that. You're obviously in a lot of pain. But I don't agree with this view you have of your life. I just don't buy it."

Cheryl threw me a glance that was half skeptical, half curious. I explained to her that there wasn't necessarily a connection between joint deterioration and pain, and that I felt she could regain much of her lost mobility with physical therapy. At this point, many arthritis sufferers recoil at the very thought of moving their painful joint, but Cheryl was tough from years of serious athletic training. She immediately agreed to any kind of plan that might get her back to the dojo.

Since she needed daily relief from the pain, I wrote a prescription for another NSAID, a COX-2 inhibitor that can reduce the risk of gastrointestinal side effects. She took glucosamine and chondroitin supplements to encourage the growth of new cartilage. And she came in regularly for physical therapy, applying heat to her elbow before each session to reduce the pain of stretching the tissue.

I was impressed with Cheryl's embrace of both conventional and alternative therapies. But there was one aspect of her chronic pain solution that daunted her: giving up inflammatory foods. For all her aikido-inspired discipline, Cheryl *loved* all things fried and crispy, especially potato chips. She understood that these snacks increase pain in nearly everyone (they act in a manner directly opposed to NSAIDs—they increase the prostaglandins that these drugs are meant to suppress) and that they promote the kind of inflammation that was probably already present in response to her cartilage damage. But she just couldn't give them up at first. Eventually, as the other therapies began to make her feel better, Cheryl felt less dependent on chips as a source of comfort, and she was able to cut back.

In about eight months, Cheryl returned to the dojo and reported that she was "almost fully rehabilitated." She couldn't perform all her old moves, but she could join practices and teach the younger children. I can't pinpoint which of Cheryl's therapies produced such marvelous results—it's likely they produced a synergistic effect. I should note that subsequent X rays revealed that her joint degeneration was still present. There was no miraculous reversal of the disease. But when you're no longer suffering, who cares what the X rays say?

PAIN PILLS AND OTHER PHARMACEUTICALS

▶▶ Acetaminophen (Tylenol and many other brands) is often touted as the best choice for osteoarthritis relief. I like acetaminophen because many arthritis sufferers need some sort of daily relief, and this drug doesn't pose the same dangers to the gastrointestinal tract as NSAIDs. However, many patients find acetaminophen too mild for their needs. If you fall into that category but can't take NSAIDs—or simply prefer not to—I suggest combining acetaminophen with some of the nondrug therapies listed in this chapter.

▶▶ Arthritis sufferers tend to have a love/hate relationship with NSAIDs. These drugs work by suppressing the release of pro-inflammatory prostaglandins. Some experts say that anti-inflammatory medications shouldn't work for osteoarthritis pain because osteoarthritis is not caused by inflammation. Preliminary research shows that low-grade inflammation occurs in osteoarthritis and may contribute to pain and tenderness. More compelling is that most people with osteoarthritis feel much better when they're taking NSAIDs—although these drugs certainly have an analgesic effect, this common experience further suggests that inflammation is a component of the pain. So why the love/hate relationship toward a drug that works? Although NSAIDs often provide steady relief, the risk of serious gastrointestinal side effects, including bleeding of the stomach lining and even death, is significant enough to give many patients pause. Most of us dislike taking them on a consistent basis, especially if multiple doses are needed throughout the day. The desire to reduce NSAID intake—without giving up the pain control they provide—is one of the most common things I hear from osteoarthritis sufferers. I usually approach this problem from a couple of directions. I often prescribe a COX-2 inhibitor, a kind of NSAID that appears to cause fewer GI problems. (If you've had trouble getting your insurance provider to pay for COX-2 inhibitors such as Vioxx or Celebrex in the past, you might want to try again. As more evidence of their effectiveness and safety is published, more providers are willing to offer coverage.) That alone can help. But if all you do for your arthritis is take a pill, you're not getting maximal relief. By combining NSAIDs (or any other pain-relieving drug) with nonpharmaceutical therapies such as yoga, a pain-control diet, acupuncture, and tai chi, you may reduce your need for medication. Perhaps you can cut back on the number of pills at each dose; or maybe you'll no longer need to take NSAIDs every day, reserving them for flare-ups or post-exercise soreness (just be sure not to take them *before* workout soreness sets in, or you won't see all the benefits of exercise).

▶ If you're having trouble sleeping because of arthritis pain, or if you feel much more pain than seems appropriate, talk to your doctor about tricyclic antidepressants or anticonvulsants. In very low doses, they improve sleep and reduce pain generated by sensitized nerves.

▶ Steroid medications can be injected into arthritic joints to reduce inflammation. Since these injections tend to weaken connective tissue, they're fairly controversial. I suggest them only when pain prevents you from getting the necessary physical therapy, or when you need to buy some time before joint replacement surgery. (For example, one of my patients received a steroid injection when she wanted to postpone surgery until after her daughter's wedding. And lots of people would prefer to wait out an icy, cold winter before an operation.) No one should receive more than a couple of steroid injections in a year.

▶ If you have knee pain, you may benefit from an office injection of hyaluronic acid. This is another controversial technique—mainly because it hasn't been solidly proven yet—but there's some evidence that the drug rebuilds knee cartilage. I've used it on patients with a medium degree of success. Some don't see relief at all, but others are able to go cross-country skiing again after receiving the injection. Hyaluronic acid may make sense if you've already used several other therapies without relief. As with any injection, you do run the risk of infection, bleeding, or an allergic reaction to the drug.

▶ Opioids are rarely used for garden-variety arthritis pain; an exception occurs when joint pain in the back or neck is compounded by other disorders. Elderly people in particular may find themselves in this situation, especially if they suffer from osteoporosis. In these cases, opioids represent a humane and sensible treatment option, one that should not be withheld because of misplaced fears of addiction.

MIND-BODY MEDICINE

▶▶ If arthritis pain is controlling your days and nights, ask your doctor about cognitive-behavioral therapy. This short-term treatment has been shown to bring down the reported pain of arthritis sufferers. It can also help you come up with ways to reduce your suffering, that is, the degree to which pain lowers your quality of life.

▶▶ Meditation and yoga can help you distance yourself from louder-than-necessary pain signals transmitted by an altered nervous system. The mental quiet and peace they bring may even help restore your nerves or production of natural painkillers such as endorphins to normal.

DEEP INJECTIONS, IMPLANTS, AND SURGERY

▶ No one *wants* to have surgery, but when arthritis is debilitating, today's joint replacement techniques can return function to your life. The most common sites for artificial joints are hips and knees, but surgeons can replace almost any kind of joint, including shoulders, knuckles, fingers, and toes. It's even possible to receive joint replacements made of metal, plastic, or bone (usually harvested from your own hip) in the spine.

IS IT TIME FOR A JOINT REPLACEMENT? AND OTHER SURGICAL CONSIDERATIONS

When patients ask me, with great trepidation and even some distaste, if it's time to get an arthritic joint surgically replaced, I tell them something similar to what my mother told me about true love: When it's time, you'll know. Most people decide to have their joint replaced when they can't move it at all, or when the pain is gnawing into their daily functioning. (Not being able to climb stairs is often the trigger for surgery.) Certainly if the joint is fully degenerated or fractured, surgery may be your best and only option. Artificial joints don't last forever, however—hips, for example, currently have a life of about twenty years—so some people in midlife delay replacements, hoping to avoid needing a second or third surgery when they're much older

(continued)

and perhaps less able to bounce back from the physical stress of an operation. That's a judgment call to be made on a case-by-case basis, depending on your current level of pain and disability.

Not everyone who wants surgery is a good candidate. If you smoke, abuse drugs or alcohol, have serious psychological problems, or are significantly overweight, a surgeon may be hesitant to operate, because all of these factors are associated with a lower surgical success rate. Anyone with a compromised immune system is at greater risk of infection from implanted foreign material.

How much improvement can you expect from the surgery? The question reminds me of that old joke in which a patient asks his doctor if he'll be able to play the piano after undergoing surgery. The surgeon assures the patient that yes, he will. "That's great!" the patient says. "I always wanted to play the piano!"

To some extent, the amount of function you experience after recovering from joint replacement surgery depends on how much function you had going in. This is a controversial view—many surgeons believe that surgery will fix the joint, end of story. But I've found that surgical outcomes are much rosier when people do *pre*surgical rehabilitation, getting the joint, and their bodies, in the best condition possible given the circumstances. I also think patients do better when they get their minds ready for surgery with relaxation exercises and guided imagery (audiotapes made specifically for those about to undergo surgery are a good choice). Of course, anyone coming out of joint replacement surgery will need postsurgical rehabilitation as well.

INFLAMMATORY ARTHRITIS

Osteoarthritis may be a normal part of aging, but inflammatory arthritis is quite another story. It can destroy joints, leaving sufferers in pain and often with severely compromised function. At its worst, it can progress from joints to attack organs such as the heart or lungs.

The term "inflammatory arthritis" encompasses several disorders in which the immune system mistakenly perceives the body's own connective tissues as foreign substances. The immune system then issues the inflammatory response, increasing blood flow and the number of immune cells in the area. Normally, inflammation is healing. If an invader were truly present in the body, the swelling and tenderness caused by the additional blood flow would, among other benefits, encourage rest of the injured site. The immune cells would destroy the substance, perhaps a virus or bacteria. But in the case of inflammatory arthritis, the "invaders" are healthy cartilage and joint lining; with time, the immune cells can go on to destroy the joints themselves and eventually attack internal organs. Most types of inflammatory arthritis follow a cycle of remission and return, although flare-ups, often triggered by intense activity, poor dietary choices, or stress, can appear at any time. There is no clearly identified cause of these illnesses; it's likely that genetics, hormones, and environmental factors are all involved.

Here are some of the disorders that fall into the category of inflammatory arthritis:

- *Rheumatoid arthritis.* Often, the first sign of rheumatoid arthritis (RA) is achiness in the small joints of the hands or feet, especially at the base of both thumbs. Unlike osteoarthritis, RA is usually symmetrical (affecting the same joints on both sides of the body). Fever, fatigue, and a general sense of malaise may be present as well. In RA, the inflammatory response initially occurs in the synovium, or lining of the joint. As the inflammation persists, the cartilage that normally provides a cushion between the bones of the joint is degraded, so that the pain intensifies. The joint may swell and stiffen; later, it may become deformed and lose its ability to function. The cartilage damage can further spur on the immune response, which may eventually spread to other body tissues. Arteries can become inflamed, and fluid may accumulate around the spleen, lungs, or heart. People with RA often experience shortened life spans as a result, but thanks to drugs developed in recent years that suppress a hyperexuberant immune system, patients are living longer and with fewer symptoms than in the past.

- *Lupus.* Officially known as systemic lupus erythematosus (SLE), lupus often starts with a red butterfly-shaped rash that spreads across the face. As in rheumatoid arthritis, another early sign is achiness in symmetrical joints (both thumbs, both ankles, and so on), especially the smaller joints of the body. As the disease moves through periods of remission and activation, these and other joints may eventually become stiff, deformed, and nonfunctional. For some, the symptoms do not progress beyond the joints. For others, the inflammatory process can spread to organs throughout the body, damaging the kidneys, lungs, heart, and even the central nervous system. Each of these effects can result not just in severe pain but in a threat to basic functioning and even life itself. However, the treatment of lupus has progressed dramatically since the early twentieth century, when it was fatal within a few years of its onset. Now, many sufferers can expect more normal life spans, as long as they take medications that slow the disease's march and are closely monitored for any threatening developments. Managing the pain and fatigue that accompany lupus is crucial to enjoying that life.

- *Scleroderma.* Also known as systemic sclerosis, scleroderma tends to attack joints at the body's periphery, mainly the hands and feet. In this disease, the immune response results in an overproduction of collagen, a protein that builds connective tissue as well as scar tissue. The excess collagen is deposited in blood vessels and the joints, producing pain and stiffness and hardening the skin that stretches over the affected joints. (*Scleroderma* literally means "hard skin.") Some people will experience no further symptoms or may even see their condition reverse. In others, scleroderma progresses. Joints may be painful and deformed, as in rheumatoid arthritis. The skin becomes so taut and hard that the joints are difficult to bend. Scar tissue may eventually appear in the internal organs, making people with scleroderma vulnerable to kidney, heart, and lung failure. They may also experience difficulty with essential activities such as swallowing.

- *Ankylosing spondylitis.* This is an apparently hereditary disorder in which the soft tissues—especially the tendons and ligaments—that support the vertebrae and joints of the spine become chronically inflamed. It usually appears in the teens or twenties and affects men more often than it does women. At the onset of the disease, the back feels stiff in the morning and gets better over the course of the day, especially with exercise. Over time, ankylosing spondylitis can cause the spinal vertebrae to fuse, and the person will develop a stooped posture. Unlike many other inflammatory joint disorders, ankylosing spondylitis does not tend to decrease the length of life—but quality of life can be considerably compromised by spinal pain and stiffness.

Needless to say, these diseases are serious and require vigilant treatment. Although there is no cure, many inflammatory disorders can be slowed down significantly and their damage reduced. If you have rheumatoid arthritis (RA), lupus, scleroderma, ankylosing spondylitis, or another inflammatory joint disease, you should be under the care of a good rheumatologist, preferably one connected with a teaching hospital. It is not the aim of this chapter to consider how best to treat these underlying diseases themselves. Instead, it discusses your options for controlling their predominant symptom: pain.

In addition to drugs for the disease itself, conventional pain treatment for inflammatory arthritis relies heavily on non-steroidal anti-inflammatory drugs (NSAIDs). These drugs suppress the pro-inflammatory prostaglandins that are normally part of the healing process but that for sufferers of inflammatory arthritis simply cause additional pain. Many sufferers find themselves taking three or four over-the-counter NSAID pills three times a day (or the prescription equivalent of this dose). The number-one pain concern of the inflammatory arthritis patients I see is the potentially harsh side effects of continuous NSAID use. Since the pain may be with these sufferers for a lifetime, they'd like to find less aggressive measures to help manage it. If you feel the same way, you're in luck. There are many alternative strategies available.

I suggest beginning with an anti-inflammatory diet. Time and again, I've seen this simple, low-cost approach make a significant difference in the pain levels of people with inflammatory arthritis, especially for sufferers whose diets were perhaps not ideal to begin with. Beyond diet, there are several physical therapies that can help you take stress off your joints and relax the surrounding tissue, which may have tightened up in a pain response. You should also have at least one mind-body therapy at your disposal. Progressive disease, especially a painful one, is one of life's most stressful experiences; you need a way to relax, reflect, and gather your psychic resources.

If you have an inflammatory joint disease, you already know the challenge it poses to basic functioning. Chores such as cleaning out the garage or staying up with a sick child can tax your system and bring on a flare-up. If you want to continue these life tasks—although it is advisable for you not to overdo activities, sometimes heavy exertion is inevitable—you'll need to develop a set of therapies for warding off pain. Here's a regimen that's helped several of my patients: After the activity, plan some quiet time. You probably know which of your joints tend to get sore; ice them down for a few minutes every hour. Eat some salmon or walnuts and drink a cup of hot ginger tea. Get a gentle massage if you can, listen to music, or see an acupuncturist. Eventually, you will find your own ideal set of therapies. Having them in place is crucial for preventing flare-ups or managing them when they do arise.

SUSAN'S STORY: WINDSURFING WITH RA

My windsurfing buddy Susan taught me something about the power of an anti-inflammatory diet. Until recently, Susan's weekend workouts were her only exercise. Although her upper body was strong from counterbalancing the weight of a fully powered sail, she was in her mid-thirties and no longer able effortlessly to maintain herself in great shape, as she'd done in her teens and twenties. Her work schedule was demanding, and she allowed herself to get a little weak and heavy. One summer, Susan noticed some soreness in the base of both thumbs, and she was diagnosed with rheumatoid arthritis. Her case was still in its early stages—she had none of the significant joint deformity that marks later stages of RA—but the pain in her hands and ankles threatened to leave her and her windsurfing board beached.

Susan received care for her RA from an excellent rheumatologist, but she wondered if I knew of any way to control the pain well enough for her to continue windsurfing. I honestly didn't know if she could surf again, but I thought that if she could turn around some of her old habits, she might feel better. She was already taking Vioxx, a COX-2 inhibitor, regularly. At my suggestion, she continued the pain medication but also took supplements of fish oil to reduce inflammation. When she complained that the fish oil was repeating on her—a feeling no one likes, especially when it's *fish* oil that you're tasting twice—she tried Fisol, a enteric-coated pill that stays intact until it gets past your stomach. This product worked better for her. More difficult was persuading Susan to give up her habit of eating fast food for lunch and rocky road ice cream every night after (and sometimes instead of) dinner. No one had ever told her that these foods are high in fats that increase pro-inflammatory prostaglandins. Somewhat skeptically, she agreed to cut back on the ice cream; when she realized that her pain level went down a bit, she embraced the experiment more enthusiastically.

Just as people can slide along downward pain spirals, in which pain and suffering build on themselves, so can they take a kind of shortcut spiral *upward* when therapies begin working and provide in-

(continued)

centive to throw more effort into pain control. Instead of eating take-out fried chicken, Susan started to make meals incorporating fresh ingredients, especially oily fish such as salmon and anti-inflammatory spices such as ginger and turmeric. She cut way back on red meat. As she noticed further improvement and began to feel generally better, she began swimming during the week for regular exercise. Even I was surprised at the improvement Susan experienced. After a month or so, she was out on her board again and even signed up for tennis lessons. The last time I saw her, she was still feeling good. She indulges in rocky road ice cream once in a while, but now that she's made the connection between lifestyle and pain, she's motivated to continue her chronic pain solution for the rest of her life.

THERAPIES

NUTRITION AND SUPPLEMENTS

For recommended doses of supplements, see Chapter 9.

►► Follow a pain control diet. Include walnuts, flaxseed, and oily fish such as salmon in your meals several times a week, and consider taking fish oil capsules (or DHA if you want a vegetarian source) to encourage the production of anti-inflammatory prostaglandins. Reduce your consumption of animal fats and partially hydrogenated oils, which make inflammation worse.

►► Since everyone's body reacts to foods differently, spend a week or two paying close attention to your diet. You may find that certain substances cause flare-ups; if so, take them off the menu or enjoy them only on special occasions. See pages 135–136, "Can Food Allergies Cause Pain?" for more information.

► Try ginger, turmeric, gamma-linolenic acid (GLA), or quercetin to inhibit inflammation. Introduce these substances to your body one at a time to determine which work best for you.

► Try capsaicin, the oil of hot chili peppers, on painful joints. Capsaicin reduces the amount of substance P in your body and may also prevent the pain signal from traveling up the spinal cord. Use the lotion three times a day for several days in a row; you need regular applications of the oil to build up the pain-blocking effect.

MIND-BODY MEDICINE

▶▶ Join a support group. Other people with your disease can provide sympathy and understanding like no one else can. Even more valuable is the down-and-dirty problem solving: You learn from one another the strategies that help you live with the pain and maintain your quality of life.

▶▶ Cognitive-behavioral therapy has been proven to reduce pain in people with RA by helping them figure out ways to handle obstacles that the disease throws in their path.

▶▶ In addition to a group or cognitive-behavioral therapy, you need a way to handle stress on a daily basis. Guided imagery and gentle yoga are both good choices. (If you're doing yoga, avoid poses that put stress on the neck.)

PHYSICAL THERAPIES

▶▶ A physical or occupational therapist can teach you techniques for joint protection. Depending on where you're most vulnerable, a therapist will show you how to grasp objects, open jars, lift heavy objects, or simply move across the room without placing undue stress on your joints. If your disease is in an advanced stage, you can learn how to use mechanical aids and body position to maintain your functioning.

▶▶ Swim, walk, or use a ski machine on a regular basis. The low-impact workout will improve pain and fatigue, even on days when you already feel tired and achy. Stay away from sports that punish your joints.

▶▶ Take stock of your posture. Pain, especially in the upper body, can send you slipping into bad form—which places additional stress on joints and surrounding muscles. Sometimes you can correct the problem simply by cultivating an awareness of your body, but if you need further help, try instruction in the Alexander Technique. Good posture is especially necessary for those with ankylosing spondylitis, a disease that affects the spine.

▶ Heat and cold therapies are reliable methods of treating joint pain. A lot of people like paraffin dips for sore hands, feet, and elbows. When you're actively inflamed, however, you should avoid heat. Instead, use cold packs to bring down the swelling. You can also use cold therapies after physical exertion to reduce your risk of a flare-up.

▶ For relaxation, pain control, and loosening of spasm around joints, get a gentle massage of your soft tissues. This is a nice therapy to use on a regular basis, but you should avoid direct massage of the joints when you're inflamed.

DISTRACTING YOUR NERVOUS SYSTEM FROM PAIN

▶▶ I highly recommend acupuncture for the pain, anxiety, and sleep disruption associated with inflammatory joint diseases. I've seen many people improve with acupuncture, and preliminary scientific evidence—we're still waiting for outcomes of large, controlled trials—points toward its efficacy.

▶▶ Cultivate the higher therapies, which draw on your mind's power to control pain. If you can get lost in books, games, or movies, you may be able to reduce your need for pain medication. Better still are expressive arts, such as painting, playing the piano, or writing in a journal, which can give voice to your problems and transport you out of them at the same time.

▶ If there's one particular joint that bothers you on a continual, long-term basis, TENS can be very helpful. I don't recommend it for pain that tends to come and go, nor do many people find it effective for pain in the extremities.

HEALING ENERGY

▶▶ Try homeopathy. A double-blind study of forty-six patients in Scotland tested homeopathic remedies on rheumatoid arthritis sufferers; those who received the remedies reported less pain, tenderness, and stiffness than their counterparts who were given a placebo. They also demonstrated increased grip strength. *Rhus toxicodendron* is the most popular homeopathic remedy for RA, but you should consult with a practitioner for an individual treatment.

PAIN PILLS AND OTHER PHARMACEUTICALS

The information below is about pain relief only, not about the many pharmaceuticals used to treat the various inflammatory diseases themselves.

▶▶ For mild to moderate daily pain, NSAIDs and acetaminophen are the pills of choice. Ask your doctor about a prescription for the new COX-2 inhibitors, which are easier on the stomach.

▶ Steroidal anti-inflammatory drugs are used to treat the disease itself; in doing so, they also undercut the pain. But although steroids are an important part of your medical program, it may not be appropriate to rely on them as your sole pharmaceutical method of pain relief. These drugs can cause serious side effects, including diabetes and bone thinning, so it's usually in your best interest to find other drugs to be used specifically for pain control. Sometimes it's wise to combine NSAIDs with a short-acting opioid such as Percocet or Vicodin for a brief but intense flare-up. When the pain goes on for months at a time, longer-acting opioids can bring it under control.

DEEP INJECTIONS, IMPLANTS, AND SURGERY

▶ When joints are truly deformed or nonfunctional, it's time to consider joint reconstruction or replacement. Although I'm not a big fan of surgery for pain, joint procedures are an exception. As surgeries go, they are effective and safe. By restoring movement, they allow you to stay active for as long as possible. For more information about joint replacement surgery, see pages 269–270.

17.

IRRITABLE BOWEL SYNDROME

Irritable bowel syndrome, often abbreviated IBS, is a common disorder that affects between 15 and 20 percent of the population. People with IBS—a population sure to include many of your co-workers and neighbors—experience a constellation of gastrointestinal symptoms: abdominal pain, bloating, gas, mucus in the stools, diarrhea, or diarrhea alternating with constipation. Although it is not a degenerative disease and will not cause harm to your digestive tract, the pain and indignity of IBS can be life-disrupting.

In a healthy gastrointestinal system, regular contractions of smooth muscle tissue propel waste matter through the colon (also known as the large intestine). In IBS, those contractions become erratic. They may be so forceful that diarrhea or even stool incontinence results; at other times, they are so weak that the sufferer is constipated. In either case, bowel movements become unpredictable and painful, and the abdomen may cramp up severely.

As yet, there is no adequate physiological explanation of IBS. It is not an inflammatory disease, nor is it associated with a progressive illness such as cancer or Crohn's disease. The colon appears normal, without any polyps, ulcers, or tumors. Because an organic cause is not clear, many doctors and alternative practitioners believe this disorder is purely a bodily response to emotional stress.

There's a profound truth to the stress-IBS connection, one that shows up in our everyday language: When we're about to give a public performance, we speak of butterflies in the stomach; when we look down from a tall building, we say that our bellies are turning flips. These clichés aren't just meaningless figures of speech. They speak to anxiety as a physical experience, one that is often felt directly in the digestive system. The lower gastrointestinal tract houses almost as many nerves as the brain does, so it's no wonder that so many of us suffer from "nervous stomachs," especially given the pressures of contemporary life.

Yet IBS is not *just* about stress. Certain foods seem to set off intestinal contractions or to slow them down. Fatty, greasy foods stimulate contractions in almost everyone; some people also react badly to dairy products, sugar, and other items. An important step in reducing your symptoms is learning which foods make you feel worse and then avoiding them.

IBS also appears to involve some disorder in nerve functioning. The exact cause or causes remain unknown, but it's clear that in people with IBS, the communication between the brain and the colon is damaged. Some experts speculate that the nerves leading to the colon are somehow sensitized, so that they send out messages of pain even when bowel movements are absolutely normal. The controversial drug alosetron (Lotronex) addresses this physiological component of IBS, although no one is precisely sure of the drug's mechanism of action—or why it helps only one slice of the IBS population: women for whom diarrhea is the predominant symptom. When it was first introduced in 2000, Lotronex improved the lives of many women, relieving their diarrhea and abdominal pain to a great extent. Later that year, it was discovered that the drug had potential life-threatening gastrointestinal side effects and it was pulled off the market, but some patients who had benefited from it were so upset that they agitated for its continued production. Through an unusual ruling by the Food and Drug Administration, it is being made available again, though at a lower dose, and with many warnings for both patients and doctors regarding its use. There is now a new drug, tegaserod (Zelnorm), which was approved by the FDA in July 2002, for treatment of constipation-predominant IBS and has been proven to speed the transit of digesting food and relieve pain. It does this by blocking the reuptake of serotonin—the chemical manufactured by nerves in the intestines that is an important factor in controlling contractions of the colon. The most common side effects are headache, abdominal pain, diarrhea, and nausea.

Some doctors prescribe antispasmodic medications in the hopes of slowing the transit time of waste through the bowel, but these drugs are losing favor among both physicians and patients because of the trade-off they present: limited effectiveness in exchange for strong side effects, including sleepiness, dry mouth, rapid heartbeat, and urinary retention. Some people find that over-the-counter diarrheal medications and laxatives help relieve symptoms, but you need to be wary of using bowel drugs on a regular basis, as it's possible to become dependent on them.

Despite the dearth of safe effective medications, the situation is not as disastrous as it sounds. Although IBS can rarely be cured, its symptoms can often be managed very well with gentle care. Treatments such as yoga, breathing, hypnosis, and biofeedback are stress-reducing; they may also have some effect on the sensitization of nerves and control of the gastrointestinal tract. Nutritional strategies that help you pinpoint and eliminate the foods that irritate your gut may surprise even long-term sufferers with their efficacy. Once you have those strategies incorporated into your lifestyle, supplements and other treatments such as acupuncture offer additional hope.

TESTING, TESTING

Lots of people with IBS are too embarrassed to see their doctor, but you really do need to rule out other causes of your symptoms, including inflammatory bowel disease and even cancer. I suggest a good internist or gastroenterologist (a specialist in the digestive system). The examination should include the following:

▶ A detailed medical history and explanation of your symptoms. This is an especially good time to use the pain diary in Chapter 4; it's smart to track IBS symptoms other than pain, such as diarrhea and constipation, in your notes. Plan to use the diary for at least a week to ten days.

▶ A stool sample. This test checks for hidden blood and will rule out colon cancer.

▶ An endoscopy, a general term for a variety of tests in which a body part is viewed through a flexible tube. (Here, the tube is inserted into the anus; how far it extends depends on the particular test. Your doctor should decide which specific test is appropriate for you.) An endoscopy will reveal any polyps, ulcers, or tumors that may be present.

BY ANY OTHER NAME, IT STILL HURTS

The symptoms of irritable bowel have always been with us, but the names of the disorder have changed several times over the years. Although "irritable bowel syndrome" is now the preferred term, you may still find some of the other names in use, including the following:

- Functional bowel disorder
- Gastric colitis
- Intestinal neurosis
- Irritable colon
- Mucous colitis
- Nervous indigestion
- Spastic bowel
- Spastic colon

THERAPIES

MIND-BODY MEDICINE

▶▶ Yoga, with its combination of physical activity and focused breathing, is ideal for IBS sufferers. If you're looking for a more portable stress-buster, learn a few breathing techniques (see Chapter 8) and use them whenever you need a mental break.

▶ Hypnosis and biofeedback can also help you control the pain and possibly your gastrointestinal functioning.

NUTRITION AND SUPPLEMENTS

For recommended doses of supplements, see Chapter 9.

▶▶ Pay close attention to your diet. You'll probably find that certain foods take the edge off your symptoms, while others lead to a flare-up. Foods that are fried, greasy, or high in fat tend to make people feel worse; so do caffeinated drinks, especially coffee, and alcoholic beverages.

▶▶ It is also possible that your symptoms are the result of a food allergy or intolerance. See "Can Food Allergies Cause Pain?" on page 135. Then check the usual suspects: Wheat and dairy are among the more common IBS triggers, but corn, soy, eggs, citrus, and nuts can also irritate the gastrointestinal tract. Some sufferers find that they cannot tolerate certain sugars: Lactose (found in dairy products), fructose (especially high-fructose corn syrup), and sorbitol (an artificial sweetener often used in gum and mints) can cause malabsorption of foods, bringing distention, diarrhea, bloating, and flatulence with it. Some people will also feel worse if they eat a large helping of fruit at one sitting. Try eliminating each of these potential triggers from your diet for a week at a time to see if you feel better. If you have difficulty tolerating dairy products, you can try Lactaid or a similar product before drinking milk or eating cheese to reduce irritation, but avoiding the offending product altogether is more likely to bring you success.

▶▶ Increase the amount of fiber in your diet. That may sound counterintuitive if you suffer from diarrhea, but natural fiber will form bulk in your digestive tract and normalize the transit time of food as it passes through your system. Vegetables, whole grains, and fruits are all good sources (but do make sure that you're not allergic to or intolerant of wheat or citrus). Since you could temporarily exacerbate your symptoms by making a sudden switch to a high-fiber diet, start slowly, adding a few extra servings a day for a week or so and then gradually increasing your intake. Most doctors as well as naturopaths will agree with me that a diet high in fiber and low in the irritating foods listed above is one of the most effective known IBS treatments. However, you should know that some people experience additional gastrointestinal symptoms, especially flatulence and bloating, when they eat cruciferous vegetables such as broccoli and cauliflower, or when they add other high-fiber products such as beans to their diet. If you're one of those people, a tablespoon of a bran fiber supplement, taken two or three times a day, may be a more pleasant solution. When buying a bran fiber product, read the label to make sure it doesn't contain potential irritants such as sorbitol or fructose.

DON'T BE AN ELIMINATION-DIET EXTREMIST

On the subject of diet, a word of caution. When food is so deeply connected to pain, it's easy to develop a fanatical approach to eating. I've seen several IBS sufferers force themselves onto unnecessarily strict diets, in the belief that nearly all foods are toxic and likely to bring on their symptoms. You may have seen extreme examples of the type—they're the ones who attend dinner parties armed with long lists of foods they can't eat, and who lecture fellow shoppers in the grocery store on their purchases. Such a pinched attitude tends to deprive people of nutritious foods they need, not to mention the pleasure of dining and good company. Do your best to walk the fine line between avoiding real IBS triggers and becoming an elimination-diet junkie.

- I suggest that most of my IBS patients try enteric-coated capsules of peppermint oil. The peppermint relaxes the smooth muscle of the colon and quiets the pain. Make sure to use the coated capsules, which dissolve only when they reach the intestines. Take three to six capsules every day, between meals.

- Some people with IBS lack enough of the bacteria that occur naturally in their lower intestines, so supplements of acidophilus and bifidus bacteria may help to normalize the gastrointestinal system. Take as directed on the package for at least two weeks.

- Herbal teas make a good substitute for caffeinated beverages and offer closure to a meal. Chamomile, ginger, mint, and slippery elm teas each have mild soothing effects on the digestive system and on the psyche. Ginger tea also eases nausea.

- If you have trouble getting to sleep, try valerian before bedtime; if it's tension that's keeping you awake, you may wish to use kava instead (but don't use kava for long periods of time).

PAIN PILLS AND OTHER PHARMACEUTICALS

- You can ask your doctor about prescription antispasmodics to relieve diarrhea, but as I've already noted, they don't have a great track record and can cause side effects that are as unpleasant as the IBS symptoms themselves. I often suggest over-the-counter preparations such as Imodium and Pepto-Bismol, tried-and-true medications that can calm diarrhea. However, it's always preferable to treat chronic diarrhea symptoms through dietary modification, since you can become dependent on bowel drugs.

▶ Be wary of laxatives and enemas. People who overuse these substances may find that they can no longer have bowel movements without them. Instead, increase your intake of dietary fiber; if that doesn't work, take a bran supplement. As a temporary remedy only, you can also try the stool softener Colace or a bulk-forming laxative such as Metamucil, both of which are available over the counter.

PHYSICAL THERAPIES

▶▶ Swim, jog, hike, walk . . . find a cardiovascular activity you enjoy and do it three or four times a week. Exercise is one of the best ways to increase the serotonin and endorphins that decrease pain; it also encourages digestive regularity.

▶▶ Gentle massage feels wonderful when your midsection is crampy and painful. The therapist can work directly over your belly if you like; some people report that massage of their lower back and hips is even better.

HEALING ENERGY

▶▶ Too many IBS sufferers don't have the chance to lie in peaceful stillness. If that sounds like you, and if you like the idea of healing touch, Reiki, Therapeutic Touch, or reflexology can provide the perfect opportunity to quiet down and relax.

▶▶ For those of you who feel too jumpy to breathe or meditate, tai chi can lend a physical, moving focus to your relaxation practice.

DISTRACTING YOUR NERVOUS SYSTEM FROM PAIN

▶▶ Most people don't think of acupuncture for IBS symptoms—and indeed there isn't yet any clinical proof of its effectiveness—but my experience has convinced me of its usefulness. One of the first things

I noticed when treating non-IBS patients with acupuncture is an unusual and welcome effect: In addition to the pain relief, patients who have been constipated before the treatment report that afterward they have their first bowel movement in days. I've also found that acupuncture can slow down diarrhea. These effects on digestive woes lead me to believe that acupuncture may regulate the gastrointestinal system (a benefit that acupuncturists have been claiming for centuries), perhaps reversing some of the nerve sensitization that occurs in the gut. Although plain acupuncture is beneficial for many people, IBS patients often appreciate the additional soothing quality of warmth during treatment. You might ask your acupuncturist about a treatment called moxibustion that combines the usual needle placement with the pouring of sand or small gravel into the navel. The Chinese herb mugwort is placed on top of the sand or gravel and then lit with a match, indirectly heating the sand, which warms your belly. (Your skin is never directly heated.) Another warming technique is to heat the needles with a stick of lighted mugwort during treatment.

▶ If you'd like to use some acupressure at home, try rubbing the inside edge of your foot, from the ankle up to the big toe, to encourage relaxation and good digestion. For nausea, try massaging the point P 6, located at the center of your inside wrist. (See Appendix C.)

▶ Aromatherapy may ease the pain. Surround yourself with calming scents like lavender, rose, sandalwood, or bergamot.

KAREN'S STORY: PREVENTING "ONE OF THOSE DAYS"

Karen, a forty-something executive, was so full of energy that she could barely sit still in my office. I'd walk in and she'd be swinging her legs from the examining table or pacing the floor, flipping through the brochures set out on the desk. Her hands constantly tapped against her thighs, as if Karen were typing out secret messages to herself.

No doubt this dynamic quality helped Karen ascend to the upper ranks of her firm at a relatively young age, but sometimes her surplus

(continued)

of energy transformed itself into anxiety, which in turn affected her gut. She experienced bouts of diarrhea, flatulence, and bloating that were sometimes merely annoying but sometimes devastating. When she was having "one of those days," she would call in sick to work, fearing she couldn't control her bowels long enough to dash from her office to a bathroom. She'd been helped by Lotronex—until it was taken off the market. She tried propantheline and Bentyl (dicyclomine), two prescription antispasmodics, but they made her dizzy and weak. Imodium helped somewhat, but not enough to control the bad flare-ups. When a previous doctor made the connection between Karen's obvious agitation and her pain, she prescribed Xanax to help Karen calm down. It worked well enough to improve her state of mind and cut back significantly on missed work days. After a few months of taking the drug, however, Karen realized that she had difficulty falling asleep without it. Afraid she'd become dependent, she was looking for another way to control her nervousness and IBS.

Karen was a hard-nosed businesswoman with no patience for acupuncture, breathing techniques, or—heaven forbid!—Reiki. She wanted a pharmaceutical to help her, and I wished I could give her one. But she'd already worked her way through the conventional drugs for her IBS symptoms.

"Taking a pill appeals to you, but I don't have any new prescription medications to offer you," I remarked. "How would you feel about taking a supplement instead?" I told her that capsules of peppermint oil might relax her spastic digestive tract. They have a very low risk of side effects and don't feel as "weird" as acupuncture or other alternatives. Karen felt more comfortable with this therapy than with any of the other possibilities for IBS. When I asked her about ways to control stress, I discovered that several of Karen's friends took a yoga class together. She agreed to join them and found that the combination of activity and relaxation soothed her restless spirit without requiring her to sit still for long periods of time.

When I last saw Karen, she was still hoping for a pharmaceutical treatment that would completely prevent her symptoms or even cure the disorder altogether. She's promised to stay in touch in case a promising new drug hits the market. In the meanwhile, it's taking no more than two simple treatments—peppermint oil and yoga—to manage her diarrhea and anxiety. She misses work now and then, but "those days" are now much fewer and farther between.

18.

NECK PAIN

MUSCLE TENSION / WHIPLASH / ARTHRITIS AND DEGENERATED DISCS

I love to see people with neck pain. Not because I'm happy they hurt, of course, but because I'm so optimistic that they can feel better. Neck pain is one of those disorders that really show what alternative therapies, especially the physical ones, can do. Special techniques for moving, stretching, manipulating, and massaging often bring pain levels down several notches. Better still, it feels great when the space between your discs opens up or when knots of neck and shoulder muscles loosen their grip. Maybe that's why these therapies remain outside the mainstream; it's hard for us to believe that such simple and pleasurable interventions can have such dramatic effects.

The neck is a highly vulnerable area of the body—a flexible structure sitting above the relatively inflexible rib cage and thoracic spine, which is a target for arthritis as well as disc degeneration. To make matters more complicated, the spinal cord runs just behind the discs of the neck. This means that an injury to the area may produce paralysis or severe malfunction, and it adds an extra element of risk to invasive techniques such as surgery.

Because the nerves leading to the arms also run through the neck, people with neck pain may suffer problems with their arms or hands. In addition, they must deal with a host of everyday consequences: If you can't move your neck and head easily, driving and sleeping pose real challenges. And it's hard to feel normal when you can't turn your head to look at someone in conversation.

There are three common sources of neck pain: muscle tension, whiplash and its aftereffects, and degenerative changes in the upper spine. Many people have a combination of these problems, so make sure your doctor doesn't rest on one diagnosis before thoroughly checking you out.

MUSCLE TENSION

The neck is where many of us deposit tension and stress, and in fact people with neck pain tend to fit the classic type A personality: hard-driving, always busy, tense and jittery. Here in New York, where the population is famously type A, I don't think I've met a person yet who had loose, supple neck and shoulder muscles. If you have neck pain, learning to manage stress is a crucial part of treatment, no matter where you live.

Stress is not the only cause of muscle tension. Poor posture and undue physical strain can send neck muscles into spasm before you can say *ergonomics*. Habitually sticking your neck out, cradling the telephone receiver between your ear and neck, or working at a computer screen that's too low are all easy ways to develop neck pain.

Most people find it hard to relax their neck muscles. You can't simply command them to loosen up—you'll probably need to draw on a combination of methods that address different aspects of the tension. Postural therapies help, as do mind-body work, acupressure, massage, stretching, and exercise.

WHIPLASH

Whiplash describes the motion that occurs in a certain kind of injury, usually an auto accident. When you're hit from behind, your neck may be thrown backward against your upper back, far beyond its range of motion. Then the neck recoils to the front—like a whip lashing—so that your chin lands on your chest. The sudden and extreme movement sprains or strains the soft tissues of the neck. You may leave the accident feeling fine but develop stiffness and pain the next day.

In a very few cases, whiplash destabilizes the neck, meaning that its injured muscles, ligaments, or connective tissues are no longer able to hold the vertebrae in place. The bones may move in directions they're not supposed to go; instead of sitting sandwiched between its neighboring top and bottom vertebrae, for example, a bone might slide forward. (If you've ever seen someone's knee shift out to the side when walking, you've seen an example of a destabilized joint.) The unfortunate people who suffer from a destabilized neck need to have their heads held rigid so that their tissues can heal and grow strong enough to keep the vertebrae in their proper alignment. This is accomplished with a halo, a metal structure attached to the skull with metal screws and secured to an upper chest brace.

However, the vast majority of whiplash sufferers do *not* experience instability. Far from requiring immobilization of the neck, most stable whiplash patients will benefit from aggressive physical therapy right away, including range-of-motion exercises, strengthening, and stretching. These exercises improve the mobility of the spine and prevent it from degenerating into a stiff, contracted, and weakened state as the injuries heal.

When the symptoms of whiplash don't disappear within a few weeks, the case is considered chronic. The neck becomes very hard to move, and you may feel like the Tin Woodsman. ("Oil can!" one of my stiff-necked whiplash patients said to me the other day, out of the side of her mouth.) The sad irony of many chronic whiplash patients I see is that their problem stems less from the injury than from improper treatment in the first place. Too often, patients respond to an acute case of whiplash with the misplaced fear that they will damage their spinal cord by moving their neck (and sometimes they are encouraged in this by well-meaning health care professionals). I can appreciate this fear—the neck is a scary site in which to sustain an injury—but patients who do not suffer destabilization aren't at risk for spinal cord injury. When fear of injury takes over, often compounded by lingering emotional upset from the accident, whiplash victims may feel too daunted or traumatized to seek the physical therapy they need. Instead, they rest in bed, or they wear one of those soft cervical collars. Both strategies further weaken the already stressed muscles and other soft tissues. As these tissues degenerate from too much rest, the pain and stiffness grow worse. Because the neck muscles aren't doing their share of the work, the shoulder muscles pull extra duty. Soon enough, they begin to hurt, too. This extra pain leads the person to treat the neck even more delicately—and the cycle continues.

The good news is that it's never too late to receive the physical therapy you should have had earlier. That, along with other chiropractic and other physical techniques, can bring many people back to normal. These therapies can feel wonderfully therapeutic, so enjoy them.

SOFT CERVICAL COLLARS: MORE HARM THAN GOOD?

Whiplash and soft collars: Sometimes it seems you can't have one without the other. But do soft collars really help the injured person? They certainly don't provide orthopedic stability or prevent spinal cord damage; for that, you need a halo or the kind of hard plastic collar emergency workers use on patients who may have sustained serious neck trauma. Soft collars may relieve some of the pain of whiplash by keeping the neck warm—but you can easily, and more comfortably, accomplish that with a hot pack. Most likely, the principal benefit of soft collars is psychological: People who've hurt their necks tend to feel fragile and frightened. Even when they are not at risk for spinal cord injury, they can't help worrying that with a turn of the neck, they could find themselves paralyzed. Soft collars offer a sense of protection from these worries, but that protection is mostly illusory. Soft collars can't prevent spinal cord injury, nor do whiplash victims with stable neck structures need protection in the first place.

If soft collars offered nothing better or worse than comfort, I wouldn't be so concerned about their widespread use. But soft collars can be dangerous. They take over the work of the neck muscles and other soft tissues; when these tissues are no longer exercised by holding up the head or moving from side to side, they weaken and degenerate—even after just a few days. When the collar comes off, the neck feels even stiffer and more fragile.

Unfortunately, most emergency rooms continue to hand out soft cervical collars to whiplash victims as a matter of routine. This practice likely persists because it's an old tradition, one that makes patients—most of whom are reeling from a car accident or other trauma—feel safe and cared for. Obviously, I discourage this habit, as it so often prolongs the pain as well as the inevitable time needed in physical therapy.

A final word on whiplash: It's well known that people with protracted neck injury lawsuits tend not to heal successfully. One study showed that of patients whose cases were settled within six months, 83 percent were completely healed a year after the accident. But of those whose cases weren't settled until eighteen months later, only 38 percent were healed after *five years*.

I doubt that these sufferers are faking their pain. Instead, I think this evidence reveals the role of the mind in recovery. It's harder to draw on the mind's healing power when you have some motivation—like money, or avoiding a difficult job or family situation—for staying sick. Moreover, the longer you think of yourself as a wounded person, the greater the chance that you will become comfortable with this notion. The initial motivation for staying sick is replaced with another one: a self-image as an invalid. Some people even find that suffering gives them a special identity, a distinguishing mark.

If your pain from whiplash seems unduly prolonged, you may wish to make an honest appraisal of your situation. Are there any factors that make it advantageous for you to stay injured? Are there any reasons your mind may be holding you back from healing? If so, then you need to change your life—maybe call off the lawyers, find a more satisfying career, seek family counseling—so that your body can mend.

ARTHRITIS AND DEGENERATED DISCS

Both arthritis and disc degeneration are a normal part of aging and occur in almost every person over forty; some people feel pain as a result, while others are not bothered at all. When it comes to neck problems, I suggest that people approach arthritis and disc degeneration in much the same way they would if it were to appear anywhere else in the body: Stay moving, keep the tendons and ligaments from binding down, and work on your range of motion. However, you should also know that degenerative changes can have more severe consequences when they appear in the neck, because of the presence of the spinal cord. If the bones shift too much, or if the soft tissues become swollen, these structures can place pressure on the spinal cord, with resulting loss of motor control, balance, or ability to walk. Most likely, you will not suffer these problems, but you should be familiar with their early warning signs: patchy numbness or tingling; numbness or tingling down the arm or hand; or loss of balance or coordination. If you experience any of these symptoms, call your doctor immediately.

A second consideration for people with degenerative disease in the neck is the possibility of misdiagnosis. Here's a scenario I see frequently: A patient feels neck pain and goes to see the doctor, who orders X rays. The films show degeneration in the upper spine, so both doctor and patient conclude that arthritis is the source of the pain.

Yet that conclusion may well be in error. As I discussed in Chapter 15, degenerative changes don't always result in pain. If you took a hundred older adults out of the general population and gave them an MRI, almost all of them would reveal wear and tear in the cartilage and discs—but only about 20 percent would tell you they felt pain. So it's entirely possible that the pain you feel is unrelated to degeneration. It may well be the result of muscular tension, or it may be that muscular tension is combining with degeneration to produce the pain. If you have not had the muscles of your neck and shoulders examined for tightness, spasm, or trigger points, you should do so, even if you know for sure that some of your pain is coming from arthritis. A correct diagnosis—which may include *both* arthritis and muscle pain—can point the way toward more effective pain relief.

NECK PAIN AND HEADACHES

Tension in the neck and shoulders can also produce a cervicogenic headache, which is often felt at the back of the head. The therapies listed here can help relieve these headaches as well as neck pain. For more information, see Chapter 14.

TESTING, TESTING

If you've had whiplash or another form of acute neck injury, you need an X ray or CAT scan to make sure the neck is stable. This procedure should be performed immediately after the injury.

In all cases of neck pain—no matter what seems to be the cause—your doctor should give you a neurological exam to rule out trouble in the nervous system. This is an important but simple procedure that involves checking your reflexes and scratching the soles of your feet lightly.

If you are elderly, then it's reasonable, although not always necessary, for your doctor to order an MRI or CAT scan, just to check for any problems in the central nervous system. You might also need X rays to look for hidden fractures or tumors.

DO YOU HAVE TRIGGER POINTS?

Trigger points are knots or taut bands of muscle that feel tender when pressed; they also produce pain that radiates to another part of your body. They are frequent contributors to neck pain. Luckily, there are several treatments that can release trigger points and significantly reduce aches and sleeplessness. For more information about trigger points and their treatment, see Chapter 24, "Myofascial Pain Syndrome."

THERAPIES

PHYSICAL THERAPIES

▶▶ Everyone with neck pain, no matter what the cause, must perform stretching and strengthening exercises on a regular basis. As long as you don't suffer from instability in the area, you can start with the exercises in Appendix A, but it's best to see your doctor or physical therapist for an individually tailored plan. If you suffer from whiplash, sessions with a good physical therapist are a necessity.

▶▶ Monitor your posture throughout the day. Lots of people hold their head forward, so that the neck and shoulder muscles strain to hold up the weight. This posture is brutal on the musculature—it's as if you're trying to pump iron while leaning sideways and standing on tiptoe. Check other habits as well. Are you bending your neck downward to see your computer screen? Carrying a heavy purse, briefcase, or backpack? Cradling the phone receiver between your shoulder and ear? All of these things can cause spasms and trigger points.

▶▶ Neck pain can feel disabling, but don't let it keep you from regular cardiovascular exercise. Swimming is a good choice, because the water lends your neck muscles support as you turn your head. (Be sure to turn your head in both directions to get the full benefit.) I *don't* recommend cycling on the road, since the forward motion tends to encourage straining the neck muscles, but stationary cycling is fine.

▶▶ Massage of the neck and shoulders helps free up the soft tissues that may otherwise bind up in response to pain. Again, if your neck is unstable, you should not receive massage.

▶▶ One of the best reasons to use spinal manipulation therapy is for chronic whiplash. See an experienced chiropractor or osteopath who will follow SMT up with stretches and exercise. (People who've just suffered whiplash should wait at least a week before receiving SMT.)

▶▶ Postural therapies will help you use your neck and shoulders without straining the muscles. I like the Alexander Technique for pain related to poor posture; the Feldenkrais Method is better suited for pain resulting from whiplash and other trauma.

▶▶ Give traction a try. It feels marvelous on compressed muscles and joints and is especially good for opening up the space around pinched nerves. Check with your doctor before using this therapy. Although it's safe for most people, it can be harmful to those with moderate to serious joint degeneration or otherwise unstable necks.

SCHLOCK THERAPY

When shopping around for a physical therapist, be on the lookout for "shlock therapy," a careless version of the real thing. A dedicated therapist may begin with heat, massage, or ice to get your neck muscles ready for action; he may employ these techniques again at the end of the session to decrease any post-workout soreness. His main focus, however, should be the active work of helping you stretch and become mobilized; he should coach you through exercises that are designed for *your* pain and *your* body. Schlock therapy, on the other hand, is characterized by the sole use of passive methods. You might receive nothing more than some electrical stimulation, followed by a hasty massage or a hot pack. Little is demanded of the therapist or of you—and "little" accurately describes the level of pain relief this kind of treatment provides.

DISTRACTING YOUR NERVOUS SYSTEM FROM PAIN

▶▶ Acupressure temporarily blocks pain signals while reducing muscular tension. I like the deeper forms for neck and shoulder pain, especially shiatsu and Jin Shin Do. For a home-care treatment, try the Catwalk for Head, Neck, and Shoulder Pain on page 151–152.

▶ Practitioners of acupuncture often notice a kind of sympathy between their therapy and pain from accidents or trauma—that is, the acupuncture appears to address components of the painful experience that go unresolved by other treatments. Perhaps acupuncture regulates elements of the nervous system that have been thrown into disorder by the trauma. If you suffer from persistent whiplash pain, acupuncture could be a smart choice for you.

NUTRITION AND SUPPLEMENTS

For recommended doses of supplements, see Chapter 9.

▶▶ Chronic muscle pain can be caused by a low-grade magnesium deficiency. Take a supplement every day and consume plenty of low-fat dairy products, green leafy vegetables, and whole grains.

▶ If insomnia contributes to your pain, try valerian before going to bed. If anxiety is keeping you up at night, use kava instead (but don't take kava for extended periods of time).

MIND-BODY MEDICINE

▶▶ When you just can't unclench your neck and shoulder muscles, biofeedback can show you how.

▶▶ Imagining that your muscles are melting or other guided imagery techniques can help you release chronic muscle tension.

▶▶ If you're one of those always-moving type A personalities, you might not like the idea of sitting down to relax and meditate. Instead, try yoga or tai chi, which are forms of moving meditation. The movements may also open up the neck and shoulder region. (If you practice yoga, make sure to do so gently. Stay away from poses that put pressure on your neck.)

▶ If you think that you might be clinging to your pain as a form of self-identity or as a way to avoid tough problems, consider cognitive-behavioral therapy. It can help you engage in more productive thought patterns. I also suggest reading *Why People Don't Heal and How They Can* by Caroline Myss.

HEALING ENERGY

▶ I've had good success with Reiki for chronic muscle tightness in the neck.

▶ Tai chi relaxes muscles and improves posture.

PAIN PILLS AND OTHER PHARMACEUTICALS

▶ Over-the-counter pain relievers such as aspirin and ibuprofen are enough for most people.

▶ When neck muscles get really tense, occasional use of muscle relaxants such as baclofen or diazepam (Valium) makes sense. You don't want to get dependent on these drugs, however, so be sure to address the root problem with physical therapies and mind-body work.

▶ If the pain you're feeling seems too high for the level of damage you've experienced, the nervous system may be sending out intensified messages of pain. Small doses of anticonvulsants or tricyclic antidepressants can help quiet down these messages.

▶ If you have moderate to severe pain from disc degeneration, anticonvulsants or opioids may be appropriate. Don't feel shy about taking opioids for severe pain if you and your doctor agree that you need them.

▶ Many neurologists like to prescribe steroidal anti-inflammatory drugs for five or seven days, when an acutely inflamed nerve or disc is suspected as a cause of the pain. This treatment will sometimes stop the pain altogether. But as always, try gentler therapies first.

DEEP INJECTIONS, IMPLANTS, AND SURGERY

▶ Pain from disc degeneration can be temporarily relieved or even halted by a cervical epidural injection of steroid and anesthetic medication. These shots are especially useful if an inflamed disc is pressing on or irritating a nerve. You should know that the risks of complications from epidurals go up when they're used in the neck region; be sure to see an anesthesiologist who is experienced in giving shots in this area.

19.

FIBROMYALGIA

"But is there anything *wrong* with you?" is a question fibromylagia sufferers must learn to field on a frequent basis. The short version of the answer is simply "Yes, there is."

Fibromyalgia is characterized by chronic, widespread—and very real—muscle pain, along with sleep disorders and general fatigue. Minor activities, such as reaching into a high kitchen cabinet, become deeply painful, and more prolonged tasks can drain away every ounce of strength and endurance, no matter how much willpower you employ. You may feel that your body is no longer under your control, as if your muscles and bones are dissolving. Headache and irritable bowel syndrome may appear alongside the other symptoms, creating additional disability.

Yet you may look perfectly healthy on the outside, nor can anything obviously wrong be found on the inside to explain the pain and weakness. There is no inflammation and no degeneration of tissues. So what's going on?

Fibromyalgia has been with us for a long, long time. Diffuse, inexplicable muscular pain is described in writings throughout history; those symptoms were first identified as a medical syndrome in the early 1800s, when it was called fibrositis. (You may still hear that term used today.) In 1990, the American College of Rheumatology officially included fibromyalgia in its canon of disorders and described criteria for its diagnosis. For a diagnosis to be made, you must experience pain in at least eleven of eighteen "tender points" throughout the body when those spots are pressed, and the additional symptom of unexplained widespread pain must be present for at least three months. Other diseases with similar symptoms, such as lupus and rheumatoid arthritis, must also be ruled out.

These criteria establish fibromyalgia as a legitimate disease, meaning that your doctor and your loved ones should take it seriously. Indeed, it's the second most common diagnosis that rheumatologists make; the National Institutes of Health estimate that 3.7 million adults over age eighteen suffer from fibromyalgia. (The disorder is more common in middle-aged women, although it can strike either sex at any age.)

Although these diagnostic criteria are helpful, they don't explain *why* the pain exists. For the most part, fibromyalgia is one of those disorders that lives in the realm of mystery. It points out how little about the body and mind we really understand, and doctors and patients alike need to accept it with a certain amount of humility and even wonder. That doesn't mean that we shouldn't continue to look for answers.

There are signs that the pain is caused by alterations in the nervous system. Abnormally high levels of substance P, a neurotransmitter that facilitates pain signals, are found in people with fibromyalgia. Certain nerve receptors may also become hypersensitive to pain. And patients, who tend to have insomnia, may be deficient in slow-wave sleep. Without this deep rest, the sensory signals just don't fire properly. In all likelihood, the nervous system has gone awry in several ways, leading to a feeling of intense pain even when no injury has been done to the body's tissues. (For more information about the nervous system's role in pain, see Chapter 3.)

A significant number of fibromyalgia patients—perhaps one-third—report the onset of symptoms after a physical trauma, illness, virus, or period of emotional stress. It may be that these events trigger changes in the nervous system. It is also true that as many as 50 percent of patients have a history of depression, which may have a similar effect.

When I diagnose a new case of fibromyalgia, I usually explain that the diagnosis is a good-news/bad-news proposition. The bad news is that there *is* something wrong, and that it will require both lifestyle changes and persistent treatment. The patient must expect flare-ups now and then, especially after high levels of activity. In addition, she will have to prepare for skepticism from well-meaning friends and even from physicians, many of whom still do not accept the disorder. The good news is that the pain is not a sign of disease or degeneration. It is real, and it must be respected, but it does usually fade with time.

If you have fibromyalgia, you can greatly improve your comfort and level of functioning with a smart integrative plan. Gentle, graded exercises that are appropriate for your tolerance level are absolutely essential; they will prevent your muscles from becoming so deconditioned with disuse that they cause more pain. Physical activity will also give you more energy, will improve your sleep, and may help to normalize aspects of your nervous system. Mind-body therapies can assist in all these functions as well. For most patients, I also suggest low doses of tricyclic antidepressants or anticonvulsants to restore the deep stages of sleep. Beyond those basics, there are plenty of other options. I'm confident that with some experimentation you'll find the combination that's best for you.

TESTING, TESTING

The tender-point exam is the only test currently available for fibromyalgia. But you'll also need a workup by a rheumatologist or a thorough internist to rule out other possible disorders. You'll need several kinds of blood work, including a complete blood count, standard blood chemistry, thyroid function studies, Lyme test, and erythrocyte sedimentation rate and C-reactive protein tests (to measure inflammation).

TENDER POINTS

The "tender points" of fibromyalgia exist in pairs (one on the right side of your body and one on the left) at the following locations:

- Base of the skull
- Base of the neck
- Upper chest, a little more than an inch below the collarbone
- Along the top of the shoulder
- Upper back, close to the spine and about an inch below the preceding set of points

(continued)

- Inside of the elbows
- Lower back, close to the dimples above the buttocks
- Upper outside edge of the thigh
- Inside of the knees

If you are testing yourself for reaction to these points, you must touch them with enough pressure to whiten the tip of your fingernail. If you feel pain—not just tenderness, despite the name "tender points"—in at least eleven of these sites, you might have fibromyalgia.

THERAPIES

PHYSICAL THERAPIES

▶▶ Low-impact cardiovascular exercise *at a level appropriate for you* is a foundation of fibromyalgia treatment. Walking, cycling, swimming, water aerobics, or working out on an elliptical trainer are all good choices. I suggest that you see a physical therapist to determine the best level of activity for you. Too little will not produce benefits, while too much can bring on a disabling, and disheartening, flare-up.

▶▶ Gentle stretching and strengthening exercises, in addition to cardio, are also necessary. You can start with the exercises in Appendix A; perform them daily. Again, though, it's a good idea to see a physical therapist for a customized routine.

▶ Cold therapy is effective at reducing achiness after exercise or other exertion. It can also take some of the bite out of a flare-up. For general, all-over soreness, you might prefer the soothing quality of heat.

▶ Try getting Swedish massage on a regular basis. This light massage feels wonderful on sore muscles, but it also helps reduce substance P, increase pain-blocking endorphins, improve sleep, and reduce stress. (Most people with fibromyalgia report that the deeper massage techniques are too intense.)

PAIN PILLS AND OTHER PHARMACEUTICALS

▶▶ Tricyclic antidepressants and anticonvulsants are two of the best ways to normalize your sleep. They also reduce pain and fatigue, perhaps as a by-product of the sleep effect. Don't use sleeping pills or alcohol at night, as they will only run down your body further.

MIND-BODY THERAPIES

▶▶ Meditation appears to improve the symptoms of fibromyalgia, and it definitely helps you cultivate detachment from the stresses of chronic pain.

▶▶ Hypnosis is another good option. A paper in the *Journal of Rheumatology* showed that it decreased both the pain and fatigue of fibromyalgia.

▶▶ If the pain is taking over your life, consider cognitive-behavioral therapy. It will help you make a mental adjustment to the disorder so that it is less disruptive and stressful.

▶▶ Yoga is a wonderful way to combine relaxation with the gentle stretching and strengthening you need. Try a beginner's class—no power yoga for you—or one that's especially designed for rehabilitation.

NUTRITION AND SUPPLEMENTS

For recommended doses of supplements, see Chapter 9.

▶▶ Fibromyalgia places the body under heavy stress. Give yourself optimal support by following the basic pain-control diet outlined in Chapter 9. Be especially sure to reduce your consumption of pro-inflammation foods, including red meat and processed items, and increase your intake of oily fish, flaxseed, and walnuts. A good diet will also help get any coexisting symptoms of irritable bowel syndrome under control.

▶▶ Sometimes an allergy or other reaction to food can contribute to the symptoms of fibromyalgia. Read "Can Food Allergies Cause Pain?" on pages 135–136 and follow the recommendations there.

▶▶ Valerian, taken just before bed, is an old-fashioned remedy for insomnia. Kava is another sedative herb that can help, especially in cases of anxiety, but use it on an occasional basis only.

▶ Supplementation with ginger, turmeric, quercetin, fish-oil capsules, or gamma-linolenic acid (GLA) can reduce inflammation. I recommend you try these one at a time, so that you know what works and what doesn't. During a flare-up, you might wish to cook with additional ginger and tumeric as spices or drink ginger tea.

▶ For mild to moderate depression, St. John's wort is a reasonable alternative to conventional medications. Do not take this herb without consulting your doctor first.

▶ There are several supplements that have shown some promise in treating fibromyalgia but that remain controversial: DHEA, 5-HTP (5-hydroxytryptophan), calcitonin, and NADH (nicotinamide adenine dinucleotide, also known by the brand name Enada). If you've exhausted other measures and want to give these a try, fine—but do so only under your doctor's supervision.

HEALING ENERGY

▶ In a double-blind study, the homeopathy remedy *rhus toxicodendron* reduced pain at tender points by an average of 25 percent. The remedies *byronia* and *arnica* are also often used. For the best results, see a homeopath for an individualized remedy.

▶ I believe there's a special connection between the energetic touch remedies and mysterious ailments such as fibromyalgia. There may be a mechanism at work that we don't yet understand—which seems likely, given how little we know about both the treatments and the illness. You may wish to try Reiki, reflexology, or Therapeutic Touch.

DISTRACTING YOUR NERVOUS SYSTEM FROM PAIN

▶ Acupuncture distracts the nervous system by temporarily closing the pain gate, and it has an energetic quality that may reduce pain. Many patients find that acupuncturists, who do not assign illnesses to the same system of cause and effect as Western doctors, respond more sympathetically to fibromyalgia.

▶ Aromatherapy can take your mind off the pain for a while, and invigorating oils such as peppermint, lemon, and eucalyptus may help relieve fatigue.

RUTH'S STORY: PERSISTENCE PAYS OFF

Ruth, a woman in her twenties, is possessed of a drop-dead chic sense of style. She's usually so pulled together that I've learned to read her external appearance as a barometer of her physical state: When her nails aren't manicured, or if her handbag doesn't match her shoes, I know she's really hurting.

When Ruth first developed the deep aches of fibromyalgia, she tried to work through them at the gym, attending her regular stationary cycling classes. It didn't take long for her to abandon this strategy. On the nights after these workouts, her upper body—mainly her shoulders, neck, and right side—burned so fiercely that she couldn't sleep through the night, even though cycling hadn't taxed those muscles at all. She dropped the workouts, but the pain and disrupted sleep continued.

A few months into her diagnosis of fibromyalgia, Ruth was achy, tired, and saddened by the extent to which the pain had cut into her social life. If she paced herself, she could make it through her daily work as a college admissions director, but she no longer had the stamina for her favored social pursuit: hanging out in trendy bars (which were often standing room only and filled with smoke) with her friends in the evening. A man she was seeing, one she liked a great deal, stopped calling when exhaustion forced her to cancel several dates in succession. But Ruth didn't feel that she'd hit rock bottom until her family asked her to spend a long weekend at their lake house. They were all going to sand and paint their old boat together. When Ruth had to decline, her sisters were furious. "What is *wrong* with you?" they asked angrily, as if Ruth were inventing excuses to abstain from hard work. "Why are you being this way?"

That's when Ruth decided to seek help from a pain specialist. She told me that the disorder was "trashing the fundamentals" of her life. I

(continued)

started to explain that graduated, gentle exercises are the best known treatment for fibromyalgia, but Ruth stopped me with a frustrated shake of her head. "Every time I do something like work out or go on a date, I pay the price in pain," she said. Her insomnia was bad enough as it was. She didn't want exercise-related pain to interrupt her sleep further.

We decided to table the issue of exercise for a short while—but only a short while. In the meantime, she started low doses of Elavil, a tricyclic antidepressant that's helped many of my patients, to regulate her sleep. The medication worked somewhat, but she felt there was room for improvement. She bought some heavy fabric to drape over her windows at night; this helped muffle the city lights and noise that made sleep all the more elusive. At the same time, we switched her prescription to gabapentin, an anticonvulsant. I'm not sure whether it was the curtains or the new drug (or both) that did the trick, but Ruth reported waking up much more refreshed in the mornings.

Now that she was less tired, Ruth agreed to revisit the issue of exercise. Instead of going to the gym for an intense workout, she began slow stretching and toning exercises as prescribed by one of the clinic's physical therapists. Usually, fibromyalgia sufferers feel better when they ice down their muscles before and after working out. Ruth discovered that she ached less when she applied heat before physical therapy and ice afterward.

Ruth has just begun to take tai chi classes. The slow, controlled movements don't jeopardize her still-fragile sense of her body, and she enjoys the peace of mind that tai chi instills. She continues to sleep through the night most of the time, and her muscles burn much less. The all-over achiness remains, but it's intermittent now as opposed to constant. She needs time—more exercise (especially cardiovascular activity), more restful nights, more care and attention to the family problems that have become explicit since her diagnosis—before she'll be ready to reengage her social life. But I'm optimistic for Ruth. She doesn't give up when a therapy such as antidepressants or pre-exercise ice packs don't work out so well; instead, she tries again. Her patience and courage are heartening to me, and I believe these personal qualities will eventually see her through.

20.

CHRONIC SPRAINS, STRAINS, AND TENDINITIS (REPETITIVE STRAIN INJURIES)

Maybe your elbow hurts when you lift packages. Or there's a sharp pain in your shoulder whenever you swing a golf club or mash potatoes for dinner. Or perhaps it's your knee, or your ankle, or some other part of your body that hurts with certain movements. If you're like most people, you've tried to treat the problem: a little rest, some ice, a few capsules of ibuprofen ... but the pain hasn't gone away. Maybe it's been hanging around for years. Friends have told you it's a sign of aging or the inevitable result of a physically demanding job. So you keep moving, trying to ignore the pain.

If an area located near a joint hurts when you move it, and if that pain has been around for a while, you may have a sprain or strain that's gone chronic. Contrary to what you might have been told, you don't need to live with this disorder. In fact, treating the problem is absolutely necessary. Without good care, your tissues may undergo further damage.

A *sprain* is a tear or other injury to a ligament, the tissue that connects one bone to another. *Strains* are injuries to the muscles or to the tendons, which bind muscle to bone. (Irritation or inflammation of tendons, often as a result of trauma, is also called *tendinitis*.) Both sprains and strains can happen as a result of trauma or an accident, but they can also occur with long-term overuse. Using one part of the body over and over again for long periods of time can lead to repetitive stress injuries such as the famous tennis elbow or jumper's knee. Don't let the sports-related nicknames fool you; most people develop repetitive strain injuries on the job. People who work on assembly lines or who lift heavy packages are especially vulnerable.

How do you know if you have a sprain or strain? Sometimes you feel a fresh, stabbing pain at the moment of injury, but often the pain develops more gradually, so that you're not sure when exactly the problem began. In most cases, you hurt when you're using the joint. At rest, you may feel very little pain or none at all. Although bad sprains and strains can lead to swelling and bruising, lower-grade injuries can fool you. It's quite possible to have a sprain or strain without the soreness, tenderness, inflammation, or discoloration that accompanies other acute injuries.

The ideal treatment for an acute sprain or strain is RICE—immediate **r**est, **i**cing, **c**ompression, and **e**levation of the joint. Modalities such as ultrasound and pain relievers may also be used. But if the pain has lasted for more than a month, it is considered chronic and will require more thorough attention. The most important aspect of treatment is complete rest of the joint; your tissues will simply not improve unless you give them extra time to heal. Physical therapy and a good look at your nutritional status may also be in order, along with some pharmaceutical treatment.

Don't let anyone tell you that your sprain or strain is just a sign of getting older. Unlike many other disorders in this book, these pains have a clear underlying disorder—damage to a ligament, muscle, or tendon—that can be treated, usually by conservative measures.

YOU MAY BE A PROFESSIONAL ATHLETE (MINUS THE $400 MILLION CONTRACT)

Don strained his forearm while at work as a beverage delivery man. Every time he lifted a pallet of sodas, he felt a spark of pain travel down from his elbow. But he kept on lifting, half wondering if the pain was permanent. He was still going to work every day when he came to see me.

In his middle age, strapping but on the heavy side, it would have never occurred to Don to think of himself as an athlete. But in truth he

(continued)

was an athlete, and a professional one at that. When I told him this, his eyes nearly popped out. Don put his body under extreme conditions for a living—that's certainly the definition of a professional athlete to me. I explained that he'd need to give his body the same kind of attention and care an athlete would after an injury: He'd need to heal and then train himself to return to the field. This proposal made sense to him, and he agreed to a course of rehabilitation.

First, Don needed to rest the arm, just as an athlete would recover from an injury. He arranged to take a new delivery man on his route for a month. The trainee would lift the packages while Don showed him the ropes and talked with the store managers. After a few weeks of rest, Don was ready for physical therapy. Like a weight lifter, his body needed strength and endurance to handle repeated stress without injury; like a long-distance runner, he needed to know exactly where his body's limits were and how to pace himself. Don came in to the office several times a week to stretch, lift weights, receive some acupuncture, and to learn strategies for lifting. In a few more weeks, Don was enjoying his old job again, with renewed pride in his athletic career.

RED FLAGS

In rare instances, a sprain or strain—or any kind of accident—can lead to a disorder called complex regional pain syndrome. If you experience a burning pain and extreme sensitivity to touch, or if the limb undergoes inexplicable discoloration, temperature changes, or swelling, see Chapter 25, "Complex Regional Pain Syndrome." You'll need a very different kind of treatment, and you'll need to receive that treatment as quickly as possible.

TESTING, TESTING

It can be tempting to diagnose yourself with a chronic sprain or strain, but you do need to see a doctor to rule out any hidden disorders or serious problems. Often, your case can be diagnosed quickly, but in some circumstances one or more of the following tests may be necessary:

▶ If you've been in an accident or experienced a physical trauma, you and your doctor should decide together if you need imaging techniques such as X rays or MRI scans to check for fractures or other injuries.

▶ If you feel pain on both sides of the body (both wrists or both ankles, for example) your doctor should perform blood work to rule out inflammatory disorders such as rheumatoid arthritis.

▶ If you experience burning, tingling, or numbness, you may need nerve conduction studies to rule out nerve entrapment (such as carpal tunnel syndrome or ulnar nerve palsy, which appears at the elbow). For more information about entrapped nerves, see Chapter 21.

▶ If you feel significant pain, your doctor might order X rays taken with your joints loaded. You may hold weights in your hands, or a technician might apply pressure to your ankle to see if X rays reveal your joint pulling apart under the strain. If so, you're suffering from a more serious injury, such as a complete tear of the tissue (as opposed to the partial tears that usually characterize chronic sprains and strains). You may need a cast or surgery to repair the damage.

▶ Sometimes it's hard to pinpoint the tendon, ligament, or muscle that's giving you trouble. In these cases, a doctor may give you an office injection of local anesthetic as a diagnostic tool. If the pain stops after a certain tissue has been injected, you'll know where the problem resides.

THERAPIES

PHYSICAL THERAPY

▶▶ The most important therapy for a chronic sprain or strain is extended rest. Although you may have eased up on the joint before, now you'll need to give it a longer break—two to four weeks at a minimum. If the problem is severe, you will need to reduce the pressure you put on the joint, which may mean altering your workout or changing the way you do your job.

▶▶ See a professional physical therapist or a chiropractor with an interest in rehabilitation. She can give you individualized exercises for strengthening and stretching the area. These exercises speed healing and will give you a better shot at going back to your old activity.

▶▶ Although ice is the preferred treatment for acute pain, chronic cases should apply heat to increase blood flow to the area. You can use heating pads, hot water bottles, or hot baths on your own; if the injury needs more attention, a physical therapist can perform ultrasound to deliver heat to your connective tissues.

NUTRITION AND SUPPLEMENTS

For recommended doses of supplements, see Chapter 9.

▶▶ Review your nutritional status. People who don't eat well injure themselves more often and have a harder time recovering. Follow the pain-control diet outlined in Chapter 9 and a take a multivitamin daily.

▶ Take an enzyme product. Both bromelain and Wobenzyme appear to improve healing of muscles and connective tissue.

▶ Devil's claw may help reduce inflammation and pain.

DISTRACTING YOUR NERVOUS SYSTEM FROM PAIN

▶ Electrical stimulation encourages healing, reduces inflammation, and distracts your nervous system from any pain you might be feeling.

HEALING ENERGY

▶ If you get lots of strains and sprains, you might benefit from a constitutional homeopathy remedy, one that addresses imbalances in your system. You'll need to consult with a professional homeopath for the best treatment. (Those of you who peruse the homeopathy aisles in the health-food store take note: You may see the remedy *Arnica montana* advertised as a treatment for sprains and strains. Although I think it's useful for acute injuries, my experience is that it's much less helpful for chronic sprains and strains. See an expert for the remedy that's right for you.)

PAIN PILLS AND OTHER PHARMACEUTICALS

► Take a low dose of over-the-counter NSAIDs such as Advil or Motrin to bring down any inflammation in the area—but don't use the pain relief as a way to keep moving on a sore joint.

INJECTIONS, IMPLANTS, AND SURGERY

► Sometimes the tendon, ligament, or muscle is so severely injured that it must be reattached through surgery. If you can't move the joint at all, your doctor may refer you to an orthopedic surgeon.

21.

PERIPHERAL NEUROPATHIES

DIABETES / POSTHERPETIC NEURALGIA / CARPAL TUNNEL SYNDROME / OTHER NERVE DISORDERS

Peripheral neuropathy is damage to a nerve outside the central nervous system—that is, any nerve outside of the brain or spinal cord. Nerve pain is unlike most others you've probably felt. It burns, shoots, or lancinates, keeping you up at night and on edge during the day. You might also get other odd sensations, such as numbness, or something called dysesthesia, in which a stimulus produces a strange response in the body. A touch on your hand might feel like running water, for example, or like heat.

Medical science has begun to understand peripheral neuropathies only recently. Recall the old model of pain, in which pain was thought to be always caused by some kind of tissue damage (such as a cut) and then to travel unedited from the site of the injury, up through the spinal cord, and into the brain. Now we know that the system of conduction—the nerves—can produce pain on its own. Sometimes nerves are hurt by disease or prolonged pressure; sometimes no cause can be found. In the latter case, the nerve may become exquisitely sensitive, firing messages of pain for no apparent reason. Chapter 3 describes sensitized nerves in detail.

Two of the most frequent causes of peripheral neuropathies are diabetes and alcoholism. Diabetes hastens nerve injury by increasing the body's levels of glycosolated hemoglobin, the same substance that can lead to plaque buildup on the walls of arteries; alcohol is a frank poison to nerves. Nerves can also be poisoned by exposure to toxins, chemotherapy, Lyme disease, and the increased urea present in kidney disease. People who suffer from metabolic disorders may experience nerve pain as a result of abnormal biochemistry in their neurons; those with autoimmune diseases or rheumatoid disorders may suffer inflammatory injury to the nerves. Sometimes the problem is not a disease but an entrapment of the nerve by bone, muscle, or other tissue. This is usually caused by an accident, repeated overuse, or continued pressure against the nerve. Despite this long list of possible culprits, it's not unusual for no cause at all to be found.

A few disorders warrant special attention here for their frequency.

Diabetes. This disease is the number-one cause of peripheral neuropathy. Most people who live with diabetes over the course of a lifetime will develop some nerve symptoms, usually numbness and pain in the feet. I see this in patients nearly every week; they shuffle across the examining room, wincing and stepping gingerly, as if walking over hot coals. These patients can no longer make short trips to the store, let alone enjoy longer walks with their spouse or friends. Their feet may burn so badly that sleep is nearly impossible; bedlinens and socks aggravate the pain.

If you have diabetic neuropathy, the first course of action is to keep your diabetes as tightly controlled as possible. You may be able to prevent further neuropathies and even reverse some of the existing damage. The suggestions below will help you relieve the pain and keep you functioning to the greatest extent possible.

Postherpetic neuralgia. A few weeks ago a lovely woman in her midsixties, with violet eyes and pale gray hair, came into my office. She told me that a year ago, she'd experienced an outbreak of shingles; the blisters from that disease had healed without a trace, but she was left with pain that she ranked an 8 on a scale of 1 to 10. She told me that the area around her right eye and upper cheekbone was exquisitely painful to the touch. When she gave me permission to run the back of my hand lightly across the skin of her face, she drew her breath in sharply. She couldn't put on makeup, she said, or tolerate the touch of a scarf around her head. It was hard for her to think of anything but the pain. She missed out on one of the great joys of her life, attending the Metropolitan Opera, because the pain would make her so antsy that she couldn't sit still for extended periods of time. Yet this woman looked entirely normal, even beautiful, aside from her worn expression.

This woman suffered from postherpetic neuralgia, a disorder caused by herpes zoster, the same bug that causes chicken pox. After a bout of chicken pox, the virus travels to nerve cells in the spine. In most people, the virus just lies there, dormant and harmless for a lifetime. But occasionally it reactivates, especially during times when the immune system is suppressed by illness, old age, or stress. In this condition, called shingles, red bumps appear along the pathway of a single nerve, usually on the head or trunk. (A tip-off that these bumps aren't just a harmless rash is that they often appear on one side of the body only.) After a few days, the bumps become painful blisters, which soon crust over and heal. Usually the pain disappears along with the blisters, but in some cases it lingers long after the bumps have gone.

This lingering pain, apparently caused by nerve damage from the virus, is postherpetic neuralgia. It's often worse at night and sensitive to changes in temperature. The burning, shooting sensations can be very hard on people whose immune systems are already run-down. For people like the woman with facial pain, it can prevent enjoyment of retirement and impede daily living—or much worse. According to one estimate, postherpetic neuralgia is the primary cause of suicide among elderly pain patients.

WHEN IT'S NOT JUST A RASH . . .

If you notice bumps or blisters that break out along one side of the body only, you may be experiencing an outbreak of shingles. If you are, prompt medical attention can reduce the chances that you'll develop postherpetic neuralgia. Shingles should usually be treated with acyclovir, an antiviral agent. If the bumps or blisters disappear but the pain continues despite treatment, an epidural injection of steroid medication may halt postherpetic neuralgia or reduce its severity.

Carpal tunnel syndrome. The carpal tunnel, a very small opening just below the base of the wrist, allows the median nerve to pass between the forearm and hand. Because the carpal tunnel is so small, it is vulnerable to pressure and swelling. People who consistently use repeated motions with a flexed wrist (typists, musicians, assembly-line workers) are at risk, as are those who sleep with their hands curled toward their inner forearms. Hormonal changes, especially during pregnancy, can also lead to carpal tunnel syndrome. The disorder begins with a mild tingling in your thumb or first three fingers; you may also feel it in your shoulder. At this stage, the pain is usually worse in the morning. Later, the pain may become constant; in the worst cases, it is crippling. If it is not treated, the nerves and muscles can weaken and degenerate.

Other entrapped nerves. Other common sites of entrapment occur at the elbow (ulnar nerve palsy) or along the forearm. Many also result from pressure by a herniated disc or sciatica; those are covered in the chapters on back and neck pain.

YOU DON'T JUST HAVE TO LIVE WITH IT

Although peripheral neuropathies are a widely recognized set of disorders, they don't get a lot of attention in general medical textbooks. The average doctor is probably most comfortable with carpal tunnel syndrome and other kinds of entrapped nerves, which are easier to understand and to treat: When the source of pressure is taken away, so is the pain. Changing lifestyle habits and stretching out compressed areas can help remove the pressure; if they don't provide adequate relief, a surgical procedure may be necessary to free the nerve.

But if you have another form of peripheral neuropathy, you may hear that nothing can be done for your pain, or you might get the old saw "You just have to live with it." True, these disorders are notoriously tough to treat, but there are several good tools for getting them under control, including drugs that were originally developed for other uses but have proven effective for nerve pain. With appropriate pain care, you won't have to let pain and sleep deprivation divert your energy, even if you can't achieve 100 percent relief. Instead, you can focus your resources on becoming and staying healthy—important for all of us, but especially for the elderly and the ill, who are most vulnerable to these disorders. I suggest that you work closely with a doctor who's experienced in treating peripheral neuropathies. Neurologists and rehabilitation doctors are both good choices, as are those who specialize in any underlying disorder you might have.

TESTING, TESTING

Get a neurological exam. This is a short, simple series of tests your doctor performs on you in the office, including a check of your reflexes and ability to feel vibration, to rule out some other progressive or serious neurological illness.

You may also need a nerve conduction study. This test is necessary only when the neurological exam reveals some kind of abnormality. The nerve conduction study, called NCV, measures how well a nerve can pick up sensations and transmit signals to the muscles.

THERAPIES

The first step is to address any underlying disorder that might be causing the pain. If your pain is from diabetes, you'll need to keep the disease under close control. Alcoholics should—of course—stop drinking, those with Lyme disease should be appropriately treated, and so on.

Beyond those basics, you also need to reduce the painful symptoms. For entrapped nerves, removing the pressure is the best treatment. For other kinds of pain, I recommend medication and possibly TENS right off the bat. No matter what kind of nerve pain you're experiencing, I hope you'll also cultivate a mind-body practice. It will help cool down the burning, quiet the jangling, and give you a safe harbor from the rough seas of nerve pain.

PAIN PILLS AND OTHER PHARMACEUTICALS

▶▶ The treatments of choice for most peripheral neuropathies are tricyclic antidepressants and anticonvulsants. Both were originally intended for other disorders (depression and epilepsy, respectively), but it turns out that they also limit pain signals and help you sleep. If you don't get relief after a few weeks, talk to your doctor about trying another drug in the same class, or perhaps combining the two types of drugs. These drugs are much less useful for entrapped nerves.

▶▶ Those with postherpetic neuralgia can try the lidocaine patch, which has demonstrated high effectiveness and low side effects. The skin around the patch may turn red or swell up a bit, but these reactions usually disappear quickly.

▶▶ If you have diabetic neuropathy, a drug called mexiletine can make the nerve cells less responsive and decrease their tendency to fire.

▶ When other drugs have failed, opioids can help. A few years ago, it was thought that opioids didn't work on nerve pain; now we know that's just not true. Opioids do indeed relieve nerve pain, but you'll need to start with a higher dose than you would for other disorders.

PRESCRIPTIONS: TAKE TIME TO GET THEM RIGHT

A smart prescription for nerve pain could change your life. A good example is my patient Frank, a retired train conductor with nerve damage in his feet. He had an aging body but a hardy soul; the day-in, day-out pain bothered him less than the interruption of his normal activities. Because warmth set off the tingling and burning, he couldn't keep his feet near the radiator or in the sun, which meant he had to be constantly mindful of where he stood or sat. He went on a tricyclic antidepressant to quiet his injured nerves and felt a little better. Since he still couldn't tolerate heat, we nudged the dose upward to give him more relief. Unfortunately, he developed intolerable side effects.

The key to Frank's success was his willingness to keep trying after the first round of medication hadn't worked. He agreed to a trial of Neurontin, an anticonvulsant, in addition to the small amount of antidepressant. Within a few weeks, I found him sitting in my office. "How are those feet?" I asked. "Right up against the radiator!" he said.

MIND-BODY MEDICINE

►► When pain flares up, try to breathe through it. The breathing techniques in Chapter 8 can make the burning pain more manageable.

►► Practice a form of meditation on a daily basis. You can meditate the traditional way, or you can try yoga as a form of moving meditation.

►► Nerve pain takes a heavy toll on both the body and the mind; it often leads to depression and anxiety. It's a good idea to visit a cognitive-behavioral therapist or psychotherapist trained in pain medicine. They can teach you skills to cope with your specific set of challenges.

DISTRACTING YOUR NERVOUS SYSTEM FROM PAIN

▶▶ TENS has a strong record with nerve-generated pain, and its virtual lack of side effects makes it ideal for people who can't take medications.

▶▶ Nerve pain can easily, and understandably, become all-consuming. But by calling in higher therapies, you can turn your focus to something more rewarding than your burning nerves. Pursue a hobby, take up painting, or just listen to your favorite music.

▶ If acupuncture appeals to you, give it a try. The scientific jury is still out about its effectiveness for nerve pain, but it's certainly worth a shot if everything else is failing. Even if you don't see a reduction in pain, you will probably feel blissfully relaxed.

▶ You can distract your nervous system by mildly irritating the painful area. Some of my patients with foot pain keep their feet under scratchy blankets and rub them against the fabric. (Just don't expose any numb areas to damage.)

PHYSICAL THERAPIES

▶▶ If a part of your body is numb, you will not feel cuts, scrapes, or burns. Take care to inspect any numb areas for damage every day.

▶▶ Those with entrapped nerves should work with a physical therapist to stretch out the area. To get started, you can practice the stretches listed in Appendix A. Do them on a daily basis. It's also possible to stretch out the nerves using a special Australian technique called Neural Mobilization or Neurodynamics, popularized by David Butler.

▶▶ The classic yoga pose called Downward-Facing Dog can relieve pressure on the carpal tunnel. This pose is described in Appendix A under exercises for the wrists. If you like the exercise, consider taking a yoga class. The basic series of movements, called the Sun Salutation, includes several poses that can stretch the wrist and carpal tunnel.

▶▶ If you have carpal tunnel syndrome, wear a wrist splint at night to keep pressure off the nerve. You can find splints at the drugstore, or your physical therapist can outfit you with one.

YOUR SLEEP POSTURE CAN CAUSE CARPAL TUNNEL SYNDROME

The way you sleep can put you at risk for carpal tunnel syndrome. If you suffer from this pain, check your nighttime posture. Do you curl your hands in toward your forearms, like a bear snuggling in for the winter, or do you habitually pull your pillow and comforter toward your body with your wrists bent inward? If so, you may be crushing your carpal tunnel. Some people can get away with these sleep postures for years until an additional risk factor, such as pregnancy, surfaces—along with pain. Wearing a wrist splint at night can correct your wrist position and reduce the hurt.

▶ When groups of nerves in your feet or legs stop working, keeping your balance can be a challenge. A physical therapist can show you how to move most effectively and safely. Some people benefit from stabilizing foot or leg braces.

▶ For a temporary but relaxing break from pain, try massage. The sensation of touch against your skin will often block out pain sensations.

▶ Chiropractic and osteopathic techniques for stretching tissue open can also help relieve entrapped nerves. Find a practitioner with experience in this area.

NUTRITION AND SUPPLEMENTS

For recommended doses and information about supplements, see Chapter 9.

▶▶ Reduce pain from nerve inflammation by following the pain-control diet in Chapter 9; be particularly sure to eat oily fish, walnuts, and flaxseed (or take a fish-oil supplement). Limit your consumption of saturated fats and partially hydrogenated oils.

▶▶ Take B-complex vitamins to keep your nerves as strong and healthy as possible. If you have carpal tunnel syndrome, vitamin B_6 may be especially helpful; take up to 200 milligrams daily.

►► Make sure you're getting enough calcium and magnesium. Eat low-fat dairy products and green leafy vegetables, and take a calcium/magnesium supplement every day.

►► Capsaicin blocks pain by reducing substance P and closing the pain gate. Apply this topical lotion three times a day. Don't use capsaicin on areas that are numb.

► If you have carpal tunnel syndrome, you may wish to try turmeric or ginger to reduce inflammation.

► Consider alpha-lipoic acid. A few studies in Europe indicate that it may help heal nerves, although it's too soon to say for sure. Take it only under the supervision of a doctor.

DEEP INJECTIONS, IMPLANTS, AND SURGERY

►► A deep injection of cortisone for postherpetic neuralgia can sometimes cure the pain.

► I'm not usually crazy about surgery for pain, but procedures to remove pressure on entrapped nerves are effective and usually quite safe when performed by an experienced doctor. Most of these surgeries simply remove the mechanical pressure of ligaments and connective tissues that may be binding the nerve as it passes near a joint or muscle. They are usually performed on an outpatient basis under regional, not general, anesthesia, and take very little time—a carpal tunnel procedure may take forty minutes at the most. If physical therapy doesn't work, and if the entrapment causes you significant dysfunction, surgery may be a wise next step.

► Selective nerve blocks and nerve ablations have been successful in some cases involving neuropathy in a single nerve. Try them if medications, mind-body treatments, and TENS fail.

SURGERY FOR CARPAL TUNNEL SYNDROME: THE DANGERS OF WAITING

Marc worked at an office job that required hours of typing every day. He developed a nasty case of carpal tunnel syndrome in his right hand; despite stretching his wrist and wearing a splint, the pain progressed. His doctor recommended surgery, but Marc passed, afraid to have anybody tinker with the delicate structures of his hand. Although I often support patients who want to avoid surgery, in this case I'm sorry that Marc put off the procedure. Now he's come to see me, but the muscles supplied by the median nerve in his hand have begun to atrophy. He no longer has the strength to lift a kettle of water off the stove, and the other day he dropped a small desk lamp when trying to move it. I'm giving him hand acupuncture for temporary pain control, but he's scheduled surgery at my urging. Surgically removing the pressure on the median nerve will help him regain some of his lost strength. However, his recovery will be much slower than it would have been earlier in the disorder, when signs of muscular degeneration first appeared, and it's quite possible that some of the weakness will be permanent. If you have carpal tunnel syndrome and find that you can no longer hold on to or lift everyday items such as pots and pans, it's time to seriously consider surgical relief.

22.

FACIAL, JAW, AND DENTAL PAIN

TRIGEMINAL NEURALGIA / TEMPOROMANDIBULAR JOINT SYNDROME (TMJ) / ATYPICAL FACIAL PAIN / CHRONIC DENTAL PAIN

Why does pain in the mouth or face hurt more than pain in other parts of the body? The answer lies partially in a medical metaphor known as the homunculus, or "little man." The homunculus is a representation of the human body according not to actual size but to the degree of attention the brain pays to body parts. Areas with the highest density of sensory nerves are biggest; those with the least are smallest. The result is a grotesque kind of caricature. His (the homunculus is traditionally a man) legs, arms, and midsection are withered, but the front of his head—where the nerves are packed in most tightly—is swollen up to several times its normal size. In this schema, the tongue is actually the largest feature on the body. (The index finger and big toe vie for second place.)

Pain in your face hurts more because the face contains more nerves to carry pain's message. This makes evolutionary sense: We need to protect our organs of sight, smell, taste, and mastication if we want to survive. But when pain is chronic, this protective feature doubles back on you. Everyday events such as eating, brushing your teeth, or walking into the wind can feel like acts of self-torture. Facial pain also tends to produce more suffering. The face is our most important means of communication and expression; it's how we present ourselves and tell the world who we are. When it hurts, our sense of self hurts, too.

The disorders discussed here are trigeminal neuralgia, temporomandibular joint syndrome (TMJ) and atypical facial pain, and chronic dental pain. Because these three categories are very different in their causes and treatments, they are presented separately.

TESTING, TESTING

Except in clear-cut cases of TMJ or tooth pain, almost everyone with facial pain needs to have an MRI to rule out some potentially nasty conditions, including infections, tumors, fractures, aneurysms, or other blood vessel disorders. I also suggest that you have a thorough exam from a good dentist, since facial pain can sometimes result from hard-to-spot dental problems.

TRIGEMINAL NEURALGIA

Trigeminal neuralgia (TN) is characterized by shocks of pain along the jaw or behind the nose and eyes. The cause is a disorder of the fifth cranial nerve. This nerve, the largest in the face, carries most of the sensations that you feel in the jaws, lips, cheeks, and forehead to the brain. Sometimes the nerve is compressed, usually by a vein or artery that pushes against it; in other cases, it becomes sensitized. When either of these things happen, the nerve shoots off pain messages, and the facial muscles may twitch or jerk (hence an old term for this disorder, tic douloureux, which means "painful tic").

The pain of TN is intermittent and unpredictable. It may last for just a second, or it can go on for a couple of minutes. This short-term feature of the pain can be confusing to those on the outside, to whom TN doesn't sound so bad. After all, it's not constant, and how bad can a little twitching be? But if you suffer from TN, you know all too well that this cutting pain is almost off the charts in its intensity. Perhaps worse, its sneak-attack quality and facial location make it deeply disturbing to the psyche.

The good news is that unlike many other pain disorders, TN is well defined. A capable neurologist should be familiar with the problem and can offer a variety of good conventional treatments. But there's a hitch: These treatments often work on a merely temporary basis, with the pain recurring after an absence of months or years. At that point, the patient must return and try a different approach. That's not so terrible, given that the doctor usually has several additional therapies at his disposal. But people who are unprepared for this cycle of remission and return are often shocked and disheartened when the pain comes back. If you have TN, try to avoid putting all your hopes into one therapy for permanent relief; instead, take comfort in the knowledge that with intelligent, persistent care, the pain can often be kept under excellent control.

Alternative therapies are best used to strengthen conventional treatments and extend their effectiveness. I usually suggest a combination of pharmaceuticals—and sometimes nerve ablations or even surgery—with acupuncture or mind-body techniques in very strong supporting roles.

THERAPIES

DISTRACTING YOUR NERVOUS SYSTEM FROM PAIN

▶▶ Acupuncture should be among the top therapies on your list. Although acupuncture doesn't have a great record with other kinds of nerve pain, I've often seen it bring the pain of TN down several notches. You may not have total success with acupuncture, but it could well reduce your need for medication.

▶▶ People who live with TN say that higher therapies allow them to feel like their old selves. One of my favorite examples is a seventy-year-old weaver, who has found that starting a new basket, working on a design and using fresh materials, turns off the pain for a while.

MIND-BODY MEDICINE

▶▶ Mind-body therapies can give you a strong, calm center, so that the pain has less power to disturb you. Find one you like and practice it daily. Guided imagery and meditation are particularly good choices for you.

▶ If you can find a support group for TN, by all means join it. There's an unsettling, foreign quality to TN that often makes people wonder if they harbor a tumor or other dread disease; meeting with other sufferers allays those fears. It's also valuable to share coping strategies.

PAIN PILLS AND OTHER PHARMACEUTICALS

▶▶ The anticonvulsant carbamazepine (Tegretol) is the drug of choice for TN; more than half of the people who take it see improvement. You'll need to start with a low dose to get your body accustomed to the drug and reduce side effects, then slowly ratchet up. Your doctor should hold the dosage at the point where you either feel relief or just before you begin to experience side effects.

▶ Baclofen is another good pharmaceutical option. Although baclofen is a muscle relaxant, it's sometimes used to reduce hyperactivity in the nerves.

▶ If neither carbamazepine nor baclofen works, then other anticonvulsant drugs, including gabapentin (Neurontin), are worth trying.

▶ Tricyclic antidepressants in small doses are next in line. They work for some people by reducing the number of pain messages. These drugs also increase dopamine and serotonin.

▶ Be willing to experiment, under your doctor's prescription, with combinations of the above drugs. Some people respond to low doses of multiple pills more readily than to single drugs. *Do not combine drugs unless you are specifically instructed to do so by your doctor.*

▶ When all else has failed, and when the pain is severe, long-acting opioids may be necessary. Don't be afraid to ask for them if your pain requires it.

NUTRITION AND SUPPLEMENTS

For recommended doses of supplements, see Chapter 9.

▶ Take a B-complex supplement to support your taxed nerves and to keep them as healthy and strong as possible.

PHYSICAL THERAPIES

▶ Engage in regular cardiovascular exercise to regulate pain-blocking chemicals and to decrease your overall pain sensitivity.

▶ Some patients find gentle facial massage quite helpful. Massage may bring down any general achiness and tension in the area; it also releases pain-inhibiting substances.

HEALING ENERGY

▶ If you are elderly, try tai chi for exercise and stress relief. (If you are younger, tai chi is still excellent for stress management, but you will need more vigorous exercise for cardiovascular benefits.)

DEEP INJECTIONS, IMPLANTS, AND SURGERY

▶ Gamma knife surgery is a reasonable, relatively low-risk means of addressing TN at its root. By directing gamma radiation at the base of the trigeminal nerve, in the pons (a part of the brain stem), the nerve is deadened. There may also be some decrease in pressure on the nerve. By at least one measure, this procedure boasts a cure rate of 90 percent; however, the treatment is still in its infancy, and we do not yet know what the long-term effectiveness might be. The risks are the kind you'd associate with other kinds of radiation exposure, including hardening of the skin. In the hands of a skilled, experienced neurosurgeon, these risks are greatly minimized. If you've used conservative measures but still need relief, I think this is a very reasonable method to try.

▶ Radio-frequency ablation, a kind of nerve ablation, is the next step up from the gamma knife. The doctor will use microwave heat to coagulate and deaden the trigeminal nerve. This therapy is most effective when the pain is caused by something other than compression by a blood vessel.

▶ In a percutaneous balloon decompression, a small balloon is inserted between the nerve and any offending blood vessel and then inflated to keep the two separated. *Percutaneous* means that a tiny puncture is made in the skin to thread something (in this case, the balloon) into the body. This is less traumatic and risky than a microvascular decompression, below.

▶ The most extreme measure for TN is surgical microvascular decompression, in which padding is inserted next to the connective tissue, vein, or artery that is pushing on the nerve. This is real surgery, and close to the brain, so the risks are higher. Use it only when nothing else has worked and the pain is unbearable. Make sure you find a neurosurgeon who makes this procedure a specialty. Expect a short hospital stay, with full recovery within a couple of days.

TEMPOROMANDIBULAR JOINT SYNDROME (TMJ) AND ATYPICAL FACIAL PAIN

TEMPOROMANDIBULAR JOINT SYNDROME

Temporomandibular joint syndrome, popularly known as TMJ, has recently been renamed TMD (temporomandibular joint disorder). It is a disorder of the jaw characterized by dull, achy pain and difficulty opening the mouth. The medical approach to TMJ has swung back and forth in the last couple of decades. At first, TMJ was considered a manifestation of stress; treatment involved sending the patient home with a few capsules of ibuprofen and a pat on the head. In the 1980s, a new theory of TMJ arose—that it was largely an anatomical disorder of joint position and formation. Patients, regarded with a new seriousness, were often sent directly for surgery. Bones were resected and repositioned, and teeth were built up or ground down. The failure rate of this approach was astronomical, and horror stories about TMJ surgery mills and unscrupulous dentists abounded.

Now, TMJ diagnosis and treatment occupy a more reasonable middle ground. Some people do indeed have malformations or disorders of the joint itself. Most, however, suffer from tension in the muscles that surround the jawbone. This tension alone is painful; over time, it can wear down the cartilage and lead to weakness in the joint.

Appropriate treatment for TMJ varies according to its cause. If your jaw makes a loud clicking or popping sound as it opens and closes, you may have a structural problem. However, if you can manage the pain and do not suffer from much dysfunction, there's no reason to operate. You can safely rely on conservative treatments alone. It's only when the disorder leads to serious, long-term life disruption—when you can't chew or laugh or yawn—that surgery makes sense.

If you have the muscle-tension brand of TMJ, you need something more than a pat on the head but something less than surgery. Resting the jaw as much as possible will help release any spasm, as will biofeedback, massage, and other gentle therapies.

Perhaps the most important treatment of this disorder is an honest assessment of your stress levels. If you're taking a beating at work, or if your home life is making you tense, you should address the problem to the extent possible. You can also use the mind-body connection to keep unavoidable stress under control.

ATYPICAL FACIAL PAIN

This is a catchall term for facial pain that's dull, throbbing, achy, and hard to pinpoint. It is also called trigeminal neuropathic pain. Here's a common scenario: You get what appears to be a toothache, but when that tooth is treated, the pain remains, so the dentist goes on to a neighboring tooth, with similar results, and then another tooth, and so on. Other manifestations of atypical facial pain include a constant burning sensation in the mouth or cheeks. What this unusual group of symptoms has in common is unwavering discomfort (although it may intensify with touch, eating, or drinking). One of the most frustrating aspects of this disorder is that other people tend to wave away your pain, not realizing how strong it can be.

If you have atypical facial pain, you need to be checked out thoroughly by an ear, nose, and throat specialist; you should also get an MRI to rule out underlying causes. If no acute disorder is found, you may nevertheless run into specialists who want to treat the pain surgically or through dental experimentation. Resist this approach. Atypical facial pain does not respond well to such techniques; too many people undergo multiple procedures that produce no benefits. (One medical textbook cites patients who've had more than seventy procedures.) I'd much rather see sufferers receive gentle care, with special focus on the mind-body relationship. If you have this disorder, take time for yourself. Support your body with good food and exercise, and cultivate a relaxation practice you can enjoy.

THERAPIES

MIND-BODY MEDICINE

▶▶ Biofeedback will teach you to relax the muscles in your jaw instead of clenching them in response to stress or out of habit.

▶▶ Gentle yoga—no headstands—relieves stress while loosening the upper body.

▶▶ If you tend to get "mind chatter" or have trouble taking your thoughts off work, try meditation.

PHYSICAL THERAPIES

▶▶ Check yourself for poor jaw and neck posture. Every few minutes, stop to ask yourself if your jaw is clenched; if it is, soften it. Proper jaw position is slightly relaxed, with your lips closed; your neck should extend straight up from your shoulders. If you've developed bad posture habits and can't correct them on your own, you may wish to get professional help from a teacher of the Alexander Technique.

▶ If you clench or grind your teeth while sleeping, see a dentist for a splint that will take the pressure off your jaw.

▶ A physical therapist can help you with stretches and strengthening exercises of your jaw, neck, and shoulders. The neck and shoulder exercises listed in Appendix A can give you a start.

▶ Craniosacral therapy, which claims to manipulate the sutures of the skull, where its bony plates meet, may be able to correct misalignments that cause pain. This technique is practiced by osteopaths, chiropractors, and others.

▶ Try getting a massage of your jaw and face to relieve muscular spasm. A physical therapist or osteopathic craniopath will be trained in this technique.

NUTRITION AND SUPPLEMENTS

For recommended doses of supplements, see Chapter 9.

▶▶ If you have TMJ, give your jaw a rest. Avoid chewy or sticky foods for a few weeks. Caramel, bagels, steak, and the like demand too much of a workout from your jaws.

▶ If you suffer from jumpiness or anxiety at night, kava can quiet your mind and help you sleep. (But don't use kava on an ongoing basis.)

▶ Examine your diet for stress-inducing products, such as coffee, tea, chocolate, and other sweets. As an experiment, stop or dramatically reduce their consumption. If you feel better, take them off the menu for good.

DISTRACTING YOUR NERVOUS SYSTEM FROM PAIN

▶ If you have painful knots of muscle in your jaw or face, acupuncture can help release them. It also temporarily blocks the pain signal from traveling up the spinal cord, *and* it's a deeply relaxing therapy.

PAIN PILLS AND OTHER PHARMACEUTICALS

▶ Teeth grinding is a side effect of certain antidepressants called selective serotonin reuptake inhibitors, or SSRIs. If you're taking Prozac, Paxil, Zoloft, or another brand of these drugs, talk to your doctor. He may wish to switch your prescription. *Do not stop taking an antidepressant without speaking to your doctor first.*

▶ Tylenol and NSAIDs can be used in limited quantities for pain relief and to relax the muscles.

HEALING ENERGY

▶ Consider Reiki. Not only is it relaxing, but it also tends to work well on ailments that can't be explained in the usual medical terms.

DEEP INJECTIONS, IMPLANTS, AND SURGERY

▶ If you have a serious case of TMJ that may be anatomically induced, you should be checked out by a specialist, preferably at an academic medical center. When the problem is truly anatomical, surgery has a good record of correcting the problem. However, you may still encounter specialists who are too zealous with their scalpels and who recommend surgery for patients who won't benefit. If an operation is suggested, get a second opinion and ask to have the anatomical problem explained to you. Be aware of the signs of a TMJ surgery mill: Ask what percentage of patients end up having surgery—if it sounds very high, be suspicious. Also be wary if the surgeon boasts of a ridiculously high cure rate, such as 95 or even 100 percent. Should two credible, reputable doctors agree that you need surgery, and you're in a lot of pain, it is very reasonable to try.

DENTAL PAIN

Strictly speaking, dental pain is rarely chronic, since it almost always is caused by tissue damage that can be fixed. A visit to the dentist will usually pinpoint the decay, disease, or injury to a structure of the mouth, and you'll leave with a diagnosis and probably an appointment for a procedure or two. Sometimes, though, it takes even the most thorough and practiced of dentists a longer time to locate the damage and even longer to fix it. During this period of waiting—which can go on for months or even years—a patient may be in serious pain. I see this problem most often in elderly people, who may suffer a great deal between dental appointments. In these cases, conservative pain management can improve quality of life until the underlying disorder is found and treated. Those same measures can also make the dental work itself a little less harrowing.

THERAPIES

These therapies are meant only to reduce pain. You must be under the care of an experienced dentist to treat the underlying cause.

DISTRACTING YOUR NERVOUS SYSTEM FROM PAIN

►► Even skeptics agree that one of acupuncture's best uses is for dental pain. A 1998 review in the *British Dental Journal* of sixteen randomized trials concluded that acupuncture does indeed relieve pain more than a placebo. Given this backing of acupuncture in a respected medical journal, your doctor or dentist may be willing to refer you to an acupuncturist, either to manage the ongoing pain or specifically to treat the pain of dental work. Your insurance company may even be willing to pay for it. On an anecdotal level, I can report that my dental pain patients who combine conventional painkillers with regular acupuncture can often bring their pain scales down from the high end (around 7 or 8 out of a possible 10) to the low end (often a 2 or 3).

►► Try massaging the following acupressure points with ice: B 2; GB 3, GB 6, and GB 9; St 3, St 5, St 6, and St 7. For a map of acupressure points, see Appendix C.

NUTRITION AND SUPPLEMENTS

For recommended doses of supplements, see Chapter 9.

▶▶ Nutritional deficiencies show up very quickly in the gums and teeth, so make sure your diet is excellent. If you've been eating lots of food that's packaged or processed, it's time to change your habits. The pain-control diet outlined in Chapter 9 is ideal for almost everyone.

▶▶ There are a couple of supplements I recommend for healthy teeth and gums. Start with a good multivitamin. Take an additional B-complex product, along with vitamin C (250–500 milligrams daily).

▶▶ Clove oil, rubbed directly on the gums, is an age-old method of treating dental pain. You can find vials of clove oil at your health-food store.

MIND-BODY MEDICINE

▶▶ Any kind of relaxation technique will help you get pain under control. Find one you like—guided imagery, meditation, breathing techniques, and so on—and use it daily. These therapies will also help reduce the anxiety that dental work often brings on.

▶ Try hypnosis. You can use it for long-term management of pain or to help reduce the short-term but intense pain of dental procedures.

23.

PELVIC PAIN

GENERALIZED PELVIC PAIN / PMS / ENDOMETRIOSIS / INTERSTITIAL CYSTITIS / VULVODYNIA

GENERALIZED PELVIC PAIN

I've said before that pain is a mystery. If I were introducing young doctors to this idea, I'd use generalized pelvic pain as the perfect example. I'd show them the patients who are frustrated from years of exams and diagnostic procedures. In particular, I'd show them the patients who have undergone extensive surgery, including removal of every single pelvic organ, even the bladder—and who still hurt. I'd show them damaged marriages and sidelined careers. I'd show them people who spend their lives doubled over in very real pain, although their doctors can find no disease to explain its origin.

An unstated bargain exists between patients and doctors. If I, the patient, feel a sign that something is wrong with my body, I go to a doctor. That's my part of the bargain. In return, the doctor gives me a diagnosis. When it comes to pain—*especially* pelvic pain—that bargain may break down. If you have chronic pain in the pelvic region, you absolutely must see a doctor, or maybe a couple of doctors, to check for disease or other underlying problems. But in a surprising number of instances, a cause for pelvic pain simply can't be found. It may even be hard to pinpoint the pain's location. In these cases, the descriptive term "generalized pelvic pain" hardly feels like a diagnosis at all. A patient might not even get this minimal satisfaction. One doctor after another may say, "I've run all the tests, and I just can't find anything."

If you have reached this point, you may feel let down by the medical system or perhaps simply exhausted by it. Assuming that you've made a good effort to find a cause (see "Testing, Testing," below), you now need to decide how you're going to respond to this diagnosis, or lack of one. Will you continue to go from doctor to doctor, looking for a "real" diagnosis or cure? Will you give up on conventional health care altogether? And how will you deal with the ongoing pain?

These decisions are personal ones, but I can tell you what's worked for the patients I've seen and what works in other multidisciplinary pain clinics. First, it helps to know that you're not alone. Generalized pelvic pain accounts for around 10 percent of consultations with gynecologists every year. It's a fact that women do suffer from pelvic pain of unknown origin, and that this pain is not a sign of cancer or another progressive illness. (This chapter is limited to a discussion of women's pelvic pain, since women represent the vast majority of sufferers. However, it is possible for men to suffer from pelvic pain, too, especially in the bladder or prostate.)

The new model of pain offers at least a partial explanation for this otherwise inexplicable disorder. We know now that pain signals do not necessarily arise from damaged tissue: Sometimes the nervous system generates pain all on its own. Even if there *is* a small amount of tissue damage, the nervous system may amplify the message as it travels to the brain. In the pelvic region specifically, one theory is that a pain message from one organ travels to the spinal cord and then is fed into the network for a different pelvic organ, resulting in pain that moves around or eventually spreads to the entire region.

Another often-ignored contributor to pelvic pain is spasm in the muscles of the pelvic floor. This is usually not the originator of the problem, but it can occur in reaction to pain that's already present—and muscle spasm can sustain pain in the pelvic region even after the initial cause or causes have disappeared.

DON'T GIVE UP: TWO LITTLE-KNOWN CONTRIBUTORS TO PELVIC PAIN

A wound-up nervous system and spasm of the pelvic floor muscles are two contributors to chronic pelvic pain that often go overlooked. If your doctor concludes that no organic cause can be found for your pain, you don't need to abandon your search for pain relief. Ask about therapies that can address these two possible factors. (You may need to see a pain specialist to get the best results.) Pharmaceuticals to calm sensitized nerves, biofeedback, or injections of local anesthetic to relax spasms, as well as gentler treatments such as yoga, breathing exercises, and supplements of calcium and magnesium, can make a real difference.

Once you've seen a couple of specialists, it's usually reasonable to turn your attention away from diagnosis. A good attitude to adopt is one that doctors call "watchful waiting." You check in regularly with your doctor, just to confirm that no sign of disease has shown up, but you cease the active search for an answer. Instead, you turn that energy toward getting back to your life and managing the symptoms.

Controlling the pain brings up additional challenges for pelvic conditions. Doctors whose specialties include the pelvic region—gynecologists and urologists, mainly—rarely have much experience treating chronic pain, even less so than internists and family physicians. This leads to the classic undertreatment/overtreatment problem. You may be told to live with the pain, or maybe you'll get one of those skeptical "it's all in your head" messages. But because there's a long medical history of removing pelvic organs for various reasons, a doctor may try to cut the pain out via hysterectomy. Although sometimes a hysterectomy is medically necessary for painful conditions—in cases of persistent bleeding that can lead to anemia, for example—I don't advise it for pain control alone.

Statistics, as well as doctors' common experiences, suggest an unusually high correlation between chronic pelvic pain and depression. As always, it's hard to say which comes first, the pain or the emotion. They tend to enlarge each other, making the zone of debility wider and wider. If you are struggling with sadness, helplessness, or overwhelming apathy, a part of your personal pain program *must* address these problems. When you ignore depression, your chances of successfully managing the pain are slim.

There is another much-publicized set of statistics that indicates a relationship between chronic pelvic pain and sexual abuse or trauma in childhood. I think a little wariness of researchers who encourage their patients to "remember" abuse is warranted, but many doctors, including myself, feel that some—but certainly not all—patients may be expressing the emotional pain of abuse through physical pain in the pelvis. If there is something in your life that you need to face, I hope you will let this pain be an opportunity for you to do so.

TESTING, TESTING

It's difficult to know when to accept a diagnosis of generalized pelvic pain and when to continue the search for a known disease. You and your doctor should work together to determine which tests are appropriate for you. Here are the basic procedures:

- A gynecological exam—one that's thorough, not rushed
- Baseline blood work, including hormonal studies, to rule out infections and other disorders
- A visit to a urologist, if the bladder is affected
- An exam by a gastroenterologist, if there are digestive problems in addition to pelvic pain

If you've had these exams and still aren't satisfied, it might be reasonable to receive a contrast-dye study of the uterus and tubes, pelvic ultrasound, or even a CAT scan if your doctor suspects a disorder of the lower large intestine. According to your individual situation, additional tests may also be appropriate. Consult with your physician.

THERAPIES

Your plan should include treatments that release muscle tension in the pelvic floor; you'll also want to settle down a wound-up nervous system (pharmaceuticals can help, and so can mind-body therapies and exercise).

MIND-BODY MEDICINE

Below are some suggestions to get you started, but feel free to try any other mind-body therapies that appeal to you.

▶▶ Basic yoga postures will help you get back in touch with your body. They also stretch the pelvic muscles and encourage deep, restorative breathing.

▶▶ On their own, breathing exercises help relax your muscles and your mind.

▶▶ Biofeedback of the pelvic floor or bladder can help you release chronic muscle tension.

▶ If the pain is controlling your life, consider cognitive-behavioral therapy to help you cope.

PHYSICAL THERAPIES

▶▶ Low-impact cardiovascular exercise releases muscular tension all over the body and may relax the muscles of the pelvic floor in particular. Exercise also increases serotonin and GABA (and possibly other neurotransmitters implicated in chronic pain, such as dopamine), as well as endorphins. Walking or exercising in water are good choices; you might also enjoy using an elliptical trainer or ski machine.

▶▶ Heat in the form of a hot-water bottle on your belly reduces flare-ups and feels comforting.

▶ Try regular Swedish massage of your belly, back, or legs. If that's not possible, reserve massage for use before an important event or for flare-ups.

NUTRITION AND SUPPLEMENTS

For recommended doses of supplements, see Chapter 9.

▶▶ Follow the pain-control diet in Chapter 9, paying special attention to foods that control inflammation. Low-grade inflammation—the kind that can be brought on by a diet high in red meat and fatty foods—can make the nervous system more reactive to pain. Try eating deep-water fish, nuts, or flaxseed to keep inflammation under control.

▶▶ Supplements to reduce inflammation include fish-oil capsules, quercetin, turmeric, ginger, and gamma-linolenic acid. Try these supplements one a time, so that you know what works.

▶▶ Read "Can Food Allergies Cause Pain?" on pages 135–136. Try eliminating the usual suspects—corn, wheat, dairy, citrus, soy, and eggs—one by one.

▶▶ To reduce muscle spasm, take magnesium and calcium. A potassium supplement may also help, but take it only under the guidance of your doctor.

▶ For anxiety that results in insomnia, try kava before going to bed (but don't use kava on an extended basis). If you're sleepless but don't suffer from anxiety, use valerian instead.

▶ Chinese herbalists have a good reputation for relieving painful pelvic conditions with their complex, individualized mixtures. But you must consult with an experienced practitioner of traditional Chinese medicine (TCM) to get the best results—what's worked for a friend won't necessarily work for you.

HEALING ENERGY

▶ I am often struck by the harmony between energy healing and pelvic pain. Perhaps that's because pelvic pain can make you feel divorced from your own body. When a compassionate healer places her hand on the place that hurts, you may feel deeply soothed. Reiki could well be a good choice for you; so might the simple touch of a loved one.

▶ Therapeutic Touch, although it does not involve someone laying her hands directly on your skin, has a similar effect.

▶ Tai chi will get your energy—and your body—moving again.

▶ For a treat, book a reflexology appointment.

DISTRACTING YOUR NERVOUS SYSTEM FROM PAIN

▶▶ It's not surprising that both acupressure and acupuncture work well for pelvic pain, since they work on the nervous system *and* manipulate the flow of energy. I especially like Japanese acupuncture for pelvic pain, which uses short needles placed along the arc of the rib cage. When it comes to acupressure, the Anmo type works particularly well. These techniques rarely cure pelvic pain permanently, but like massage, you can use them for flares or anytime you need to get the pain under temporary control.

▶ When pain is crippling, consider TENS to get you functioning again.

▶ Aromatherapy may help. Add a few drops of lavender oil to a hot bath to help you relax and take your mind off the pain.

SELF-ACUPRESSURE FOR PELVIC PAIN

This easy ritual follows the same basic idea as a professional treatment. The initial upward motion takes you along the Conception Vessel meridian, an energy channel that governs the pelvic region.

Lie down in a comfortable, quiet spot. Take a few moments to breathe deeply. Start by pressing your fingers firmly (but not so hard that it hurts) in the center of your lower abdomen, just above the pubic bone. Hold the pressure for one or two minutes as you continue to take deep, slow breaths. Then move your fingers up about half an inch and repeat the process. Continue moving up in a straight line until you reach the sternum. Then move out and down along the right inside edge of your rib cage. Repeat on the left side. With your hands at your sides, relax for a few more breaths.

PAIN PILLS AND OTHER PHARMACEUTICALS

▶▶ Constant tension in the pelvic floor can cause trigger points, which are knots or taut bands of muscle. They are painful in and of themselves, but they also send pain shooting into another part of your body, usually a nearby area. Office injections of local anesthetic into these points is a new treatment for pelvic pain, and one that shows real promise. Make sure to work with a physician who is experienced in both treating chronic pelvic pain *and* injecting trigger points.

▶▶ NSAIDs can ease mild to moderate pain. If you need to use them daily or in high doses, ask your doctor about the COX-2 inhibitors, which are less irritating to the stomach than other NSAIDs.

▶▶ When muscle tension or spasm is a large component of the pain, muscle relaxants, especially diazepam (Valium), can help.

▶ If the pain is moderate to severe, opioids may be used. The drug with the best reputation for easing pelvic pain is methadone. Don't let methadone's association with drug rehab clinics (it's used to help heroin addicts kick the habit) put you off. It is a fully legitimate opioid that is excellent for easing chronic pain.

DEEP INJECTIONS, IMPLANTS, AND SURGERY

▶ You can get a nerve block of something called the superior hypogastric plexus, which is the cluster of nerves that transmit information to and from the pelvic region. For some people, the procedure provides temporary but long-term (a few months or more) relief.

▶ If you get some relief through TENS but not enough to manage a high level of pain, you might benefit from a spinal cord stimulator implanted at the base of the spinal cord.

▶ In rare cases, a presacral neurectomy (a kind of nerve ablation) may help. In this major surgical procedure, some of the sensory nerves that feed into the pelvic organs are removed. Presacral neurectomy has a fair to middling record of success, with the usual risks that attend abdominal surgery: infection, damage to the organs, reactions to anesthesia, and so on. I include it here only because some people have in fact been helped by the surgery. If you do wish to consider a presacral neurectomy, make sure you've tried all the other options available to you first, and find a neurosurgeon who is experienced in the procedure.

▶ For severe, intractable, disabling pain, your doctor or surgeon may discuss a selective cordotomy with you. Chapter 13 covers this extreme but sometimes effective procedure in more detail; if you choose to undergo it, make sure that you understand the very real risks that are involved—including the risk that you won't feel any better.

DO HYSTERECTOMIES HELP?

Of all hysterectomies in the United States, 12 to 16 percent are performed not to treat disease but to relieve chronic pelvic pain—that's about eighty thousand hysterectomies a year. These surgeries rarely achieve their goal, probably because the pain exists less in the organs themselves than in the nervous system. *About a quarter of women who are referred to doctors for chronic pelvic pain have already undergone a hysterectomy, with no relief from their symptoms.* A wiser pain-control plan looks to more conservative measures.

PMS

Premenstrual syndrome, more commonly known as PMS, is characterized by a wide range of symptoms, including (but not limited to) pain, bloating, breast tenderness, mood changes, and fatigue. These symptoms appear in midcycle, usually a week or so before bleeding begins, and disappear with its onset. Almost 75 percent of menstruating women are affected to some degree, but an unlucky few are stricken with severe abdominal pain every month. Many of them schedule their lives around their predictable days of disability.

The cramping pains of PMS are linked to the monthly surge of estrogen, which allows the uterus to thicken and engorge with blood. Estrogen also kicks in an increase of prostaglandins, the inflammatory hormone. In addition to hormonal fluctuations, a woman's level of physical activity appears to affect PMS pain: Sedentary women are much more prone to cramping than active women are. And it's long been suspected that there is a genetic component to all symptoms of PMS.

If you have serious recurring abdominal pain, you need to be checked out by a doctor. If she determines that you do not have an underlying problem, such as a hormonal imbalance, then you can bring your focus to a plan for keeping your pain levels in check.

TESTING, TESTING

You'll need a thorough gynecological exam, with blood work to check your hormone levels. If you are not satisfied with this level of testing, you can see an endocrinologist (a specialist in hormones).

THERAPIES

The therapies listed for generalized pelvic pain starting on page 336 will also work for PMS; below are a few more. There are four therapies that I consider essential: cardiovascular exercise throughout the month, to regulate hormones and reduce muscle tension; a pain-control diet, especially when you usually experience pain; supplementation with magnesium and calcium; and a mind-body therapy. A good rule of thumb for PMS is to stay ahead of the pain. You probably know when in your cycle to expect the symptoms; try to use your therapies—whatever they are—*before* you are curled up in agony.

NUTRITION AND SUPPLEMENTS

For recommended doses of supplements, see Chapter 9.

▶ Take a B-complex supplement during the time you usually feel pain.

PAIN PILLS AND OTHER PHARMACEUTICALS

▶▶ For PMS, pain, Motrin is the NSAID many women prefer, although other preparations of ibuprofen may work just as well or better for you. Although it's not as effective, acetaminophen (Tylenol) is an option if you don't want the stomach-irritating ingredients.

▶ Oral contraceptives can regulate hormones. Some doctors will prescribe low doses on a continuous basis—meaning that you won't experience menses—for cramping and other symptoms.

▶ If the pain is intense, your doctor might prescribe codeine, a short-acting opioid, to use only on an occasional basis.

ENDOMETRIOSIS

Endometriosis is a condition in which tissue from the lining of the uterus (called the endometrium) attaches itself to other organs. The uterine tissue usually appears elsewhere in the pelvic cavity, often in the fallopian tubes or ovaries, or it may implant itself on the outer walls of the uterus itself. In rare cases, the tissue travels outside the pelvic regions and appears in the intestines or even as far away as the brain.

These masses of tissue can be painful in and of themselves, but to make matters worse, they continue to fill up with blood over the course of the menstrual cycle, and every month, they slough away blood and other material, just as the uterus does. Unlike normal menstrual blood, however, the blood from the abnormal growths has nowhere to go. Instead, it accumulates inside the pelvic cavity, where it often forms cysts. As menstrual cycles repeat themselves and the tissue continues to bleed each month, the cysts may grow so large that they bind organs together. Sometimes a cyst ruptures and leads to agonizing pain.

Endometriosis does not always cause symptoms. But when it does, those symptoms include pain in the pelvis and lower back; this pain usually varies with the menstrual cycle and is at its worst during ovulation, menstruation, or sexual intercourse. If the growths occur in the intestines, they can obstruct the bowel or lead to other digestive problems. In some women, these symptoms are mild to moderate, but in others they are so intense as to be incapacitating. In addition, endometriosis can lead to infertility; sometimes the only warning sign of this disorder is difficulty conceiving. Awareness of endometriosis has grown in the last several years, but not all primary-care doctors are trained to look for it. As a result, women with this condition may go undiagnosed for years.

Like so many of the disorders in this book, what causes endometriosis is unknown. But unlike those other disorders, there are effective medical treatments for endometriosis, including synthetic hormones and a kind of laparoscopy (a procedure performed via the insertion of a scope outfitted with a tiny sterile camera into the belly) in which growths are removed but not any pelvic organs themselves. While pursuing these treatments, you can use the therapies suggested here to manage the pain. With good medical care and a little luck, the growths and your pain will disappear.

But you should also know that treatment does sometimes fail—the endometrial tissue returns after laparoscopic removal, or the pain continues for an unknown reason despite the absence of growths. In those cases, your doctor may recommend a hysterectomy. Exercise caution here. Although this extreme procedure may indeed be helpful for some women, I am suspicious of its use at this stage for two reasons. First, it may fail just as the aforementioned medical treatments did, and you may experience new tissue growth or unexplained pain. Second, it may simply be unnecessary. By employing gentler methods, you may well get control over pain *and* keep control of your reproductive organs.

TESTING, TESTING

Laparoscopy (the insertion of a scope into the belly) can be used as a diagnostic tool, not just for removal of growths. It is the gold standard of diagnostic testing for endometriosis. In this minor surgery requiring general anesthesia, your doctor will make a small incision in your abdomen (usually around the navel), and insert a telescopelike tube into your pelvic cavity. She will also use carbon dioxide to expand your abdomen and make visual inspection easier. By looking through the tube, she can see the size, location, and number of the growths.

Your doctor will also need to rule out ovarian cancer, irritable bowel syndrome, pelvic inflammatory disease, and a few other disorders.

THERAPIES

Most gynecologists will prescribe hormonal therapy for endometriosis, often birth control pills but also GnRH (gonadotropin-releasing hormone) agonists (Lupron and Synarel are the most common preparations), synthetic progestin, or danazol (Danocrine). In addition to these pharmaceuticals, the therapies listed starting on page 336 can help you handle the painful aspects of the condition. You might also consider massage, mind-body techniques for relaxation, and acupressure or acupuncture.

INTERSTITIAL CYSTITIS

Interstitial cystitis, or IC, causes symptoms that are similar to garden-variety cystitis: severe bladder pain, pelvic pressure and tenderness, and a constant urge to urinate. Unlike cystitis and other acute infections of the urinary tract, however, no bacteria can be found to explain the symptoms, nor do the symptoms retreat after a few days of discomfort. Instead, the pain persists, sometimes to the point of being disabling. It also tends to flare up with menstruation, certain foods, and sexual intercourse. The peculiar nature of this pain makes normal activities such as riding on the subway or bus, sitting at a desk for eight hours a day, or having sex extremely difficult.

One of the most challenging tasks for someone with IC is receiving a proper diagnosis. Although an awareness of the disorder is growing among doctors, it still takes an average of four to six years between the onset of symptoms and a diagnosis of IC.

IC is puzzling to many doctors because there is no apparent infection or damage to the urinary tract, nor is there any obvious cause. (A common scenario is for a doctor to test the urine for bacteria; when none can be found, the patient is told, "There's nothing wrong with you.") This absence of explanation is deeply frustrating to patients, whose pain and symptoms are most definitely real. However, it is also comforting to know that IC is not progressive or destructive. It also tends to fade with time.

If you have IC, or think you might, it's essential for you to work with a specialist who understands your disorder—and who believes it exists. A urologist or urogynecologist (an OB-GYN with a specialization in the urinary tract) associated with a teaching hospital is your best bet. You can also check the Web site of the International Cystitis Association (http://www.ichelp.org), which lists qualified doctors. However, doctors who are excellent at managing this disorder are not always trained in managing the pain that comes with it. You may need to consult a pain specialist or even take matters into your own hands. Although there is no known cure for IC, an integrated plan can minimize or even completely relieve the pain.

TESTING, TESTING

See both a gynecologist and a urologist (or a urogynecologist) for a thorough physical exam. From there, your doctor may wish to conduct further tests, including urodynamics, in which your bladder is emptied and filled so that the doctor can measure its ability to function; a cystoscopy, in which the doctor examines the bladder via a fiber-optic scope; or a bladder biopsy. Before you agree to any of these tests, which can be uncomfortable and invasive, talk to your doctor and find out why she feels they are necessary. As always with pelvic pain, you'll need to walk that line between conscientious testing and a never-ending series of exams.

THERAPIES

See the list starting on page 336. Bladder and pelvic floor biofeedback are especially valuable, as are other mind-body therapies, a pain-control diet, and gentle exercise. Below are some conventional treatments used specifically for IC.

PAIN PILLS AND OTHER PHARMACEUTICALS

►► The drug pentosan polysulfate sodium (Elmiron) leads to improvement in about 40 percent of the patients who use it. It may work by repairing microscopic defects in the bladder lining. Side effects include gastrointestinal discomfort and possible liver problems. You'll need to give Elmiron a trial of six months before coming to a conclusion about its usefulness.

► A bladder wash with DMSO (dimethyl sulfoxide, made from a substance that holds the cells of trees together) can help. A 50 percent solution of DMSO is flushed into the bladder with a catheter and held for ten to fifteen minutes before emptying. This procedure should be performed every week or two for a total of six to eight weeks. You may have a garliclike odor on your skin and breath for up to seventy-two hours after each treatment.

► Antihistamines are another pharmaceutical option for IC. Low-grade allergic responses, perhaps to food or other substances, can irritate and inflame the bladder; antihistamines can stop or ease this process. You should know within two weeks whether they are helping.

NUTRITION AND SUPPLEMENTS

For recommended doses of supplements, see Chapter 9.

►► In addition to following the pain-control diet and checking for food allergies, you should avoid any food that irritates your bladder. Spicy and acidic foods or caffeinated beverages are most likely to make your symptoms worse.

►► Smoking also irritates the bladder, so avoid places where you're likely to encounter secondhand smoke. And if you smoke, quit.

DEEP INJECTIONS, IMPLANTS, AND SURGERY

▶ For severe pain that can't be controlled in any other way, a pump implant or spinal cord stimulator may give relief.

▶ Avoid bladder reconstruction or removal for IC; these surgeries rarely help, probably because the pain is more at home in the nervous system rather than in the organ itself.

VULVODYNIA

Vulvodynia is a little-understood painful syndrome characterized by burning, searing, or stinging pain in the vulva. Pain during sexual intercourse may also be present. In women with vulvodynia, there are no visible changes to the organs themselves, and possible acute causes of pain such as infection, irritation from soaps and hygiene products, and sexual trauma have all been ruled out. Although the pain is restricted to a small area of the body, it can seriously cut into the normal activities of life, from sex to sports to sitting down. It's hard to estimate how many women suffer from this disorder, because vulvodynia has been recognized as a medical syndrome since only 1983, and because many women may be prevented from seeking treatment out of embarrassment or fear that they will be disbelieved.

The exact cause of vulvodynia is unknown. Just as with many pelvic pain syndromes, both pelvic floor muscle spasms and nervous system alterations (including hypersensitized nerves, discussed in Chapter 3, and injury to the pudendal nerve) may be implicated. Low-grade inflammation—in response to allergies, recurrent yeast infections, unlubricated sexual intercourse, and other acute sources of pain and irritation—may play a role in rewiring the nervous system, sending so many pain signals to the spinal cord that the nerves no longer distinguish between gentle touch or movement and horrible pain. Sometimes, if the vulvar pain—whatever its initial source—has continued for long enough, the nerves can produce pain all on their own. Another possible contributor to vulvodynia is a diet high in oxalates. This chemical, found in many foods, is made up of crystals that may trigger pain in the vulva as urine passes through the urethra.

(continued)

Some doctors believe that herpes, human papilloma virus (HPV)—a disease that causes cervical cancer and warts on the vulva—or yeast infections are causes. Low levels of estrogen may also trigger some vulvar pain.

If you suspect you have vulvodynia, the core member of your pain team should be a gynecologist who makes a specialty of treating this disorder. The National Vulvodynia Association (see Appendix E for contact information) can help you find a practitioner in your area who is interested in treating vulvar disorders. A pain specialist can help, too, especially if your pain is severe and your coordinating doctor is uncomfortable prescribing opioids.

As with other painful syndromes, especially those whose causes are unknown, you may need to try several therapies before finding a combination that keeps your pain under maximum control. The therapies listed starting on page 336 may help; of these, I especially recommend tricyclic antidepressants or anticonvulsants (to calm misfiring nerves), pelvic-floor biofeedback (to relax muscles in spasm), a pain-control diet (to reduce any low-grade inflammation that may trigger vulvar pain and sensitize nerves), and mind-body therapies (to help you distance yourself from the pain). Reduce your consumption of foods that are very high in oxalates, including berries, chocolate and cocoa, peanuts, beer, tea, pecans, and beverage mixes. If you notice a difference after a week or two, keep these foods off your menu. But if you don't feel any better, there's no need to deny yourself. Other treatments that vulvodynia experts often prescribe include topical local anesthetics, estrogen creams, and interferon (a treatment for HPV).

As a very last resort, some doctors may recommend a vestibulectomy, in which a piece of tissue is removed from the vestibule, between the labia minora. This option, which does not interfere with sexual intercourse and rarely affects childbearing, may make sense for those patients who have exhausted *all* other avenues of pain control, but the vulvodynia patients I see prefer to manage their pain with opioids and other drugs rather than have this surgery.

24.

MYOFASCIAL PAIN SYNDROME

You've probably never heard someone say, "My goodness, this myofascial pain is really acting up again!" Although myofascial pain syndrome, or MPS, is one of the most common painful disorders in existence—some doctors I know say that two-thirds of the pain they treat is caused by MPS—most people have never heard of it, nor have physicians been trained to recognize it. That's a shame, because this muscular pain is highly treatable. In the pain clinic where I work, a diagnosis of myofascial pain is cause for excitement among the staff, since we know that the patient is likely to feel better within weeks or even hours.

The term "myofascial pain syndrome" may sound obscurely technical, but it's actually based on the familiar concept of muscle tension. *Myo-* refers to muscles; *fascia* is the fibrous sheet of connective tissue that surrounds and supports each and every structure of the body. (If you've seen the filmy, whitish sheath that covers a piece of raw steak or chicken, you've seen fascia.) MPS usually occurs after an injury or alongside another painful condition, such as arthritis or a pinched nerve. In response to the injury or pain, the muscles brace themselves tightly. This is a natural reaction meant to immobilize a damaged area and to protect it from further harm. But if the muscles stay tensed for a long period of time, they can generate their own problems. Localized pain and spasm develop, along with a limited range of motion and a sense of weakness.

It appears that what happens is a kind of auto-strangulation: Constant tension within the muscles impedes blood flow or even prevents it completely. Oxygen can't get to the cells, nor can the cells get rid of lactic acid and other metabolic wastes. The nerves in the area become irritated and send amplified messages of pain to the brain—which responds by clenching the muscles even more tightly. This vicious circle of pain-tension-pain expands into wider and wider areas. The collagen fibers that make up the myofascia can thicken or stick to one another; when the fascia around one muscle tightens, it can pull on the fascia of neighboring muscles and make those muscles hurt as well. Or the pain may lead to sleeplessness or inactivity, both of which lower the body's resistance to pain.

But myofascial pain syndrome goes beyond tensed muscles. For a diagnosis to be made, you need to have something called a *trigger point.* A trigger point is a knot or taut band of muscle. The knot or band feels tender or painful when pressed, and it also produces pain that radiates to another part of your body. The trick to trigger points is that they often exist in places *other* than where you feel your day-to-day pain. For example, I see many patients with neck pain who have trigger points in their shoulders; when I press on these shoulder points, the patients actually feel their familiar pain in the neck.

Trigger points can develop anywhere you have muscle tissue, but they usually appear in the shoulder, neck, and lower back. (President Kennedy suffered from agonizing low back pain as a result of his World War II injuries. He was treated by a revolving series of top-notch doctors without relief. Then he met Janet Travell, the doctor who first described trigger points and their treatment. After she worked on the president, he said that he was pain-free for the first time since the war.) Trigger points frequently pop up in clusters, although it's possible to have just one.

I like to tell my patients that they have the right to more than one painful condition. This is especially true for myofascial pain, which often crops up as a defensive reaction to other problems, most especially—but not limited to—arthritis, whiplash, chronic sprains and strains, headache, pelvic pain, and pain in the low back, shoulders, and neck. By treating the trigger points, you may find that much of your pain vanishes. In a few cases, *all* of the pain will disappear.

Myofascial pain can also develop on its own, often through poor posture or overuse of a muscle. This happened to my father, a devoted fisherman who spent hours bent over a table tying flies and who developed burning pain in his neck and shoulders as a consequence. Long periods of immobility are another way to cause trigger points; they appear frequently in people whose pain has kept them inactive. And of course, we can't forget that emotional stress often deposits itself in the muscles.

Plenty of good treatments exist to break the myofascial pain cycle, but far and away the best is stretching of the area. To make stretching less painful, you and your doctor can use injections of local anesthetic, a coolant spray, or ice. Special deep-tissue massage techniques are also quite helpful, as are mind-body therapies that relax the muscles.

TESTING, TESTING

You can check for trigger points on your own or have a friend do it for you. Examine the painful region (for head and neck pain, make sure to include the shoulders) for a lump or knot of muscle. If a knot feels tender when pressed *and* if it sends pain radiating to another location, you have a trigger point. (If a knot doesn't cause pain to radiate, it's not a trigger point, although you will probably still benefit from massage, stretching, and relaxation.) Continue to check around the area for additional trigger points.

THERAPIES

PHYSICAL THERAPIES

►► The best way to stop myofascial pain is to stretch it away. You can use the exercises in Appendix A; you might also want to see a physical therapist for a customized plan.

►► Heat and cold therapies were made for myofascial pain. A technique known as spray-and-stretch, which uses a vapocoolant to numb the muscles, is excellent and well known to physical therapists. You can also use ice massage before or after stretching. Heat and ultrasound will help dissolve tension.

►► Moderate cardiovascular exercise is another good way to loosen up muscles and work out emotional tension. It also produces chemicals that reduce pain. Try Pilates, a good workout that lengthens the muscles.

▶▶ If you sense that poor posture is at the root of your myofascial pain, take steps to correct it. Cultivate an awareness of your back, head, and shoulders, and watch out for a tendency to slump or hunch over when you work, drive, or engage in hobbies. If self-help doesn't work, try the Alexander Technique, Feldenkrais, or Hellerwork.

▶ Sometimes trigger points can be pretty stubborn, even when you've stretched and stretched. In these cases, deep-tissue massage (such as trigger point work, myofascial release, or Rolfing) is a great addition to other physical therapy. It works out the kinks, stimulates endorphins, reduces emotional stress, and boosts your resistance to pain. Don't forget to keep stretching! If you want to learn about a home massage technique for myofascial pain, see Appendix B.

PAIN PILLS AND OTHER PHARMACEUTICALS

▶▶ I often use trigger point injections as a first-line technique for myofascial pain. These office injections of local anesthetic numb the pain and allow you to stretch out the muscle. The needle itself may also help break up the tension by stimulating the point. Remember that you absolutely must stretch after the injection; otherwise, the effect will be only temporary.

▶ NSAIDs can keep the pain down as you pursue other treatment.

▶ If the pain is disrupting your sleep, low doses of a tricyclic antidepressant can help you get a good night's rest.

▶ Muscle relaxants are a good choice when spasm is a strong component of the pain.

MIND-BODY MEDICINE

▶▶ It matters less which mind-body technique you use than that you find one you like and use it regularly. You might employ guided imagery—you could imagine your muscles melting from the inside out, for example. Or use the breathing techniques in Chapter 8 to soften the tissues. If you're having a lot of trouble unclenching the muscle, EMG biofeedback can help.

DISTRACTING YOUR NERVOUS SYSTEM FROM PAIN

▶▶ Acupressure, especially Jin Shin Do, is a form of deep-tissue work that addresses trigger points as well as the flow of energy through your body.

▶▶ Acupuncture is another choice treatment for myofascial pain.

▶ Electrical stimulation temporarily blocks pain signals from moving through the spinal cord, giving you a window in which to stretch and exercise. (But stimulation is useless without proper stretching afterward.) It also sends the muscles into a brief spasm, so that they exhaust themselves and release.

▶ If the pain just won't go away, you can try TENS to block the pain signals. People tend to have the most success when the electrical nodes are placed *not* on the trigger points themselves but off to the side of the trigger points or farther down the body from them.

NUTRITION AND SUPPLEMENTS

For recommended doses of supplements, see Chapter 9.

▶ If tension and anxiety are keeping you up at night, consider taking kava before you go to bed (but don't use kava for extended periods of time).

25.

COMPLEX REGIONAL PAIN SYNDROME

It was one of those freak summertime accidents. Deirdre, an engineer from the Midwest, was walking out onto her back deck when she slipped and tumbled over the low railing. She fell into the pool a story below, smacking her foot hard against the metal ladder. At first, she was thankful that she hadn't been more seriously injured; she made off without even a broken bone, just some bruises and a hairline fracture. Her doctor put her into an air cast, and everyone assumed she'd be fine, aside from missing out on some seasonal fun.

After a couple of weeks Deirdre began to wonder if she'd been so lucky after all. The pain, instead of gradually subsiding to a faint ache, had changed character. Her foot had become hot, prickly, and exquisitely sensitive to touch. When X rays revealed that her injury was healing on schedule, the orthopedist prescribed more rest. After another couple of weeks, her foot hurt nearly all the time. She walked with a pronounced limp and wore her shoes without laces, since they put too much pressure on her feet. Although she visited several orthopedic specialists and racked up thousands of dollars' worth of tests, no one could explain her unusual symptoms. She couldn't sleep well, and she found it difficult to manage her three children. Plainly speaking, she was crabby. Soon her husband and kids were crabby, too. Then a dark thought occurred to her: Could this pain, which her doctors were at a loss to explain, be a symptom of bone cancer?

Deirdre did not have bone cancer, nor was she crazy. She was suffering from complex regional pain syndrome (CRPS), a disorder that is not yet well understood but that is most definitely real. The condition was first identified in 1864 by Weir Mitchell, a doctor who treated Civil War veterans at the Philadelphia Stump Hospital. He noticed that some patients suffered from a burning sensation that couldn't be explained by their wounds; these same patients went to extreme lengths to avoid touching the area or exposing it to air. Mitchell gave this syndrome the name "causalgia." Since then, complex regional pain syndrome has been called by many different names, and you may still hear doctors use the terms "causalgia" or, more likely, "reflex sympathetic dystrophy." But the disturbing, apparently inexplicable symptoms remain the same.

Complex regional pain syndrome usually begins after an operation or an accident—even a relatively minor one such as Deirdre's. (It's also possible, but unusual, for CRPS to occur spontaneously.) After the precipitating event, the damaged tissues heal, but the pain doesn't stop. Instead, a burning pain develops and spreads throughout the limb. The skin of the affected area may become extraordinarily sensitive, so that a breeze or the touch of clothing, even a bright light, delivers a bolt of pain. These symptoms are classic signs of pain originating in the nerves.

In a majority of cases, CRPS affects the sympathetic nervous system, which regulates involuntary body activities. This often (but not always) causes odd changes in the limb in addition to the pain. The skin may become mottled or blue, or feel unusually cold or hot. The limb may shed its body hair, sweat, or swell. And it doesn't stop there—the pain and other symptoms can sometimes spread to other parts of the body. Because the person hurts so much, he rarely exercises. The muscles atrophy, and before you know it, general weakness and fatigue overtake the body and mind. If CRPS is not treated, it can result in long-term disability and loss of function in the affected limb.

Exactly what causes CRPS is unclear. The only thing that's certain is that the nervous system is somehow rewired, either by the trauma that caused the original injury or by some unknown mechanism. The nerves become unusually sensitive, and the neurochemicals that regulate pain are altered. One leading theory is that the receptors for adrenaline, a neurotransmitter that puts your body on a heightened state of alert, develop an increased ability to receive and pass on signals that lead to pain, making you hurt even when there's no obvious damage. The tissues of the affected limb, bombarded by nerve input and vascular constriction, also appear to go into a kind of overdrive and contribute to the pain. In yet another example of pain's vicious circles, the increased pain tends to increase the abnormal neurological activity.

Although complex regional pain syndrome is an accepted disorder, one that's described in all the neurological textbooks, it's not the kind of thing that many primary-care doctors are taught about in school. For that reason, its bizarre symptoms may be mistaken for something else entirely, perhaps a hairline fracture, an entrapped nerve, or an emotional problem that's manifesting itself in the body. (One of my patients received *four* unsuccessful operations on his foot before he was diagnosed with CRPS at the pain clinic.) That's a pity. Despite the mysterious workings of CRPS, there are tried-and-true treatments available—and the earlier you get them, the better your chances of healing. Even if you've been suffering for years, however, you can still benefit from appropriate medical attention. If your doctor is not experienced in treating CRPS, ask for a referral to a neurologist or to a pain clinic.

When it comes to treatment, nerve blocks are at the top of the list. They temporarily halt the barrage of heightened sensation and give your sympathetic nervous system and body tissues a chance to quiet down. These nerve blocks must be followed by physical therapy to return function and normality to the limb. I also strongly recommend mind-body work, which may affect the limbic system and help it control the nerves that are haywire. As secondary therapies, medications can help, and both distraction and energetic methods encourage the nervous system to heal.

TESTING, TESTING

A medical history and physical exam are sometimes all you need to identify CRPS, especially if you show the telltale signs of discoloration, swelling, and temperature changes in the limb. You and your doctor should keep in mind that CRPS can develop in the absence of these changes; sometimes the only symptom is pain.

If the diagnosis can't be made from the history and exam, you might get one or more of these tests:

- *Sympathetic nerve blocks.* These are a first-line therapy, but they are also a diagnostic tool. A feature of these blocks is that they produce immediate relief of pain that is sympathetically maintained—that is, pain whose source is in the sympathetic nervous system. So if your pain is significantly reduced after this block, your doctor will probably make a diagnosis of CRPS. However, failure of a block does not necessarily rule out CRPS.

▶ *Triple-phase bone scan.* Too much activity from the sympathetic nerves stimulates the bone to turn over its tissue more frequently than normal. This test determines if such activity is present.

▶ *Intravenous lidocaine drip.* If this drip cools off the nerve pain, there's a good chance you have CRPS. You are also likely to respond well to treatment with the drug mexiletine (discussed below).

THERAPIES

DEEP INJECTIONS, IMPLANTS, AND SURGERY

▶▶ The grade-A treatment for CRPS is a sympathetic nerve block. If the pain is in the hand, arm, or elsewhere in the upper body, the block is performed on the stellate ganglion, a cluster of sympathetic nerves at the base of the neck. When the pain is at the hip or below, the nerve group called the lumbar sympathetic plexus, which resides in the lower spine, is blocked. When the sympathetic neurological input is shut down in this way, your nervous system has the chance to reset itself, much as a computer gone haywire may behave perfectly normally after you shut down and reboot. You may get immediately noticeable relief from a sympathetic nerve block, or it may take a day or two. Although a few lucky people will experience permanent pain control, the effects are usually temporary. This pain-free window should be used for intensive physical therapy.

▶▶ If blocks, alternative therapies, and drugs don't work, your next choice might be a spinal cord stimulator or a pump implant. Both stimulators and morphine pumps have been used with success for CRPS.

▶ Another procedure—but a much less common one—is a pump implant filled with clonidine, a drug that helps to block sympathetic nervous system activity. Rarely, baclofen (a muscle relaxant) may be used instead.

▶ When CRPS is intractable and resistant to all other therapies, a sympathectomy may erase the pain. The first kind of sympathectomy is a nerve ablation, in which a knot of sympathetic nerves is deadened.

(This is different from a nerve block, in which the nerves are simply numbed for a while.) In the second and even more drastic brand of sympathectomy, the nerves are actually cut. I think of both forms as treatments of last resort, as they are major neurosurgical procedures. A vast majority of the time, the surgery will go smoothly. But as any neurosurgeon will tell you, there are always risks. If the wrong spinal nerves are deadened, or if nervous tissue is accidentally cut, you are in serious trouble. Should your circumstances require sympathectomy, make sure you work with a surgeon who is experienced in this procedure. Sympathectomies are far less effective for people who've had CRPS for more than two years.

DEIRDRE'S STORY CONTINUED

Deirdre was so wary of nerve blocks that she initially refused treatment. Instead, she saw a chiropractor. The spinal manipulation helped her get around a little more comfortably, but when the pain didn't stop, the chiropractor encouraged her to give conventional medicine another try. Deirdre agreed to the nerve block—and felt better within minutes. She performed physical therapy exercises with her foot immersed in a whirlpool bath, received massage, and practiced guided imagery to relax and to improve her mood. She eventually required two more blocks to give her extra time to continue the physical therapy. After about three weeks, her limp—and her pain—were nearly gone.

PHYSICAL THERAPIES

►► After receiving a nerve block, you need to receive a thorough round of physical therapy, including range-of-motion and strengthening exercises. Working out in water can feel especially good.

►► Moving around is not always possible with CRPS, especially if it's your foot or leg that's in pain. But if you are not debilitated, get cardiovascular exercise at least three times a week. You'll increase your endorphins, the pain-blocking chemicals, and ward off weakness, fatigue, and depression.

MIND-BODY THERAPIES

▶▶ Mind-body therapies are especially important for you, because they plug directly into the limbic system, a part of the brain that helps direct both the emotional response to pain *and* the sympathetic nervous system. When you calm down the limbic system, you may accomplish two things: loosen pain's control over your emotions, and pacify your out-of-control sympathetic nervous system. Biofeedback, hypnosis, and meditation are all good choices.

▶ If the pain is dominating your life, try cognitive-behavioral therapy. It helps you find ways to maintain an active, satisfying life despite the pain.

DISTRACTING YOUR NERVOUS SYSTEM FROM PAIN

▶ I recommend a combination of nerve block, physical therapy, and mind-body work as the best set of treatments. But if that approach hasn't worked so well for you, or if for some reason you can't have a nerve block, you may wish to move on to acupuncture. It's not always successful, but from time to time it really turns patients around.

▶ TENS is another alternative when blocks don't work.

NUTRITION AND SUPPLEMENTS

For recommended doses of supplements, see Chapter 9.

▶▶ CRPS places huge demands on the body. By supporting yourself with the pain-control diet, you can reduce your chances of developing fatigue, weakness, or other illnesses.

▶ Take a B-complex supplement to support nerve health.

▶ Take a calcium and magnesium supplement daily, and be sure to include low-fat dairy products, soy foods, and green leafy vegetables in your diet.

ENERGY HEALING

▶ I've seen CRPS patients greatly improve with Reiki, although I'm hard pressed to explain why. My guess is that for some people, this and other energy treatments soothe the nervous system, perhaps helping it return to normal.

▶ For the same reason, you may also wish to try homeopathy or tai chi.

PAIN PILLS AND OTHER PHARMACEUTICALS

▶ Anticonvulsants and tricyclic antidepressants inhibit pain signals from firing. Remember that you and your doctor may need to experiment until you find the right drug and dosage.

▶ Another drug that has a particularly good record with CRPS is mexiletine (Mexitil), an adrenaline-blocking drug; it's often used as a supplement to antidepressants. You may also need to use an anticonvulsant and tricyclic antidepressant in combination with mexiletine. *Do not combine drugs unless you have specific instructions from your doctor.*

▶ Calcium channel blockers may quiet down your nervous system. The generic drug verapamil or its brand-name counterpart, Calan SR, is often prescribed for this purpose. A significant side effect of calcium channel blockers is that they lower blood pressure, so you'll need to be checked out by your doctor before you can take them.

▶ Tizanidine (Zanaflex) is a muscle relaxant that also opposes adrenaline in the nervous system. It may have some moderating effects on CRPS and is often worth a try.

▶ Opioids, especially methadone, often provide relief when other drugs fail. Once, it was thought that opioids did not affect nerve pain; however, this idea has been discarded. You may need a higher dose of opioids for nerve pain than someone with a different disorder.

PART V

SPECIAL CONSIDERATIONS

26.

PAIN MANAGEMENT FOR CHILDREN, PREGNANT WOMEN, AND THE ELDERLY

PAIN MANAGEMENT FOR CHILDREN

Not so long ago, it was thought that infants couldn't feel pain. Surgery, from circumcision to complex procedures, was routinely performed without anesthesia. Even older children were deemed less vulnerable to pain than adults—many of us can all too clearly recall the acute, untreated pain that lingered after the requisite tonsillectomies of the 1950s and 1960s. Today, it is widely understood that infants and children feel pain as intensely as anyone else does and that they deserve appropriate treatment. What constitutes "appropriate," however, can sometimes be confusing for concerned parents.

WHAT DOES YOUR CHILD FEEL?

It is a challenge for most children to describe the severity and quality of their pain. They lack the vocabulary and ability to put pain in context; very small children may not even understand the need to communicate about what hurts them. Since you and the doctor need some way of measuring the pain, the usual methods of communication—ranking the pain on a scale from 1 to 10 and employing descriptive adjectives—must be modified for children.

The Faces Pain Scale, below, is one way for children ages six or seven and older to rank their pain effectively, since it doesn't require an abstraction to numbers. For the best results, you or the doctor need to calibrate the scale for the child. The child is asked to think of the worst pain he's ever felt—usually from a fall or perhaps getting shampoo in their eyes. That pain is assigned to the sad, crying face at the right end of the scale. Then the child thinks of the smallest amount of pain he's felt, like having shoes laced too tightly. This pain is associated with the neutral face on the scale's left end. Only after this calibration is performed is the child asked to point to the way the pain feels right now. It's a good idea to remind the child of the extreme ends of the scale and the painful events associated with it each time he uses it.

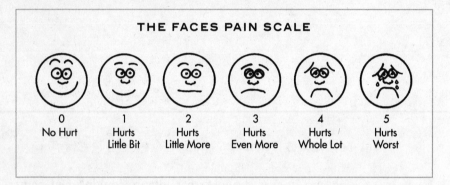

THE FACES PAIN SCALE

Older children may use a thermometer scale, in which the pain rises like the red line on a hot day, or a shortened number scale from 1 to 5.

Although children are rarely skilled at using traditional pain descriptors such as *stinging* or *aching,* they are adept with metaphorical or imaginative language. Here are some questions that can elicit helpful responses:

- Can you show me how big the pain (or *ouch, owie, boo-boo,* or *hurt*) is?
- Can you use your crayons to show me what color the pain is?
- What kind of animal would cause this pain?
- What kind of sound does this pain make?

In addition, many kids are more willing to talk about their pain through dolls, puppets, or teddy bears than directly to an adult. Other children may be encouraged to show you where the pain hurts and how it feels by coloring an outline of a human figure.

TREATING YOUR CHILD'S PAIN

TLC. Children are highly sensitive to their emotional environments. They need more reassurance and tender loving care than adults, and it might be argued that these things also bring them more pain relief. By believing your child, remaining calm, cuddling her, singing songs, and holding her close, you relieve some of the distress and fear that come with pain. You may also help reduce some of the pain itself, by stimulating endorphins and other body chemicals that block pain.

Another component of TLC is respect. As the adult, you of course must make the decisions about what kind of care the child receives, but it's usually a good idea to prepare the child for any kind of procedure or treatment he's going to face. Explain to the child what's going to happen to him—a toy doctor's kit can come in handy here—and explain what you or the doctor is doing when the child must be physically handled. Being "surprised" with a visit to the doctor or with having one's pants pulled down for a shot is as degrading to children as it is to adults. It also compromises the trust that you and your child will need to share throughout any extended painful ordeal.

Finally, be on the lookout for depression or anxiety. Our culture assumes that kids don't suffer from these problems, but chronic pain may well bring them on. Common signs are listlessness or lack of appetite, but nothing is better than your parental judgment when it comes to spotting unusual behavior in your child. If you suspect a problem, talk to your doctor or to a children's psychotherapist.

Pharmaceuticals. Don't be afraid of judicious pain medication for children. If your child is experiencing moderate to severe pain, painkillers and other medications are an essential component of compassionate care.

That said, it must be acknowledged that prescribing any medication at all for children is a tricky business. Most pharmaceuticals are not tested on kids—for the obvious reason that no one wants to make guinea pigs out of small children—including the common drugs for coughs and colds as well as NSAIDs and opioids. Doctors need to rely on basic guidelines regarding the child's age and weight, and on their own experience prescribing for children. Therefore, it's wise to work with a doctor who has spent several years treating children in pain. Many family pediatricians and family practitioners fall into this category, but in cases of severe or long-lasting pain you may wish to find a pediatric pain specialist. Be aware that an inexperienced physician is likely to err on the conservative side.

Touch. Many kids, and almost all infants, respond to therapies that involve a loving touch. Simply holding your child and stroking her head or back can reduce pain, depression, and anxiety. If your child is willing, you can also try massage, reflexology, Reiki, or Therapeutic Touch. Be sure to find a practitioner who has experience treating children, and never force your child to undergo a touch therapy if he doesn't want to.

Breathing, guided imagery, hypnosis, and biofeedback. Kids take to these simple mind-body techniques like ducks to water, especially if you give them a little help. While sitting close to your child, you can show him deep breathing to use before bedtime or whenever he needs to relax. Most kids also enjoy being taken on an imaginary trip to a relaxing place, perhaps a favorite vacation spot or their grandmother's house. Younger children may need you to guide them every time, but older children enjoy contributing to the images and can mentally replay them on their own. If your child likes, you can make a tape of your voice describing the relaxing scene in great detail, which she can play whenever she needs to unwind and take her mind off the pain. This technique can be especially helpful during an unpleasant procedure.

Hypnosis, with its reliance on the client's trust and imagination, has an exceptional track record with children. Stories abound of hypnotized kids who have undergone long dental or surgical procedures without anesthetic and reported no pain or discomfort. I don't recommend you send your child under the knife without adequate conventional pain control, but you might try hypnosis in addition to anesthesia, or for postoperative pain. Again, be sure to find a therapist who knows how to work with children.

Finally, consider biofeedback, especially for headache and pain that features muscle tension or emotional stress as a major component. Kids who like computers and video games enjoy the high-tech, interactive quality of this therapy.

Acupuncture. Acupuncture may reduce severe pain and anxiety in children. Obviously, this therapy is not appropriate for children who are fidgety or who are afraid of needles. Make sure the acupuncturist is experienced with children and uses kid-size pins.

Higher therapies. Children are geniuses at taking their minds off pain. Laughter, books, painting, music, and even video games help them enter another, pain-free world for a while. (One caveat here: I advise against distracting kids with a video or jokes in order to give a doctor time to sneak up with a needle. Let the child know what will happen; *then* help him to distract himself.)

If you'd like to learn more about pediatric pain control, I highly recommend the book *Soothing Your Child's Pain* by Kenneth Gorfinkle, Ph.D. Dr. Gorfinkle has many specific suggestions for interacting with kids in pain and especially for helping them through painful procedures. I am indebted to him for several ideas I've presented here.

PAIN MANAGEMENT DURING PREGNANCY

Pregnancy itself can bring on chronic pain—for example, hormonal changes can induce temporary carpal tunnel syndrome and back pain—or it can make existing conditions more trying. In either case, most conventional pain medications are inadvisable, as well as most herbal preparations. (In severe situations, it's possible to take certain opioids in the second or third trimester, with the agreement of your physician.)

You need not go without pain control, however. Alternative medicine provides many gentle techniques that can keep pain in check during your pregnancy. Some of the best bets for keeping pain in check are listed here. Don't forget to follow the basic plan of eating well, exercising regularly, and managing stress.

If you have a preexisting painful condition, it's a good idea to create a strategy and build your pain team in the very early stages of pregnancy. If you don't already have relationships with practitioners of gentle therapies such as massage or acupuncture, now is the time to start—you don't want to wait until you're in a pain crisis to find someone you like and trust. I also recommend that you learn some additional mind-body techniques as soon as you discover that you're expecting. They'll come in handy throughout the pregnancy (not to mention those sleepless months after the delivery).

GENTLE PAIN-CONTROL METHODS DURING PREGNANCY

THERAPY	BENEFITS	BEST FOR . . .	CAUTIONS
Mind-body therapies	Promote relaxation, reduce muscle tension and "nerve noise"	Any pain condition	
Exercise: swimming, prenatal yoga, Pilates, stretching	Helps block pain signals, reduces muscle tension, strengthens and stabilizes	Any pain condition, especially back pain, neck pain, and headache (certain yoga poses are good for carpal tunnel syndrome)	Avoid aquatic exercise during the very last stages of pregnancy. (If your water breaks while you're in the pool, you might not be aware of it.) Pilates can be difficult, if not impossible, to do during the last trimester.
Acupuncture and acupressure	Reduce pain, stress, and nausea	Any pain condition as well as nausea	Be sure your practitioner is experienced in working with pregnant women.
Massage	Promotes relaxation, reduces muscle tension	Back and neck pain; myofascial pain syndrome; fibromyalgia; and most other pain conditions, as well as general discomfort	Again, find someone experienced in prenatal massage. Positioning is very important, so that you don't put pressure on the baby.
Aromatherapy	Distracts your nervous system from pain, soothes the mind	Any pain condition	
Higher Therapies	Lifts your mind off the pain temporarily	Any pain condition	
TENS	Blocks pain signals from traveling up your spinal cord	Most pain conditions, especially back pain (TENS is less helpful when pain occurs on the body's periphery.)	Don't place a TENS unit over the belly or pelvis.

NAUSEA DURING PREGNANCY

Strictly speaking, nausea isn't a pain problem. But alternative medicine offers a number of ways to reduce the queasiness that so often attends pregnancy. Consider the following techniques:

- *Acupuncture and acupressure.* A full professional treatment is probably most effective, but for an at-home treatment you can work the front of the hip, the instep of the foot, and especially the inside base of the wrist (some health-food stores sell wristbands that provide continuous stimulation of this point, called Pericardium 6 in acupuncture terms).
- *Ginger tea.* Buy a commercial preparation, or make your own: Peel and finely chop fresh gingerroot and steep in a cup of hot water. Peppermint tea also eases nausea in some people.

PAIN MANAGEMENT FOR THE ELDERLY

Advanced age doesn't just put people at risk for pain. It also increases the chance that the pain will be poorly treated. The many complicating factors of age, including other illnesses and medications, altered metabolism, and a changed social environment, pose a challenge even to health professionals who are highly knowledgeable about pain. Here's a look at some of the mistakes most often made in pain management for the elderly and how to correct them.

FIVE MISTAKES IN PAIN MANAGEMENT FOR THE ELDERLY

1. ***Overlooking malnutrition.*** Older people may lose their sense of taste and with it their appetite, making malnutrition a very real problem. Do your best to eat a variety of foods, and make sure to take adequate supplements as recommended in Chapter 9, especially the B-complex vitamins. Get a careful workup by a good physician to look for malnutrition and for malabsorption syndromes, in which nutrients are not properly extracted from food.

2. ***Overmedication.*** Reduced levels of body fat and metabolic changes make overmedication of the elderly all too easy. Many older people suffer from sedation even on very low levels of painkillers, and I've seen people sleep for days after taking the tiniest dose of tricyclic antidepressants. This effect is compounded by the long list of drugs most elderly people are taking for other conditions. The result is patients who are drugged into a stupor, or who miss out on pain control altogether because side effects have scared them away from medications.

You don't have to accept heavy sedation or other serious side effects just because of your age, nor do you have to walk away from pharmaceuticals in general. You and your doctor should plan to tinker with your prescriptions for a while to hit on the right drug and dosage for you. If you've tried a pain medication before, only to have it knock you out, consider trying it again (with your doctor's agreement) in a smaller dose or using a slightly different version. Explain to your doctor that you want to "start low and go slow" with your pain medication. Should you experience unacceptably strong side effects, don't hesitate to give her or the nurse a call.

Finally, remember that alternatives such as massage, mind-body techniques, TENS, acupuncture, and others can reduce your need for pain medications.

3. ***Giving up on exercise.*** A lot of older people have led amazing, fascinating lives—and now they'd like to rest and reflect. But a sedentary life can lead to pain. If you're in your seventies, eighties, or nineties, you don't need a grueling workout to see results. Gentle exercises such as tai chi, yoga, walking, and aquatic exercise can improve your health and reduce your pain.

4. ***Not getting enough touch.*** This tends to be true for people living on their own or in nursing homes. If you miss the feeling of caring human contact—not just the medical, clinical kind—consider getting a massage, volunteering at a hospital to massage and hold premature babies, or adopting a furry pet. If you're a caregiver to an elderly person, don't underestimate the value of holding hands or giving a light massage.

5. ***Missing an opportunity to make meaning.*** Skeptical family members and caregivers are often surprised at how enthusiastic elderly people are about mind-body therapies. As they get older, many people develop a stronger interest in reflecting on their lives, shaping their stories, and making meaning from their experiences. If you're religious, prayer can be of great value in these endeavors. So can meditation, gentle yoga, writing in a journal, playing music, painting, and drawing. Even the act of looking at art made by someone else, reading books, or listening to music can engage you on a higher plane. On a more practical level, these therapies can also turn the mind's attention away from pain—an important strategy for isolated people who may have little else in their lives. When a person has art class or a good book to look forward to, the pain loses some of its overwhelming quality.

27.

PAIN AND TERMINAL ILLNESS

Death and pain used to be nearly inseparable: To die meant to die in pain. This is no longer true, thanks largely to medications such as opioids and steroid drugs. These and other pharmaceuticals allow people a much more comfortable transition out of this life.

But pain management for terminal illness is about much more than drugs. Too often, compassionate pain relief is confused with massive doses of narcotics, so that a patient is doped up beyond recognition. Current pain-relief strategies also may fail to take nausea, depression, and anxiety into account. The sick person, treated with heavy opioids and little else, isn't in pain, but it can't be said that he's fully himself, either. Friends and family members lose the chance for meaningful goodbyes. And the terminally ill person loses the opportunity to reflect on his life, to put his affairs in order, and to face death as he's faced life, not just as a body but as a complete human soul.

SOME PRACTICAL MATTERS

S*tart with conventional pain medicines.* Throughout this book, I've emphasized the importance of using gentler techniques first, saving the more aggressive ones until it is clear that they're necessary. This approach is less appropriate for pain at the end of life. Diseases such as cancer, AIDS, and other disorders can cause great pain; it is often immediately obvious that medication or injections are necessary. Nor is there time to experiment with alternative methods in their various combinations. Finally, the long-term health risk from strong drugs is obviously less pertinent here. Although I consider alternative medicine an important part of treating terminal pain, it can rarely replace conventional methods completely.

Build your pain-management team as soon as possible. Studies show that cancer patients whose pain is controlled live longer than those who don't receive adequate treatment. I wouldn't be surprised if this is true for other diseases as well. As soon as you know that you have a terminal illness likely to cause pain, ask your doctor for a referral to a pain specialist, and start looking for appropriate alternative therapists—even if you're not hurting much now. Should you find yourself in a surprise pain crisis, you'll appreciate having a team already in place.

THE HOSPICE MOVEMENT AND PALLIATIVE CARE

The hospice movement, which was begun by Dr. Cicely Saunders in England in the 1960s, provides a caring environment for the terminally ill. In hospice care, physicians, nurses, psychologists, clergy members, social workers, and volunteers look after the patient's full set of needs, including pain control and emotional support. Conventional medicine has responded to the popularity of hospice with something called *palliative care,* which is practiced by pain-management specialists as well as some gerontologists and neurologists. In the best situations, these doctors pull in the same kind of varied team available at a hospice. A dying person may still elect to go to a hospice, but it is growing more and more possible to receive this kind of complete care in a hospital or even at home.

Remember that anxiety and depression add to pain. Fear and sadness are natural responses to both pain and dying. The patients I've known to have the most peaceful deaths are those who have not denied these difficult emotions. But sometimes normal fear and sadness turn into the extremes of anxiety and depression, and the person's final days are spent in deeper pain of both the physical and spiritual variety. If this happens, you should know that there are prescription drugs as well as alternative methods that can help. Don't hesitate to take advantage of them. You have the right to die feeling like *yourself.*

THE MOST POWERFUL PHARMACEUTICALS

For more detailed information about pain medications, consult Chapter 12. If you want to learn more about deep injections, see Chapter 13.

Opioids and how to manage them. Opioids are the mainstay of terminal pain treatment; nothing else relieves severe pain quite like them. For pain that is nearly constant, moderate to high doses of a long-acting opioid are usually necessary to deliver smooth, continuous relief.

Make sure, however, that your pain strategy doesn't stop there. Opioids in the kind of doses used for terminal pain will produce side effects, including sedation, nausea, and constipation. A good pain plan will encompass therapies to reduce these effects. By changing the delivery system of the drug—receiving medication either through a patch placed on the skin or via a pump implanted at the base of the spine—you can cut back on the dosage and consequently the side effects. If sedation is a particular problem, your doctor can create a drug cocktail, combining the opioid with other pharmaceuticals to keep you alert. Use acupuncture to alleviate the nausea; massage therapy and ginger can help as well. If you're given a prescription for opioids, it's a good idea to start an anti-constipation program right away, since this side effect is more difficult to treat once it has become entrenched. For suggestions, see page 174.

Steroids to keep you up and about. Steroidal anti-inflammatory drugs are rarely used in managing long-term chronic pain, as these strong drugs can lead to serious health problems down the road. But at the very end of life, there's no reason to avoid them. Steroids reduce inflammation drastically; for cancer patients, they shrink tumors that are pressing painfully on other tissues. Steroids also pep you up—an effect that might well be desirable when pain, illness, or medications (such as opioids) leave you sedated or exhausted. Used properly, they can help even a gravely ill person participate in important duties or pleasures, such as attending a wedding.

Controlling spasm. If the pain has pushed muscles into spasm, a muscle relaxant is appropriate. Don't forget that a spasm can happen in the belly or chest just as easily as in the back. These drugs are especially helpful for diseases such as multiple sclerosis or when a tumor has expanded and is pushing on other tissues.

Drug cocktails for more relief and less sedation. Drug cocktails sound exotic, but they are simply combinations of pharmaceuticals. Opioids often form the base of a cocktail; steroids or muscle relaxants might appear as well. To counteract the sedating effects of opioids or certain muscle relaxants, you may also receive a stimulant, an antidepressant with an activating effect, or even an amphetamine. Anticonvulsants, which appear to quiet down the nervous system's reaction to pain and to improve the effects of other pain medications, may be included. For certain people, antianxiety medication or antidepressants such as Prozac or Paxil may be useful.

Deep injections for visceral pain. Pain in the viscera is a common result of terminal illness. Selective nerve blocks anesthetize the nerves that carry pain signals to the chest, ribs, abdomen, and pelvis. My aunt, who had pancreatic cancer, received something called a celiac plexus block, which targets the bundle of nerves that receive pain signals from the upper belly. It gave her three and a half pain-free weeks before she passed away. These blocks are the realm of the seasoned pain injection expert.

Cordotomy. An extreme but powerful procedure is the cordotomy, which severs nerves that carry pain signals from the spinal cord to the brain. It's used for intractable pain below the neck and is probably best used at the end of life, since the pain often returns after several months or years. Before you agree to a cordotomy, make sure you understand all the risks involved.

Medical marijuana. At the time of this writing, federal law prohibits using marijuana for any purpose, even though it reduces pain and—maybe even more important—relieves the nausea associated with opioids, chemotherapy, and other medications. Without it, many people can't keep food or drugs down. That we ban marijuana for this compassionate use is nothing short of an outrage.

ALTERNATIVE MEDICINE: INCREASE THE COMFORT

REDUCING SIDE EFFECTS

Some of the most common side effects of pain medications are constipation, nausea, dry mouth, and sedation. Alternative therapies and home-care measures can make these problems more tolerable. See the chart on page 174 for detailed information.

MAKING A CONNECTION

People who are very sick are rarely touched in a loving way. Without touch, we are all more vulnerable to depression, anxiety, insomnia, and pain. A therapeutic massage can be a profound experience for the terminally ill, but any caring person can deliver massage's benefits as well. A light back rub or leg massage is often welcome; a foot rub may even impart some of the effects of reflexology, helping a distressed person quiet down. And none of us should underestimate the simple act of holding hands.

HEALING

Terminal illness can't be cured. However, it is possible for a dying person to be healed. "To heal" means not to cure but to make whole. What wholeness means will vary for each one of us, but most people have some personal understanding of the concept. For some, it means forgiveness, of ourselves or of loved ones; for others, it involves weaving a meaning from life and death; for still others, the term has an intimation of grace. The greatest opportunities for wholeness arise in the face of challenges, including pain and dying. By allowing yourself time to be still, to breathe and to meditate, or to pray, you are likely to diminish the physical pain as well as anxiety and depression. You may need fewer medications or find that the pain just doesn't have as much power over you as it did before. Quietude and reflection in the face of death may even hold the power of transformation.

If you would like to read further on this topic, I recommend *Choices in Healing* by Michael Lerner. It is primarily for cancer patients who wish to explore the options of alternative medicine—and for that alone it is valuable—but its chapters on living and dying with illness have helped many people, regardless of their specific disease, arrive at a personal approach to the mysteries of death and healing.

28.

"IS THERE SOMETHING I CAN DO?" FOR LOVED ONES OF PEOPLE IN PAIN

In China, where traces of traditional ancestor worship linger in contemporary society, care for the sick remains in the hands of the family. When someone is hospitalized, the family supplies scented oils and clean linens. The sick person can expect her loved ones to change her sheets, massage her limbs, and bathe her with hot towels. The hospital staff welcomes family members as an essential part of the medical team. What a contrast to Western hospitals, where caregiving has become professionalized. Family and friends are relegated by their amateur status to the gift shop, where they can buy artificial flowers (real ones trigger allergies) or a box of processed candy—hardly items to inspire healing. Both the loved ones and the sufferer are cheated of opportunities: to express caring and to receive it, to deepen their connection.

The practical and personal value of doctors, nurses, and other medical staff cannot be underestimated. But you do not need to be a professional to give care. This is true no matter whether your loved one is in the hospital, homebound, or carrying on the daily routine. You know better than anyone else what makes your loved one feel better, how to encourage him to follow his medical routine, and what, for him, constitutes signs of distress.

That said, pain is not an easy condition to care for. It's invisible, quirky, often defiant of explanation. And continuing pain makes people behave differently—they are sadder, more anxious, less spirited. I think the best way to help a loved one is to learn as much as you can about the nature of the pain. Talk to the sufferer and, if appropriate, to her doctor. You might also read Part I of this book as well as the chapter that homes in on your loved one's disorder. Beyond that, here are some additional thoughts for those in the important but undervalued role of caregiver.

"BUT HE LOOKS FINE!"

Pain sufferers often look perfectly normal, both on the outside *and* on the inside. Countless scans, X rays, and blood tests may fail to show anything "wrong." That's because chronic pain often occurs when the nervous system—normally responsible for conducting messages of pain—actually creates pain all on its own or exaggerates existing pain messages. (For more information about the nervous system's role in pain, see Chapter 3.)

People just don't lie about chronic pain. In all my years treating pain sufferers, the number I've thought might have been faking could be counted on one hand. That's just a couple of patients out of thousands. Most other pain specialists will tell you the same. So believe your loved one, and keep in mind the words of Samuel Johnson: "Those who do not feel pain seldom think that it is felt." Without trust, the caregiving relationship itself becomes a lie.

PAIN DOESN'T TURN PEOPLE INTO SAINTS

We'd all like to believe that pain and illness have the power to bring a family together, that everyone will rally in loving support around the noble sufferer. When this idyll of family togetherness fails to appear, we're crushed and bewildered.

Pain doesn't suddenly turn sufferers or family members into selfless angels. The person in pain may become depressed, angry, or anxious. Under the pressure, the quirks of family members are also magnified. Some people will wrest control of medical decisions from the sufferer; others will wail over the bedside; and still others will ignore the most basic of their own needs to wait on the sick person hand and foot.

I do believe that pain, like other life crises, offers the possibility of transformation, but such a change usually occurs gradually, and results in something more subtle than sainthood. Bear in mind that a person in pain is a person under duress: The sufferer may be upset, especially during a flare-up. Look out for odd behavior from well-meaning friends and family, and try to protect the sufferer from power games and pity parties. And don't expect perfection from yourself, either. Just watch out for the tendency to go to extremes: A sufferer is not helped by controlling perfectionists or sacrificial lambs.

GET QUIET

Sometimes we're so eager to help that we run over sufferers like steamrollers of advice and action. Take this imaginary scenario between two friends:

JAN: I heard about your horrible back pain! How awful!

NAOMI: It does hurt quite a bit.

JAN: That's an understatement! My grandmother's sciatica nearly drove her insane.

NAOMI: Well, I'm not crazy—yet [she laughs]. The worst part is that I can't lift up my kids anymore.

JAN: That's terrible. You know, my grandmother tried these herbs and they really worked for her. I bought some of them for you. I can make them into a tea right now. . . .

Jan wants to help Naomi, but she's so caught up in her own response to the idea of pain that she's just not listening very well. For one, she's giving the pain tragic dimensions ("horrible," "insane," "terrible"), when Naomi seems to prefer a lower-key approach. What Naomi would really like to talk about is what the pain means for her as a parent of small children. Jan, in her desire to offer advice, misses this cue. Now Naomi may feel obligated to try herbs she'd really rather not take, just to satisfy her friend.

A better example of listening comes from Lillian, who was frightened by her chronic pelvic pain. Her father, a doctor, would call her up and let her vent her fears over the course of long conversations. Looking back, Lillian realizes that her father was probably in the grip of strong emotions himself—frustration that he, a doctor, couldn't cure his daughter; anxiety for Lillian and her small child. But he also realized that his panic would only add to Lillian's wound-up emotional state. So he just listened quietly. His calmness soothed Lillian, and eventually the worst of her fears spent themselves.

You can't help a friend without listening to her. And sometimes the calm, quiet act of listening is a help in itself. So before you go to see a pain sufferer, take a few moments to get quiet. You might meditate, or take some deep breaths. (Some breathing exercises can be found in Chapter 8.) Prepare yourself to receive whatever the sufferer would like to offer you, be it her distress, her laughter, or her silence.

ASK THE SUFFERER WHAT HE WANTS

One of the ways we try to help people is to imagine how we would feel, what we would want, in their situation. This is a natural and compassionate mental exercise. But sometimes it results in forgetting to ask the sufferer an obvious question: "What do you want?"

So ask the person directly if there is anything that might make him feel better. If he isn't forthcoming, it might be appropriate to offer suggestions based on your knowledge of that person's preferences: "Would you like some ginger tea for your nausea?" "How about if I play some quiet Brahms, maybe that piano piece you like so much?"

If you don't get a positive response after a question or two, it's time to back down. You don't want the sufferer to feel obliged to accept your form of assistance.

I've mentioned my patient Gwen elsewhere in this book. Gwen suffers from a severe case of interstitial cystitis, a painful bladder condition. After work, Gwen's husband comes home and rubs her back with lavender-scented oils. That's probably not what he would choose if he were in pain, but he's discovered that it makes her feel much better. And the massage helps them both wind down after the day and prepare for a closer evening together.

NO PITY PARTIES: SUPPORT ACTIVITY AND GOOD HABITS

When I was a medical resident, an internist asked me to see his patient, a sixty-six-year-old woman who might have had a stroke. I was rushed that night, so instead of carefully reading her chart, I tucked it under my arm and entered her room.

I was totally unprepared for what I saw. Lying on the bed was a five-hundred-pound woman. She was alert, talkative, and pleasant, but she was too weak to lift her legs off the bed, and she could hold her arms up for no more than a moment. Eight years before, she had been a bit overweight, but she was holding a job and getting around without difficulty. Then she broke her left ankle and required surgical placement of pins in the bone. She was supposed to enter physical therapy after the surgery but found it too painful. After a couple of months of hobbling around, she decided to put herself to bed, and she had been there ever since.

Her husband fully supported her surrender to pain. He put plastic sheets on the bed and placed a small refrigerator on a stand next to it, so that she could eat whenever she wanted. He would wash her when he got home at night and change her sheets and clothes. She had not left her bed in eight years. It was remarkable that she was still alive.

Why did I tell you this story? Because there is a little bit of this person in each of us. It's very difficult to face the pains and disabilities that dog us. Sometimes it seems best just to succumb to gravity and go downhill. That can be true for caregivers, too. It may be easier to let the sufferer give up—to make her the guest of honor at a pity party—than to get her to go to physical therapy or take her medication.

But someone who lets go of her life is only going to feel more pain, disability, and depression. As a caregiver, you can encourage the sufferer to stay engaged with pain-relieving habits, and, on a wider scale, with the activities of life. Without being controlling, support a good diet, exercise, and relaxation. Try to get the person to a doctor on a regular basis and to take any medications as prescribed.

The road to pain control can be a long one, and there are no miracle cures. Some treatments fail, and others produce intolerable side effects. As a caregiver, you can remind the sufferer not to give up, to contact a doctor if a medication isn't working, to see a therapy through a full trial before rejecting it, to rest when appropriate, to laugh, to see friends, to keep up hobbies, and to live as fully as possible within the limits of pain.

KNOW SOME SIMPLE TOOLS FOR PAIN CONTROL

These easy therapies come in handy during a flare-up or sleepless nights:

▶ *Touch.* You can rub the sufferer's hands or feet; when someone is bedridden, a leg massage can greatly increase comfort. For nausea, you can rub the inside base of the wrist, along the instep of the foot, or the front of the hip. You might also gently place your hand on the spot that hurts. Or you can just hold hands. (See Appendix B for instructions in home massage. Make sure to get permission before touching someone.)

▶ *Guided imagery.* Try taking the person on a mental journey to a favorite vacation spot or to a relaxing place. Use as many sensory details as you can to conjure up the most effective image. You might say: "Dad, remember when we went on that trip to the beach together? Remember how we rented that cottage that smelled like bread baking, and Mom made you piña coladas every night in that rusty old blender? There were pine trees all around the yard, and there was a terrible storm that lasted all night, so the next day you took all of us kids out to play in the ditch that flooded. I was wearing my favorite green-and-white-striped bathing suit, and we all wore white stuff on our noses. . . ." This kind of psychic vacation can take the bite out of a flare-up, and it offers a chance for the two of you to relive some pleasant moments together. For more information about guided imagery, see Chapter 8.

▶ *Breathing exercises.* When the pain gets bad, you can hold hands and take deep breaths together: "Okay, I know this pain is rotten, but let's try to get you through it. Can you breathe with me?" Then you take a big breath in, encouraging the sufferer to do the same. Then let the breath all the way out. Continue for as long as necessary. Further breathing exercises are in Chapter 8.

▶ *Distraction techniques.* Guided imagery and breathing, above, are two methods. But you could also play board or card games, read aloud, watch a good movie, listen to music, or just share some gossip. This is especially important for people who live alone or in nursing homes, who might have nothing to think about all day except their pain.

▶ *Heat and cold therapies.* They're awfully simple, but a hot-water bottle against an aching back or a cold cloth for a headache are highly effective.

▶ Make the sufferer's environment relaxing. Scented oils or sachets, a pretty photograph, or some fresh flowers will all contribute to a calming atmosphere.

LOOK FOR SIGNS OF DEPRESSION OR ANXIETY

Pain is rigged up to the part of the brain that governs emotions, so it's only natural that living with pain for a long time can lead to depression or anxiety. These mental states also contribute to pain, creating a vicious circle. If the sufferer appears listless, hopeless, constantly drained, apathetic, or inexplicably fearful, or if he suddenly loses interest in food or starts eating uncontrollably, he might be suffering from depression or anxiety. Encourage him to talk to his doctor. Medication or therapy can help people cope with the changes that pain brings.

TAKE CARE OF YOURSELF

The effects of pain aren't restricted to the patient. Long-standing pain can also bring down family and friends with it. When someone close to you is disabled or constantly distraught, your life changes radically. You need to develop coping techniques, and you need to take care of yourself. Eat well, exercise, and take time to relax. (The mind-body techniques in Chapter 8 may help.) Join a support group for caregivers. Ask friends if they can take over for an hour or two.

You and the sufferer need to build a life together in the face of pain. You will need to find ways to bring down the physical hurt as well as to handle pain's emotional component—the fear, the anxiety, the anger, the grief for your old ways of life. But it is our worst times that offer the most opportunities for learning and connection. If you can, I hope you will create time for stillness, to ask yourself if there is a way you can use this difficult event to some purpose, and to search for any meaning that might lie in the suffering.

CARETAKER WARNING SIGNS

No doubt about it: Prolonged caretaking is one of life's most stressful events. Consider talking to a doctor or therapist if you experience any of the following:

- You're feeling anxious, sad all the time, listless, helpless, or apathetic.
- You're taking care of a spouse, but you're beginning to feel like his or her parent.
- You sense that you're being manipulated by the sufferer. Maybe you are and maybe you aren't, but mistrust is a clear sign that something in the relationship is amiss.

29.

THE LESSONS OF PAIN

In avoiding all pain and seeking comfort at all costs, we may be left without intimacy or compassion; in rejecting change and risk we often cheat ourselves of the quest; in denying our suffering we may never know our strength or our greatness.

—RACHEL NAOMI REMEN,
Kitchen Table Wisdom

Pain is a gift. Without pain there is no joy. No pain, no gain. Clichés like these, deprived of the hard philosophical thought behind them, take a profound idea and boil it down to a sweet, sticky syrup, one that's hardly palatable when you're in the grip of suffering. No wonder so many pain patients are visibly sickened at the sound of them.

But when pain, despite your best efforts, just won't go away, you may find yourself wondering about the meaning of your suffering. You may ask yourself why the pain has happened to you; how God could let this happen; even whether there is any way you can learn from your experience. At these times, it is worth trying to look past the clichés and to recover their meanings in their wholeness and difficulty. Although I can't accomplish such a task here—that's a lifetime's worth of work—what I can do is share some ideas that my patients and colleagues have brought to me. I have found them useful in my practice and in my personal life; I hope they bring you some comfort as well.

WHO'S TO BLAME?

Many people who are willing to contemplate divorce, unemployment, or other kinds of emotional suffering in terms of personal growth or lessons learned will reject the idea that physical pain may also have something to teach us. Joseph Loizzo, M.D., Ph.D., founder and director of the Center for Meditation and Healing at Columbia-Presbyterian Medical Center, notes that Western medical attitudes prevent us from thinking of pain as a teacher. Instead, we are coached into believing that a pain-free life is nothing less than a birthright. In this view, pain has no meaning outside itself; it is merely a symptom. And who among us doesn't feel entitled to diagnosis and removal of symptoms?

But as we have seen, pain is stubbornly unyielding to such a mechanistic approach. When medicine fails to cure or even to diagnose our pain, we don't just hurt—we suffer from a philosophical upset. Our sense of how the world works is violated, so we cast about for a source of blame: The doctor must have done something wrong; the employer should have instituted a wellness plan; our families should have been more supportive; the universe is out to get us; we are being punished. Deprived of a sophisticated cultural response to chronic pain, unable to place it within a philosophical, medical, or religious context, our psychic resources for handling it are limited.

If you find yourself looking for someone to blame, you might ask yourself how much good this exercise is doing you. Does blame relieve your suffering? Does it deepen your understanding of your life and the people in it? If not, then you may wish to ask yourself an entirely different question: Given that pain is in your life, what can you learn from it?

Not everyone wishes to see their pain as a gift, nor is it appropriate for me or anyone else to tell you what to think or how to feel. But I do want to tell you a few stories of people who have indeed found some use for their pain, because they have helped me adjust my own relationship to the practice of pain medicine and to pain itself.

I want to point out that looking for meaning in pain does *not* require you to sacrifice good treatment. The people below are not saints or martyrs; even as they recognized value in their pain, they continued to seek out means of alleviating it. (Note that while some of the people discussed here are religious, by no means all of them are. Religion can be an important element in coming to terms with pain, but it is not necessary for everyone. Philosophy, a more informal worldview, or simple reflection may be just as helpful.)

PAIN AS A PROTECTOR

Lillian had been married twice, both times to angry, explosive men. After her second divorce, she dated an alcoholic with a mean streak. When he left her, Lillian knew that she should have been glad to see him go. His departure could have been an end to her cycle of hurtful relationships. But the change Lillian needed to enact in herself seemed beyond her reach. Instead, she pursued her ex-boyfriend and spent months in anguish. Lillian, a lifelong Christian, finally decided to pray for help: "I got on my knees and said, 'God, I cannot heal. But I don't want to be like this. Would you heal me in any way you can? I leave it up to you.' "

A week later, Lillian developed crippling pelvic pain. Terrified at first, she made the familiar rounds of doctors and specialists, none of whom could identify a physical cause. Then a friend stepped in. "Start examining what you think you're supposed to be learning from this," the friend suggested, and Lillian for the first time made a connection between her prayer and the pain.

What others would see as the pain's worst effects, Lillian has come to view as its gifts: "This pain has kept me away from relationships. I hurt more at night, I can't go to dinner, I can't sit down, and so it's really isolated me." Lillian says that the pain has prevented her from continuing her pattern of destructive relationships and especially from pursuing her alcoholic ex-boyfriend. She uses the solitary time forced upon her by pain to reflect on her life and to enter psychotherapy. It has been hard work, but gradually she is reentering life with a more solid sense of herself, and soon she hopes to return to school. Of course, she continues to visit medical doctors and has found considerable relief with nerve blocks, relaxation techniques, cognitive-behavioral therapy, and acupuncture. But as long as the pain is there, Lillian intends to keep using it. "You know," she says, "even when I'm really scared about the pain, I go, 'Okay, God, if you're taking me to a new place, I want to go there.' And that's really what keeps me going. I'm still in the process. And I have to say, it's been the most painful and scariest time in my life—and the most enlightening, all at once."

PAIN AND TRANSFORMATION

When I was practicing acupuncture in California, before I went to medical school, I had a patient named Noreen. She was an attractive woman, with long, thick hair and high cheekbones; in fact, she'd been a socialite before breast cancer and a mastectomy had changed her life. She'd been married to a philanthropist and took great pleasure—too much, she'd say later—in driving a nice car, lunching, and shopping, especially for shoes, her particular weakness. Life-threatening illness often stokes dramatic change in people, and Noreen's experience led her to abandon recreational shopping in favor of volunteer work. When she came to me, she was studying toward a degree in public health.

Noreen's cancer was in full remission, but the mastectomy (of a more aggressive sort than is now usually practiced) left her with lymphedema in her right arm, which caused painful swelling. She received acupuncture and massage to reduce the symptoms, and yet I recall that Noreen confessed to me that she wasn't ready to let go of the pain completely: "I don't really want to feel entirely normal yet. I'm afraid that if I felt entirely normal I would forget this gift, this thing that has been taught to me. The fact that my arm was swollen and my shoulder always hurts a little bit is a constant reminder to me of how precious my time is. How thin my time is." For Noreen, pain was a mark of her transformation from a sweet but frivolous young woman to a seasoned, mature adult. It was a reminder of who she wanted to be.

The Culture of Pain, a provocative, scholarly work by David B. Morris, weighs in on pain as a badge of honor or symbol of change. Morris observes the connection between pain and rites of passage. Consider the pain of childbirth, which some women experience as transformative; the pain schoolchildren feel when cutting a finger in a blood-brother ritual; the pain inflicted in sports, secret fraternity rituals, and military training. All of these rites include an exchange of comfort for the responsibilities of parenting, friendship, or membership in a community. As Morris says, "Pain is a kind of tunnel through which one passes to a new stage of being."

Again, this view represents just one way of thinking about pain, and it's not right for everyone. But as long as you have the pain, you might want to really *know* it—the darkness, the cliffs, the deserts, the blinding light. These metaphors, so often used to describe pain, describe a strange, discomforting land. But they also represent the landscape of adventure. In this terrain, pain is not an enemy but the setting for revelation.

EVERYDAY GIFTS

Pain's gifts are sometimes subtle. They may not effect revolution or transcendence; sometimes they serve as nothing more than a nudge toward common sense. Pain in the knees might be telling you to lose some weight; neck pain might be a reminder to exercise or to manage stress. "It's time to take care of yourself," pain often says, and we'd be smart to listen.

Pain may also bring us a new way of seeing, or strengthen a connection already in place. This happened to Duane, an office manager who had hurt his back while skiing. He required several months at home to recover, and this loss of income and occupation threatened his sense of the place he held within his family. I was worried about him. But he progressed nicely, and when it was time for him to return to work, he actually expressed some regret. Then I grew even *more* worried, since it's my experience that people who don't want to go back to their jobs tend not to heal very well. I asked Duane to talk about his regret.

"I know I've been so itchy to get back to work," he admitted, laughing. But he explained that the temporary cutback in income had forced him to take his four-year-old daughter out of day care (Duane's wife worked full time) and look after her himself. Duane had always loved his daughter, but during his recovery he discovered her personality in its fullness. He read to her, played with her, and found that she was eager to hear stories about his own childhood. "I discovered something so amazing," he said simply. "I'm really going to miss my daughter when I go back to work. Our relationship has been permanently changed. I know that I'm going to think about this person differently for the rest of my life because of this thing that happened to me."

I have also had some experience with pain as a gift. I have a stomach condition that gives me some pain on a regular basis—nothing to prevent me from working or any other activities, but enough that it stops me in my tracks for a moment or two. My father, who died when I was a teenager, had the same condition; in a funny way, I think of him whenever I get the pain. It keeps me in touch with him and reminds me of what he must have felt and how he must have come to terms with it in *his* own way. Sometimes I even laugh—I can imagine him, with his particular brand of humor, saying to me, "Take my stomach—please!" So my stomach still hurts, but I can't say that I really suffer from it much. The pain is transformed into a daily connection.

PUTTING PAIN TO SPIRITUAL OR ARTISTIC USE

Harriet Beinfield, an expert in traditional Chinese medicine, uses the story of Dr. Tenzin Choedrak as an example of a remarkable response to great pain. Dr. Choedrak began the study of Tibetan medicine as an adolescent, at a time when medical students were required to memorize thousands of pages of text and to engage in at least eleven years of strict mental and physical discipline before matriculating. He eventually became the Dalai Lama's personal physician, and when the Chinese army invaded Tibet, Dr. Choedrak was captured, imprisoned, and starved. He refused to denounce his spiritual leader and was tortured and beaten, his shoulders torn out of their sockets repeatedly. He was imprisoned under vile conditions for twenty-two years.

It is a testimony to Dr. Choedrak's resilience that he survived his ordeal. What is harder for many of us to comprehend is his controlled response to the pain. As a Buddhist and a Tibetan doctor, Tenzin Choedrak had already been trained to focus his mind, to cultivate compassion for his patients, and to put his own suffering to spiritual use. In prison, he maintained this focus and drew on his disciplined memory to recite hundreds of mantras daily. Instead of allowing anger at his captors to take over his mind, he used the pain as a means of developing compassion for the soldiers who were torturing him, and to nurture his desire to treat them for their own illnesses.

Dr. Choedrak's level of compassion is probably not a realistic goal for most of us. His story, notes Beinfield, is one of an "extraordinary training of mind, extraordinary infliction of suffering, extraordinary capacity to transcend." Accounts like this one are valuable not so much because we are able to precisely emulate them but because they stretch our sense of what is humanly possible in the response to pain. They make us ask: By controlling the response to pain, is it possible to develop a kind of mastery or resilience? Can we bring that strength to other areas of life?

There may also be something to learn from people for whom pain is closely linked to art. Again, in *The Culture of Pain,* David Morris describes the close link between dancers and their pain:

> Dancers sometimes speak of riding into their pain, as if it were a source of energy they could tap. The worst relation to pain for a dancer or athlete is simply to resist it: to stiffen the body, however slightly, in compensation.... In a very practical sense, the dancer must accept pain, come to terms with it, and the dancer's use of pain thus lies in this willing acceptance.... Perhaps the dancer's simultaneous acceptance and forgetfulness of pain offers a useful model. The art would lie in discovering how to avoid merely stiff, passive resistance and how to use the pain as the medium for a fluid, creative performance, even if the performance were limited to walking downstairs for dinner or climbing behind the wheel of a car.

These uses of pain don't suggest that we go out looking for suffering. But if it appears and cannot be fully alleviated, it might not be helpful to think of it as an enemy that must be fought at all costs. Instead of fighting it, we might try learning how to live inside it, letting it inspire us to new levels of spirituality, art, or focus.

THE NEXT STEP

The disrupting effects of pain may lead you to a deeper consideration of the world, and of the location of you and your pain within that world. Pain is intimately joined to philosophy and religion, and undertaking the study of either (or both) may lead you to fruitful thought. The great rational and mystical traditions alike have sprung in part from this question: If there is a moral order to the universe, how can we explain the presence of suffering? In some traditions, suffering is to be cultivated as a tool of transformation, a sensation that pushes us past the ordinary and into the sublime. In others, an understanding of suffering is beyond mortal knowledge, and a proper response is to suppress easy cause-and-effect hypotheses (for example, we hurt because God is angry) in favor of a more challenging exploration of the world's character. Buddhism in particular offers an interesting approach to pain: According to the Buddha's teachings, "to live is to suffer." In other words, pain simply is; it is a truth of the universe. By learning to detach ourselves from a panicked reaction to pain (often through meditation, prayer, or reflection), we can develop resilience that can be applied to other challenges in life.

It is beyond the scope of this book—and my talents—to address the nature of suffering more fully. But I believe that the human experience of pain naturally spurs us to some of the profound questions: Why are we here? Why do we suffer? Does pain have meaning? Can it lead us to a deeper meaning in our lives? You may wish to engage in formal philosophical study of those questions, to do your work within a religious group, to talk things over with family or friends, or to spend time writing in a journal or in quiet self-reflection. When you shape the role pain plays in your life, when you use it as a tool of understanding or transformation, then you will have control of your pain in the truest sense.

APPENDIX **A**

SUGGESTED EXERCISES

These basic stretches and exercises can be used by almost everyone in pain, although if you have unstable joints or a very serious medical condition, you should always contact your doctor before beginning an exercise plan. I advise going through the entire routine daily for maximum relief, but if you like, you can focus on the parts of the body that affect you the most. Of course, you will also need to perform some kind of cardiovascular exercise several times a week.

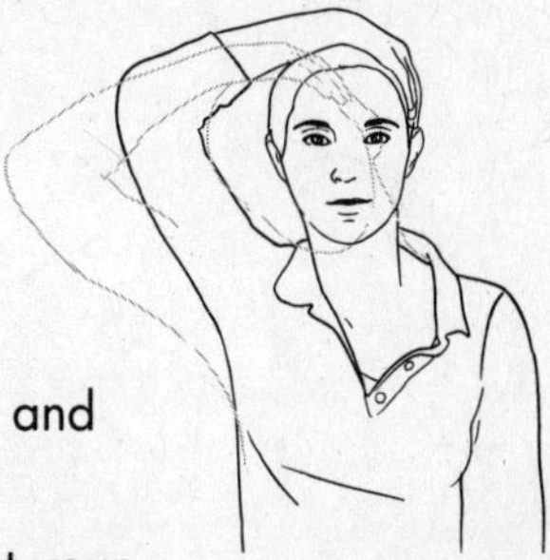

fig. 1

NECK

For each of the neck exercises you should be seated comfortably with your shoulders, neck, and jaw as relaxed as possible.

1. Reach your right arm over your head so that your palm is on top of your skull, your fingers resting just above the left ear. Allow the weight of your arm, along with light fingertip pressure, to gently bend the head toward your right shoulder **(fig.1)**. Do not strain. Check to make sure your shoulders are still relaxed. You should be looking forward. Hold the pose for 30 seconds. Move your fingers toward the back left corner of your skull, this time allowing your head to bend forward and to the right, about 45 degrees in front of your shoulder **(fig. 2)**. Hold for 30 seconds Now place your fingers at the back of your skull and gently pull your head straight forward, toward your chest **(fig. 3)**. Hold for 30 seconds. Switch hands and repeat the stretches in reverse order: Pull forward, then 45 degrees in front of your left shoulder, and finally directly over your left shoulder. Do *not* push your head backward.

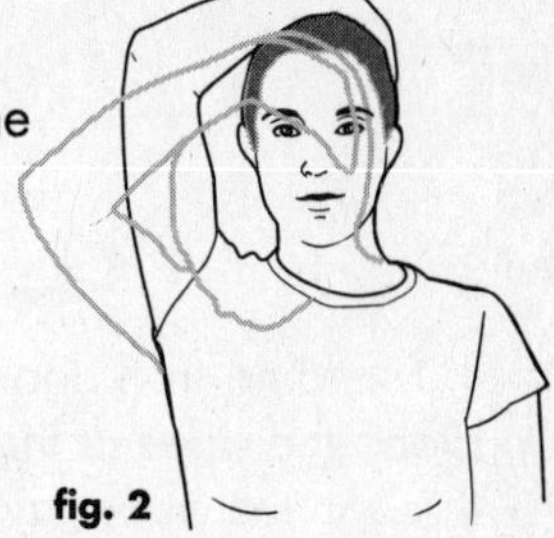

fig. 2

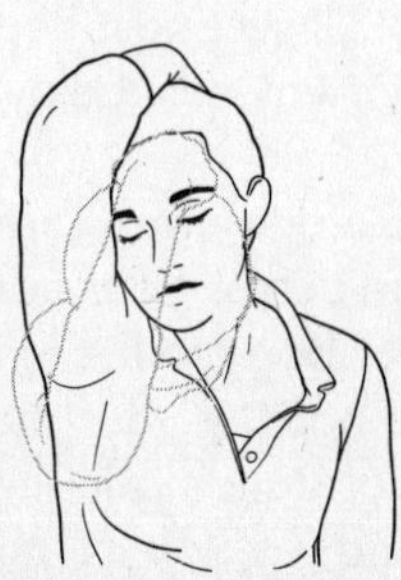

fig. 3

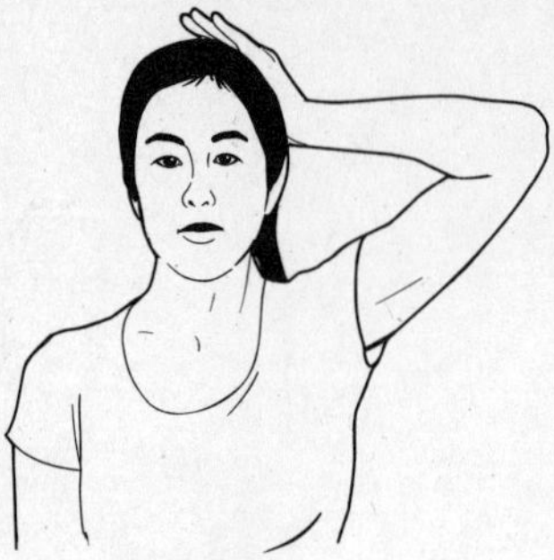

fig. 4

2. Do an isometric push against your hand to strengthen the neck. Hold your left palm against the left side of your head **(fig. 4)**. Push your left hand against your head while also pushing your head toward your left hand at about half strength. Hold for 30 seconds. Repeat with your right hand on the right side of the head. Do the same exercise, using either hand, with the back of the head **(fig. 5)** and the forehead **(fig. 6)**.

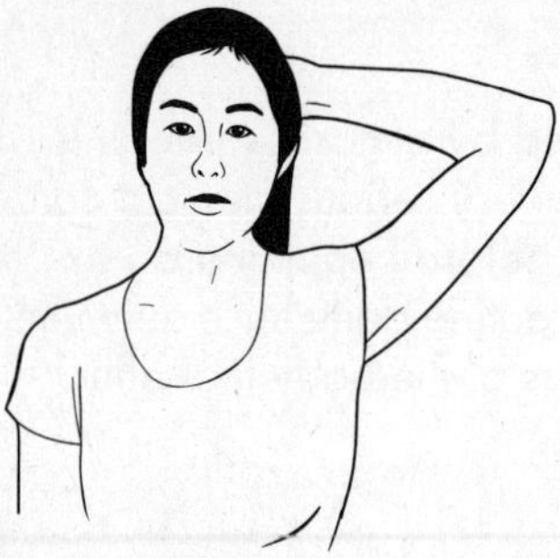

fig. 5

3. Do a chin tuck. Keeping your chin parallel to the ground, bring your head straight back until you feel a pull at the top of the back of the neck where it connects to the base of the skull **(fig. 7)**. Hold for 10 seconds. Repeat this exercise 10 times and perform it twice a day.

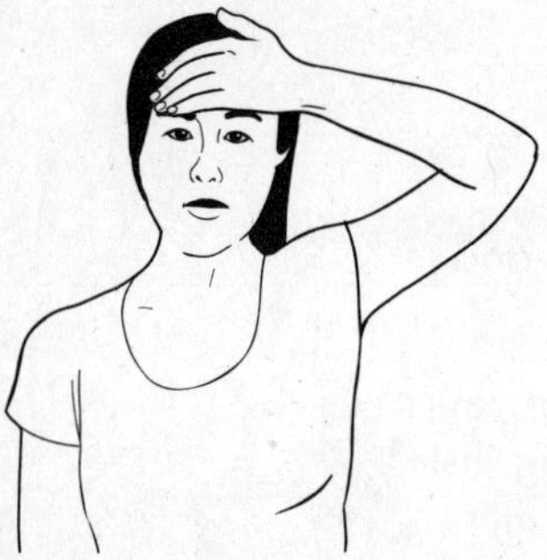

fig. 6

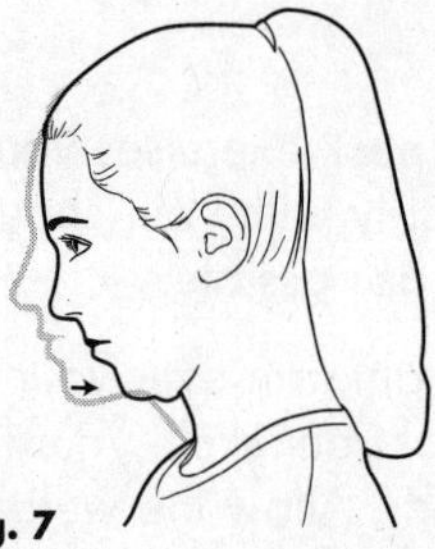

fig. 7

SHOULDERS

1. Standing in a doorway, reach your hands up to the lintel (or as far up along the sides of the doorway as they will go **(fig. 8)**. Lean forward through the doorway to stretch your inner arms and shoulders and hold for 30 seconds. Repeat with your hands positioned at the side of the doorway, just below your shoulders **(fig. 9)**.

2. Stand arm's distance to the right of a doorway. Reach your left arm across your body and grasp the doorway **(fig. 10)**. Now gently turn your body to the left, away from your hand, so that you feel a stretch in the back of your shoulder. Hold for 30 seconds and repeat on the other side, standing to the right of the doorway and reaching with your right hand.

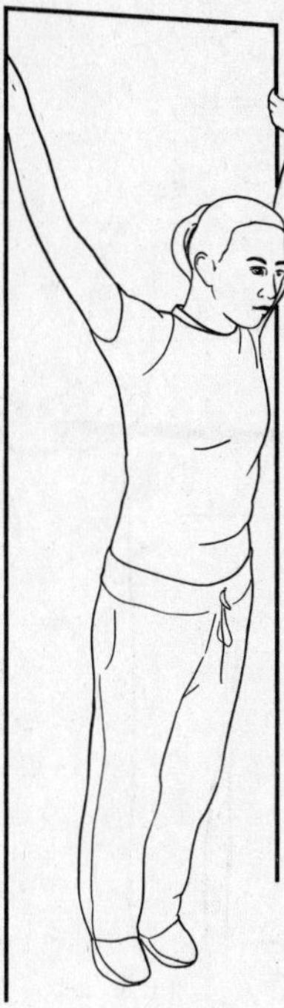
fig. 8

fig. 9

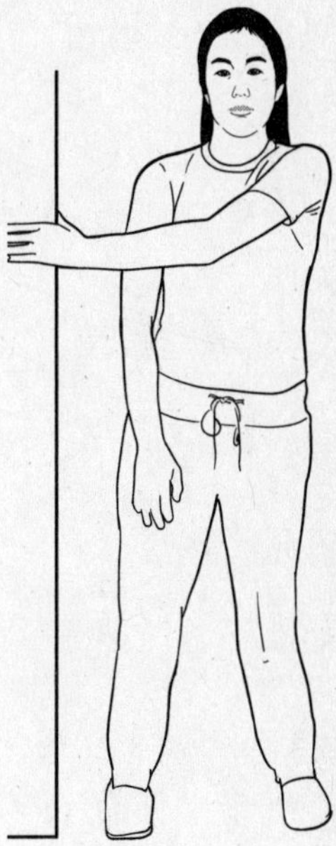
fig. 10

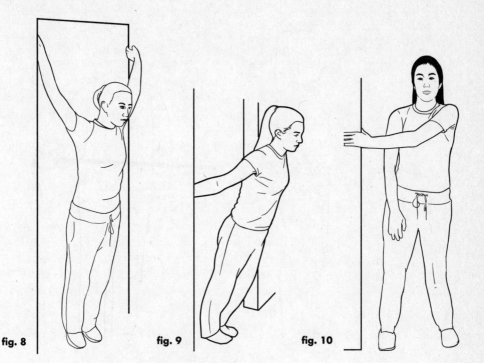

3. Sit with your legs in a comfortable position. Tuck your left hand under your buttocks, the palm facing up **(fig. 11)**. Then, keeping your back straight, lean your torso toward the right as far as you can. Hold the stretch for 30 seconds and repeat on the opposite side.

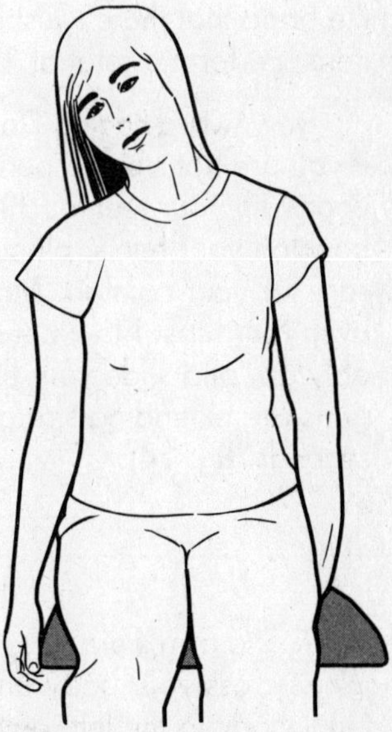
fig. 11

4. This exercise requires the use of a stretchy exercise band, the kind available at most sporting-goods stores. Place one end of the band around the knob of a closed door and stand perpendicular to it, holding the other end of the band taut. Your thumb should be pointing upward. Lower your hand so that your forearm is parallel to the floor. Keeping your elbow close to your waist and holding your wrist straight, pull your hand toward your body, so that it traces an arc **(fig. 12)**. Then stretch the band out to the side of your body as far as the band will allow,

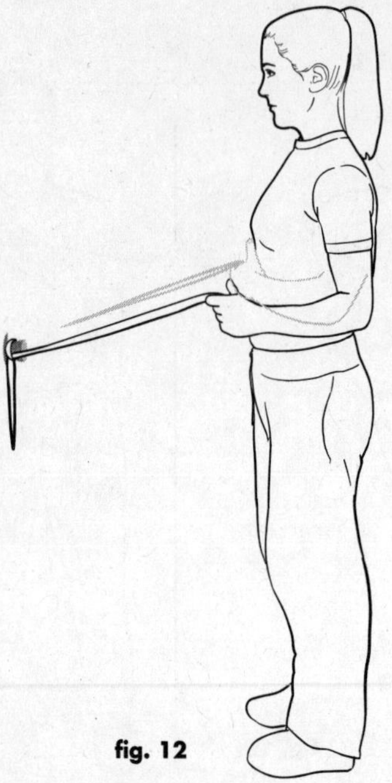

fig. 12

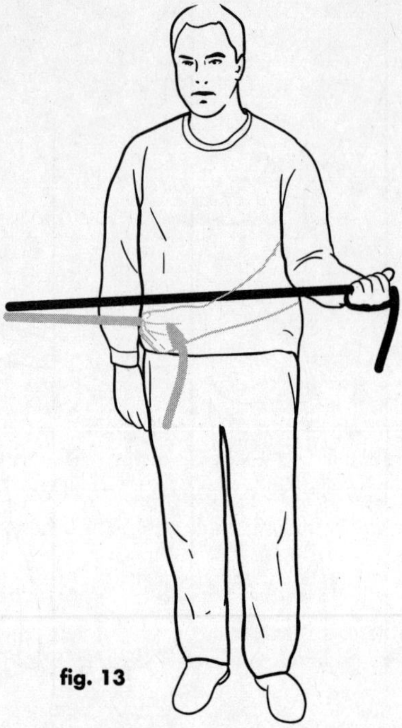

fig. 13

again in a smooth arc **(fig. 13)**. You should feel enough resistance from the band that there's just a bit of a burn in the muscle after ten repetitions. Perform a total of 10 reps.

5. Downward-Facing Dog (under "Wrists") also eases shoulder tension. If you are not able to perform it, try Child's Pose instead. Kneel on the floor with your feet touching and your knees spread slightly apart. Sit back on your heels, placing a blanket or pillow under your hips if necessary for your comfort. Make sure that your weight is evenly distributed over your hips. Now bend your torso forward as far as you can comfortably go, and slide your hands in front of you on the floor, so that your arms are extending straight out from the shoulders. Hold this pose for 30 seconds **(fig. 14)**.

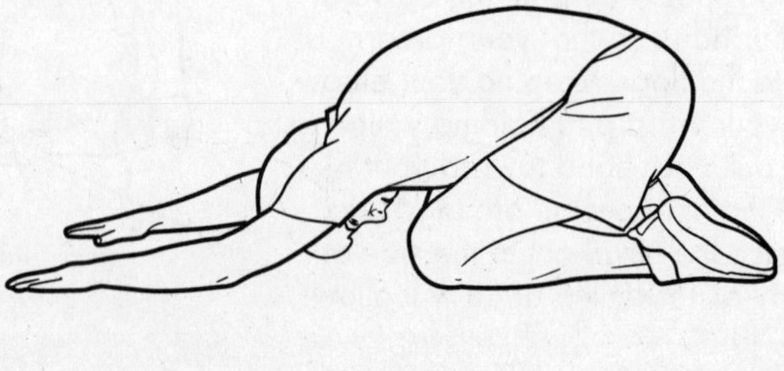

fig. 14

WRISTS

This yoga pose, called Downward-Facing Dog, is a staple of yoga practice and can help reduce pressure on the carpal tunnel nerve. It is also useful for shoulder and back tension.

Get down on all fours. (It helps to practice on a mat.) Your hands should be directly underneath your shoulders, and your knees under your hips. Look at your hands: Each finger should be extended, with your middle finger pointing straight forward. Feel the pressure at the roots of your fingers. Make sure the weight is evenly distributed across your hands, including the outside of the hands and the pads of flesh between your thumb and forefinger. Reposition your feet so that the balls of your feet are on the floor. Then lift up your hips and straighten your legs. Check your hands again—is the weight balanced evenly throughout? Keep the hands pressed down as you imagine lifting the forefingers and arms out of the wrists. Be sure that your neck and head are in line with your spine and arms. You should be looking down, not out.

Hold the position for 30 seconds **(fig. 15)**.

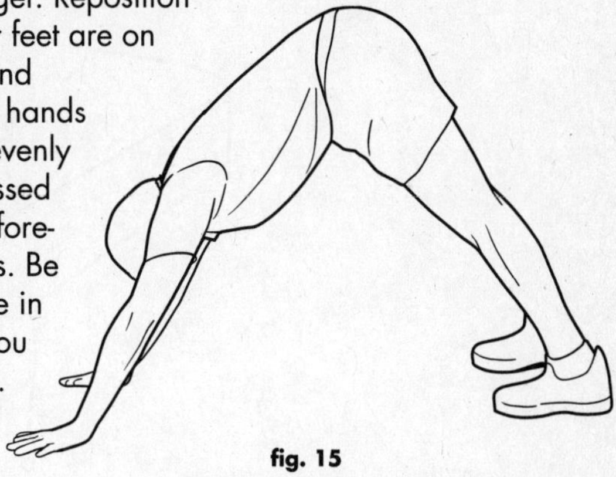

fig. 15

UPPER BACK

1. Lie down on your bed, face up, positioned diagonally, so that your head and upper back are at a corner. Let your arms drop to either side and hold for one minute **(fig. 16)**.

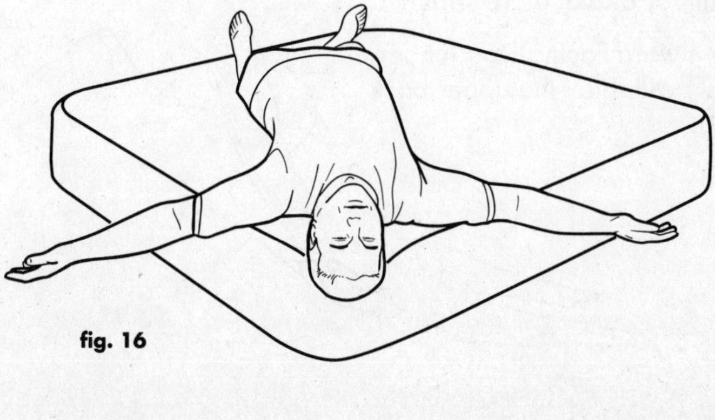

fig. 16

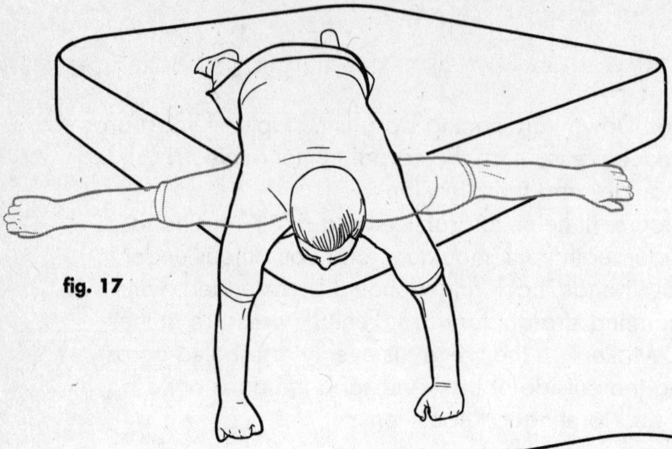

fig. 17

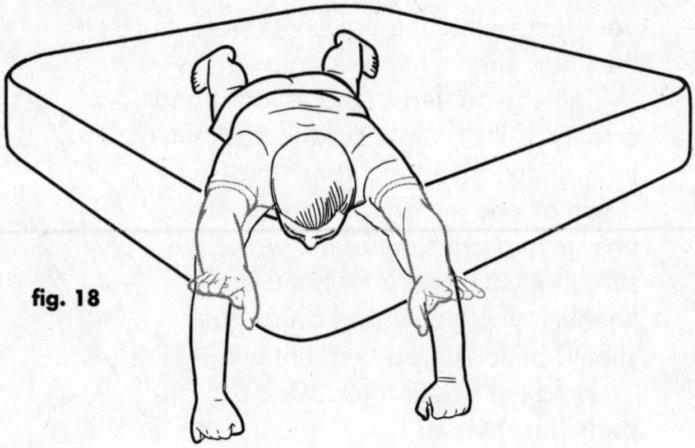

fig. 18

2. Lie in the same diagonal position but turn over so that you're on your stomach. Let your arms fall to the sides and then raise them so that they are straight and parallel with your shoulders. Hold for five to 10 seconds **(fig. 17)**. Repeat, this time bringing your arms straight in front of you **(fig. 18)**. Do this set of exercises (arms to the side, arms to the front) for a total of 10 reps.

3. Downward-Facing Dog (under "Wrists") will relax the upper back **(fig. 19)**.

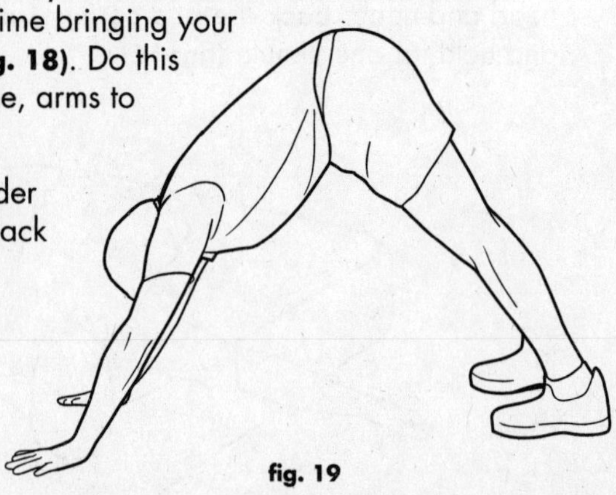

fig. 19

LOW BACK

These exercises work best on the floor or other very firm, stable surface. Most mattresses are too soft.

1. Lie down on your back with your legs straight. Bend one leg and use both arms to pull your knee up to your chest as far as it will go. Hold for 5 seconds and release. Repeat for a total of 10 times **(fig. 20)**. Switch legs **(fig. 21)**. Then pull both legs up to your chest simultaneously and hold for 10 seconds **(fig. 22)**.

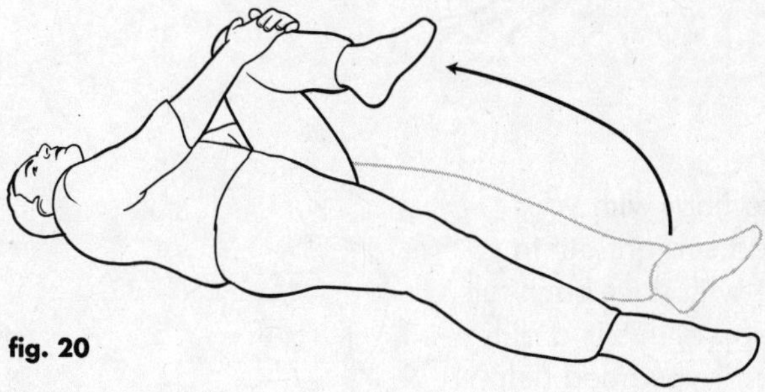

fig. 20

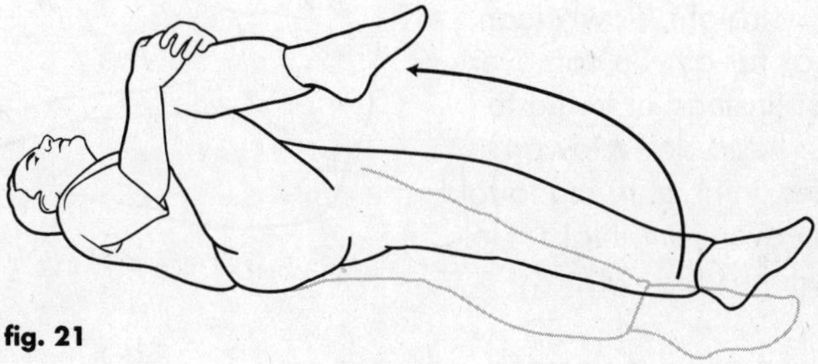

fig. 21

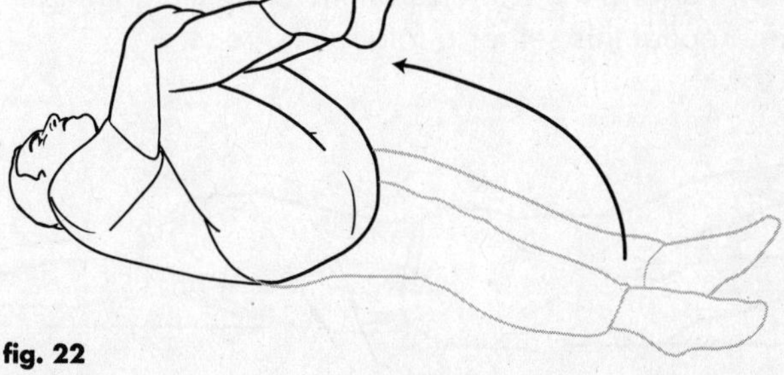

fig. 22

2. Lie on your back with your legs straight. Swing your left leg over your right to gently twist your low back, keeping your shoulders flat on the floor. Allow the right leg to turn out slightly. Hold for 10 seconds and release **(fig. 23)**. Repeat on the opposite side.

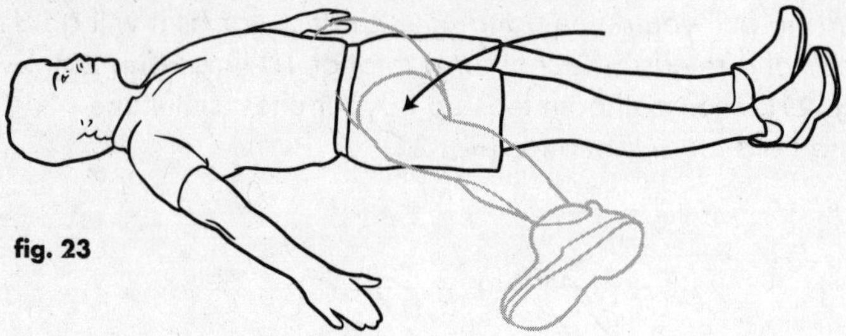

fig. 23

3. Sit on the floor with your legs extended straight out in front of you, with your back tall. For some people, this is a difficult exercise; if you need help, prop yourself up with a pillow under your buttocks. Keeping your back straight, slowly lean forward as far as you can over your legs. (Instead of trying to push your head down toward your knees, think of trying to fold your belly over your thighs. Hold for 30 seconds **(fig. 24)**.

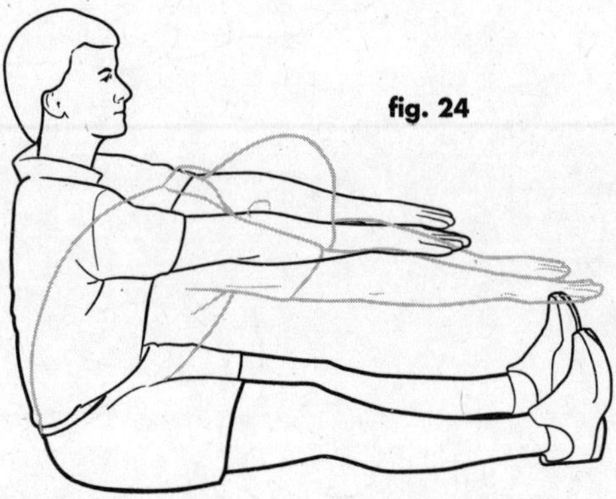

fig. 24

4. Lie down on your stomach with your arms extended straight in front of you. Prop your chin up slightly on the floor. Lift your left leg and your right arm straight off the floor as high as you can go. Hold for 10 seconds **(fig. 25)**. Perform the exercise on the other side, lifting the right leg and left arm. Repeat this set for a total of 10 reps.

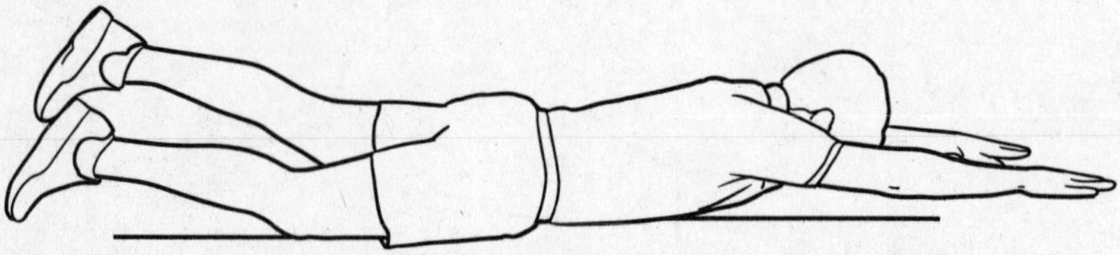

fig. 25

5. Do partial sit-ups. Lie down with your knees bent and the small of your low back pressed firmly into the floor. Lace your hands behind your neck and keep your elbows straight out as you use your abdominal muscles to lift yourself several inches off the floor **(fig. 26)**. (Do *not* go all the way up.) Do as many as you can, building up to 20 reps.

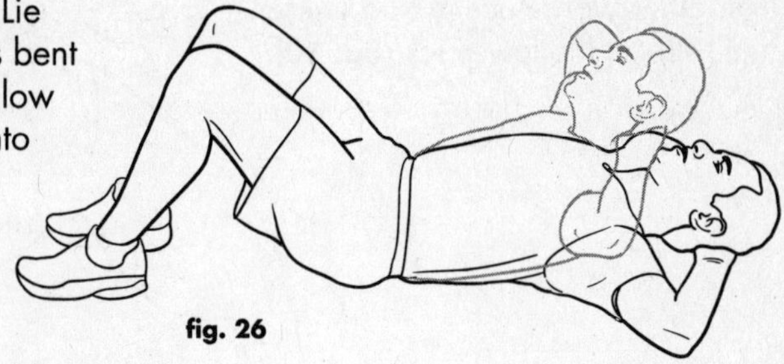

fig. 26

6. This set of yoga poses is called Cat and Camel. Get down on all fours. Slowly round your back and tuck your head down **(fig. 27)**, then lower yourself so that your back and neck are in a neutral position. Then slowly arch your back, bringing your head slightly upward **(fig. 28)**. Return to a neutral position. Repeat for a total of 10 times.

fig. 27

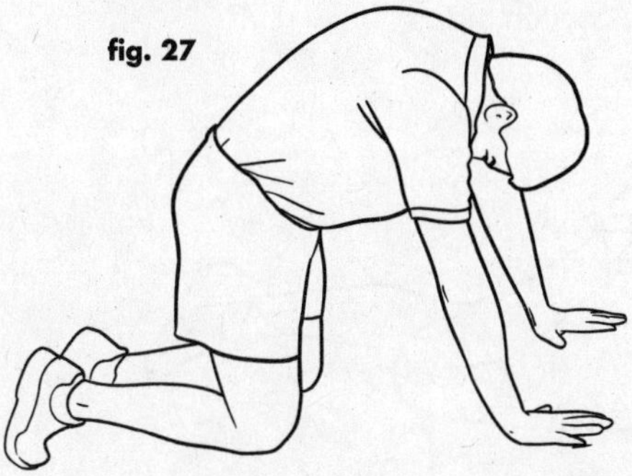

fig. 28

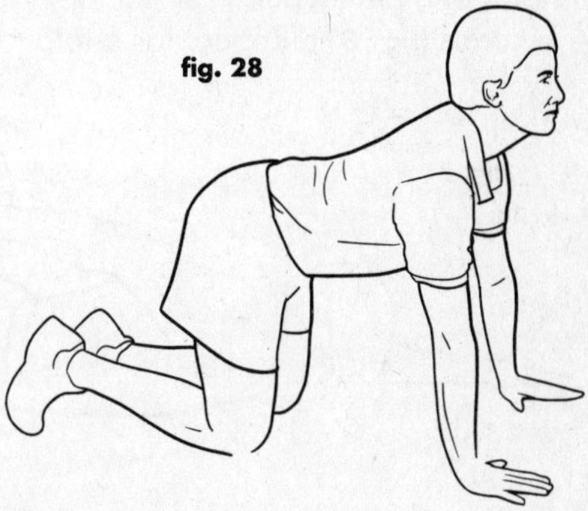

7. Lie on your back. Bring your straight left leg up as far as it will comfortably stretch. Place a belt, strap, or folded towel over your heel and hold the ends in your hands. Use these ends to pull the leg—which is still straight—closer toward your body **(fig. 29)**. Don't jerk the leg forward; just pull smoothly and gently until you feel the stretch. Hold for 5 seconds. Repeat with the right leg. Do a total of 10 reps on both sides.

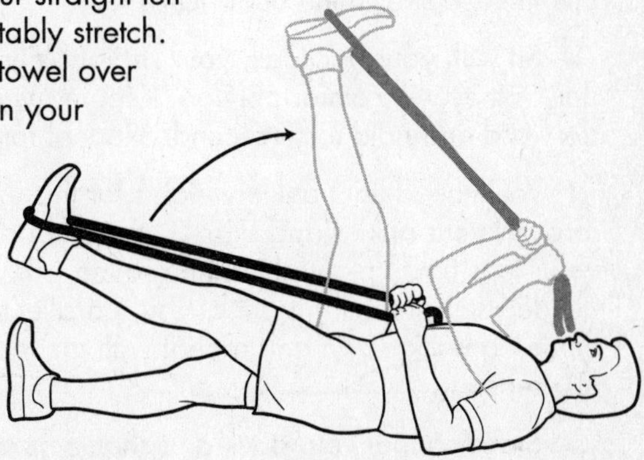

fig. 29

8. Downward-Facing Dog (under "Wrists") will stretch the low back **(fig. 30)**.

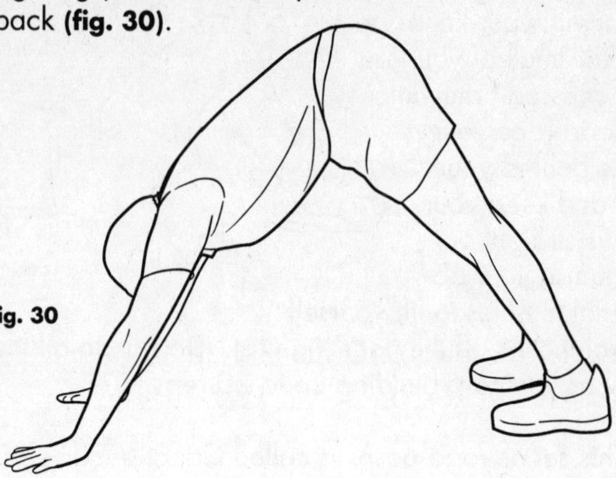

fig. 30

KNEES

1. Lie down on your stomach. Bend your left knee. Reach back with your hand and gently pull your left foot toward your buttocks and hold for 10 seconds **(fig. 31)**. Repeat for a total of 5. Switch sides.

fig. 31

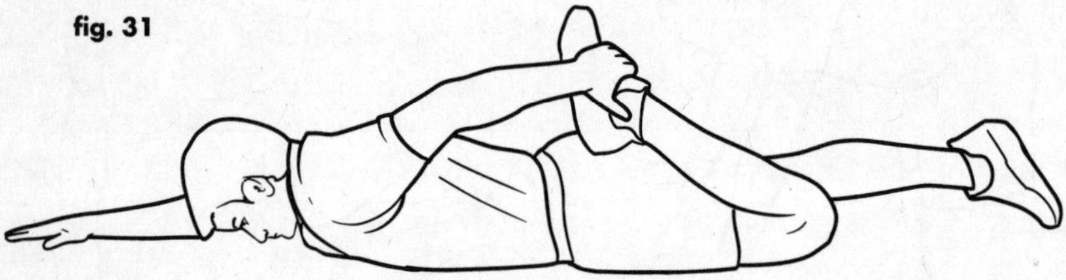

2. Perform the first exercise again, this time with a pillow placed under the knee to stretch the quadriceps fully.

3. Sit with your back tall, your straight legs extended out to the sides as far as they will comfortably go. Keeping your back straight, lean forward and hold for 5 seconds. Repeat for a total of 10 reps.

4. You'll need light ankle weights for this exercise. Wrap the weights around your ankles and sit in a straight-backed chair, your back tall and your legs firmly planted on the ground. Lift your right leg so that it is extended straight out in front of you, parallel to the floor **(fig. 32)**. Bring your leg back down and repeat with the left leg. Repeat for a total of 10 reps.

5. Stand so that your back and shoulders are touching the wall. Your feet should be shoulder width apart and slightly out in front of your

body. Bend your knees and slide your back down the wall so that your knees form a 90-degree angle. (If you are not able to go this far at first, just bend your knees as far as you can and work up to a 90-degree angle.) Do not go farther than 90 degrees, and do not allow your knees to go out over your toes—if you do, you risk injury. Hold for a count of 10. Repeat for a total of 5 reps at first, slowly working up to a total of 10 reps.

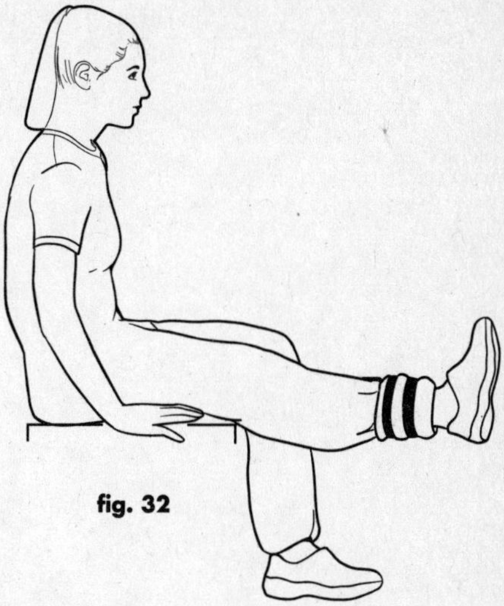

fig. 32

APPENDIX B

HOME MASSAGE TECHNIQUES

Home massage is not just relaxing; it can be truly therapeutic. If a spouse, friend, or relative is willing, here are some suggestions for working out kinks, encouraging restful sleep, and reducing pain.

GENERAL PRINCIPLES FOR THE MASSAGE GIVER

It's obvious that the person receiving a massage should be in a comfortable position, usually lying down (although sitting will often work for shorter treatments). But if you're giving a massage, *you* must be comfortable as well; otherwise, you may tire quickly or even hurt yourself. You should be seated, and you should not have to bend, twist, or strain. The body part you're working should be easily accessible, at the same level with your body as a computer keyboard should be.

Make the environment as safe, quiet, warm, and comforting as possible. This is a good time to light a scented candle or to use a scented oil (lavender, rose, geranium, sandalwood, bergamot, and clary sage are some good choices) or to turn on the person's favorite soft music. By adding a few thoughtful extras, you can turn a ten-minute massage into a real treat.

When you are giving a massage, always ask the person if you are using the right amount of pressure. Most people prefer a firm touch, and studies indicate that a firmer touch does indeed bring greater benefits. Of course, you never want to bruise or otherwise hurt anyone.

HEAD MASSAGE

A head massage is best performed with the person lying down; you should be seated next to him. (If you want to do a quick seated rub, have the person sit below you, perhaps on the floor with you in a chair.) Remember that the person's head should be easily accessible to you and that you should not need to strain to reach it.

1. Begin by rubbing your hands together to warm them. (Most people prefer not to use oil on the head.)

2. While cradling the head with one hand, use the fingertips of the other hand to make sweeping motions along the underside of the neck, from the base of the neck toward the head **(fig. 33)**.

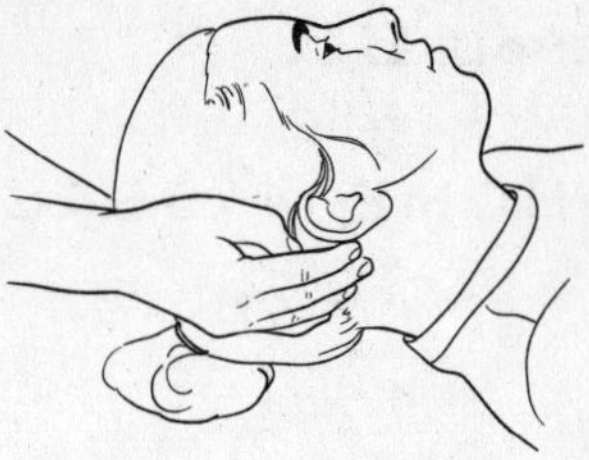

fig. 33

3. Then begin to focus along the line between the skull and the neck, using gentle fingertip pressure. If you encounter some tender spots, strum the spots with your fingertips, rubbing back and forth over them.

4. When you're done with the neck, move to the temples and the flat plates that run along the front sides of the head. Start at the top of these plates (next to the sides of the forehead) and work down to the ears, keeping your fingertips spread apart and moving in little circles **(fig. 34)**. In general, you don't want to stay on one spot for a long period of time, as the constant pressure will begin to feel irritating. Instead, keep moving around the area—up, down, and along the sides of the head. If you find a spot that is particularly tender, you can stay on it, lightly, for a little while.

5. Continue moving in small circles over the top of the head, then to the back, and then around the back sides so that the rest of the scalp is covered. This should feel like a really nice, slow shampoo.

6. The next area you'll work is the face. Begin at the hairline and rub in small circles, working your way down to the eyebrows **(fig. 35)**.

7. Move to the jaw joint, in front of the ear. Bring your fingers closer together and work down along the angle of the jaw. Avoid the throat **(fig. 36)**.

8. Make small circles at the sides of the nose, the sides of the chin, and just over the eyes **(fig. 37)**.

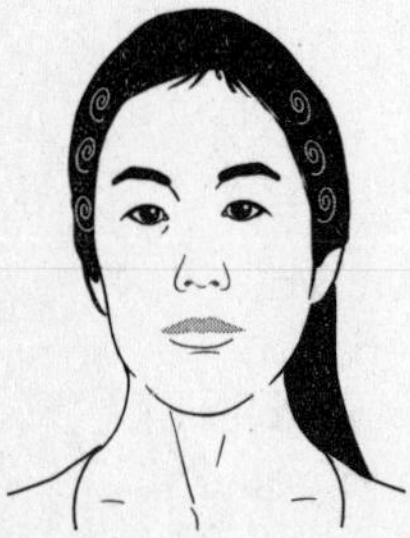

fig. 34

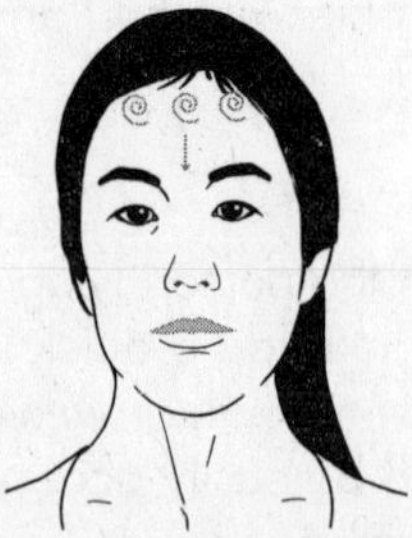

fig. 35

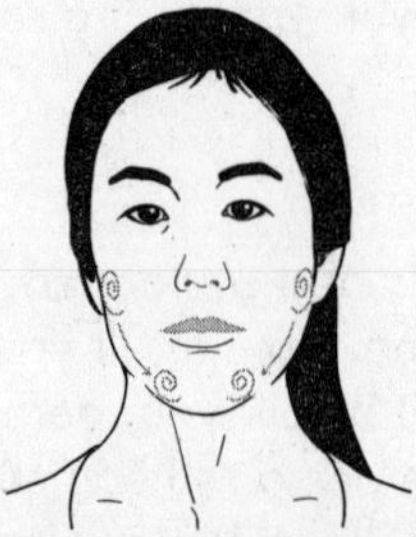

fig. 36

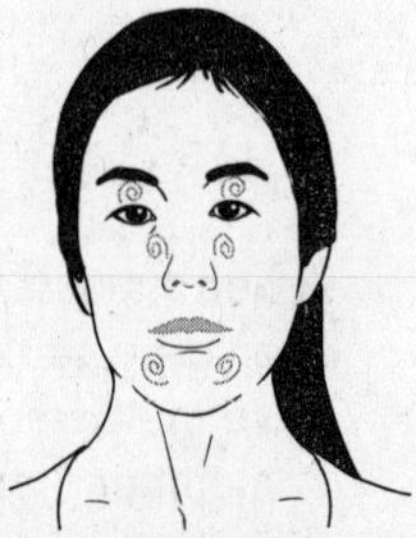

fig. 37

9. End the massage by sweeping the flat of your thumbs across the forehead in a windshield-wiper motion, one at a time in each direction—a slow, soothing finish.

NECK AND SHOULDERS

Have the person lie on her back, perhaps in bed with you seated alongside. Make sure you're low enough; you might even want a footstool for this massage. If you're using oil, place a towel beneath the person's neck and shoulders.

1. Rub your hands together to warm them; if you're using oil, rub a little between your hands.

2. Begin with the tops of the shoulders. Your thumbs should be at the back of the shoulders and your fingers at the front. Use a kneading motion to rub along the length of the shoulders, starting at the outside and working in toward the spine. If you feel knots in the shoulders, you can stop the rubbing and simply hold the area for a moment. Then resume the kneading motion.

3. Using alternating hands, use a cupping motion to sweep from the base of the neck toward the skull. Repeat several times.

4. Now squeeze the neck lightly, again moving from the base toward the skull.

5. Finish by using gentle fingertip pressure to work along the line between the base of the skull and the neck. If you locate any tender spots, move over them with a back-and-forth motion.

LOW BACK

Have the person lie facedown. It's often best if the person lies on the bed, with you sitting on the bed next to him. The shirt should be off. If you're using oil, place a towel or two beneath the person.

1. Rub your hands together to warm them; if you're using oil, rub a little between your hands.

2. Place your hands on either side of the low back **(fig. 38)**. In a long, slow sweep, move them in toward the center and then up the sides of the spine. Repeat several times.

3. Place your thumbs on either side of the spine and use them to knead the area. If you find a tender spot, you can rub

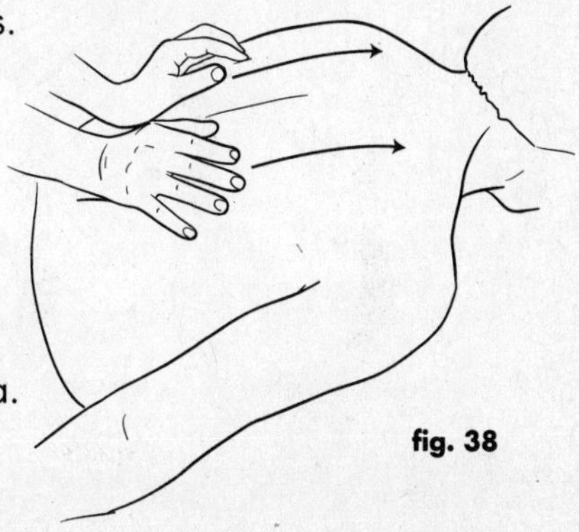

fig. 38

your thumb back and forth over it. Otherwise, don't stay in the same spot for long; instead, work across the entire low back. If your thumbs tire easily, ease up on the pressure so that you can last longer.

HANDS

I love hand massage in the hospital, as it's a caring but nonintrusive way to help someone relax. Always use oil or lotion on the hands.

1. Rub a little oil between your hands to warm it.

2. Turn the palm faceup. Your thumbs should work the palm as your fingers provide stability under the back side of the hand.

3. Place your thumbs in the center of the palm. Slowly sweep the flats of your thumbs outward, so that you're opening up the palm and stretching it a bit **(fig. 39)**. Use the whole thumb, not just the fingertip. Lift up your thumbs and move back to the center; repeat several times.

4. Work the fingers. Begin at the top of the finger and use a gentle twisting motion until you reach the base **(fig. 40)**. The finger should twist slightly; you should also be twisting the skin of the hand a bit. Move back up the finger and then down once more. Proceed with the next finger, and continue until all fingers and the thumb have been worked.

5. Return to the palm. Run the flats of your thumbs across it several times and then start making small circles with the tips of your thumbs **(fig. 41)**. Spend extra time on the fleshy parts of the hands. If you find a sore spot, stretch it gently and work it with your thumb tips.

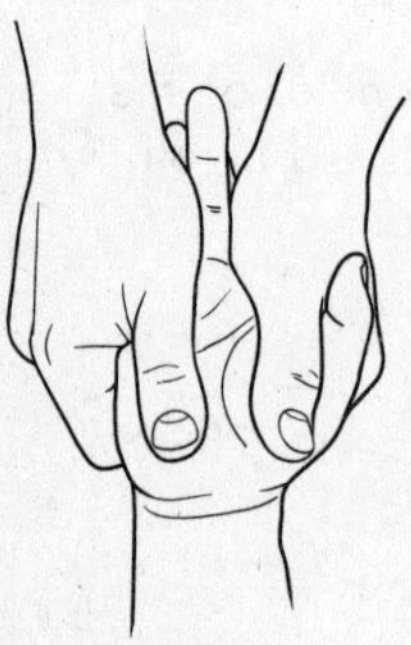

fig. 39

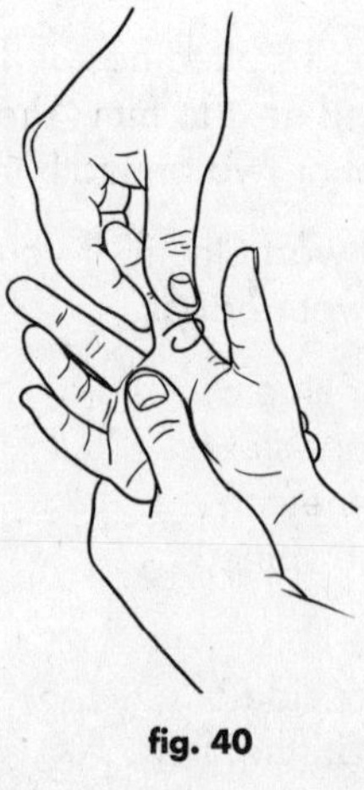

fig. 40

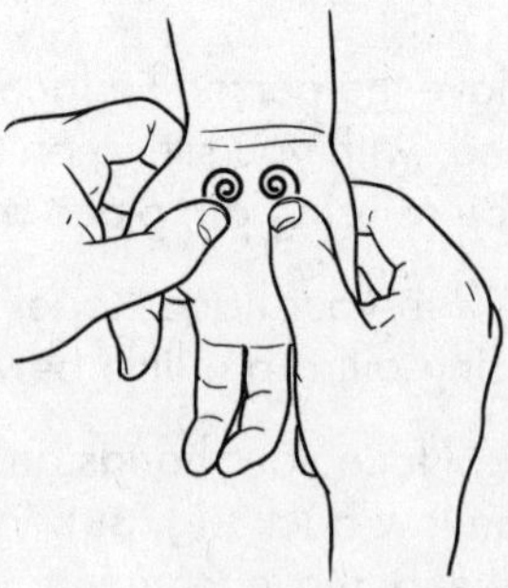

fig. 41

FEET

If you're using oil, place a towel below the person's foot.

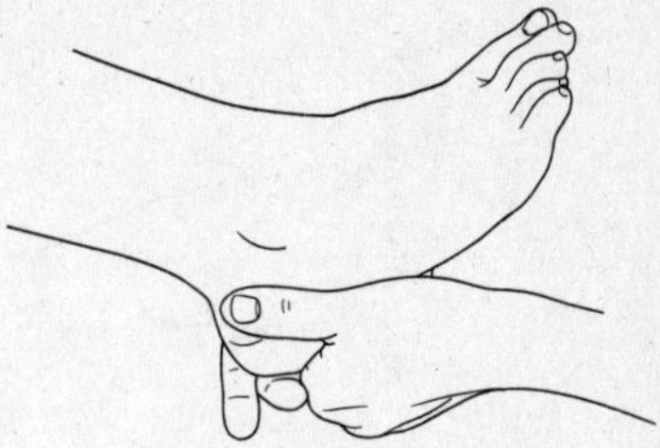

fig. 42

1. Rub your hands together to warm them; if you're using oil, rub a little between your hands.

2. Begin by squeezing the upper part of the heel, working your way down. Repeat several times **(fig. 42)**.

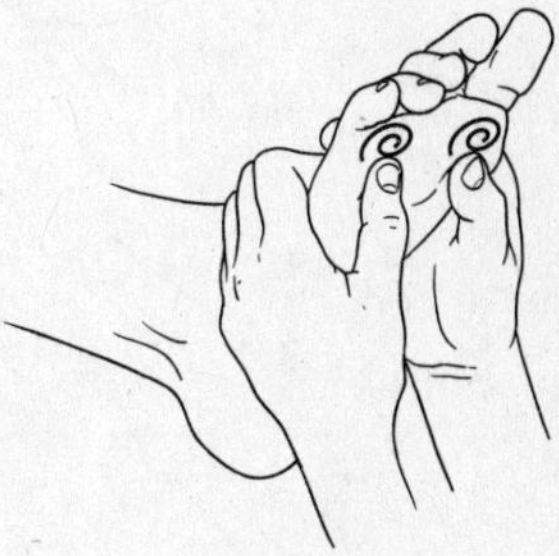

fig. 43

3. Rub along the sole of the foot. Work from the bottom of the heel to the ball of the foot, making small circles with your thumbs. Concentrate most of your efforts along the arch **(fig. 43)**. If you find a sore spot, stay there for a moment and work it with your thumbs. If your thumbs tire at any point, press your fingertips in sequence along the arch, under the ball of the foot, or along the foot's inner edge.

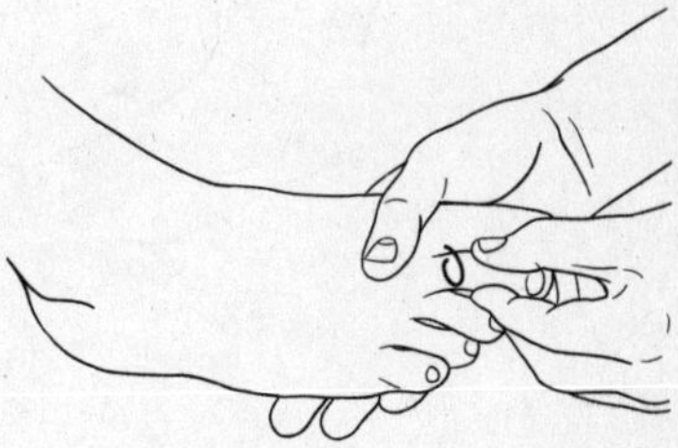

fig. 44

4. Work the toes. Begin at the top of the toe and use a gentle twisting motion until you reach the base **(fig. 44)**. The toe should twist slightly; you should also be twisting the toe's skin a bit. Move back up the toe and then down once more. Proceed with the next toe, and continue until all toes have been worked.

5. Return to the ball of the foot and work your way down, making little circles.

6. Finish by squeezing the heel again, this time working up from the base and toward the ankle.

MYOFASCIAL PAIN

In this technique, you're looking for trigger points—tender knots or bands of muscle that radiate pain to another location when pressed. This massage works for trigger-point pain in any area of the body. Oil is optional for this massage; if you're going to use it, make sure to put down towels wherever the person's skin might touch. (For more information about trigger points, see Chapter 24.)

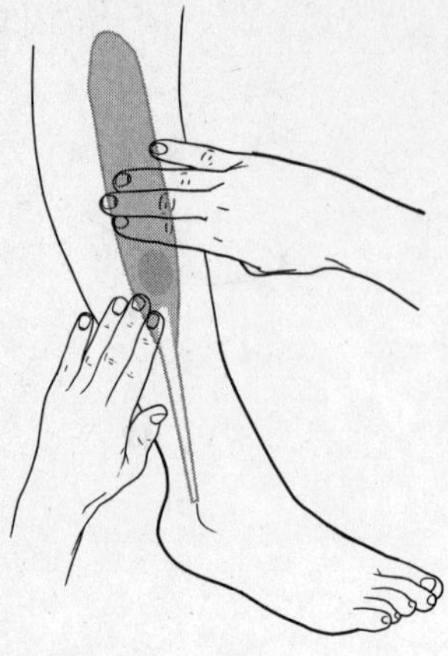

fig. 45

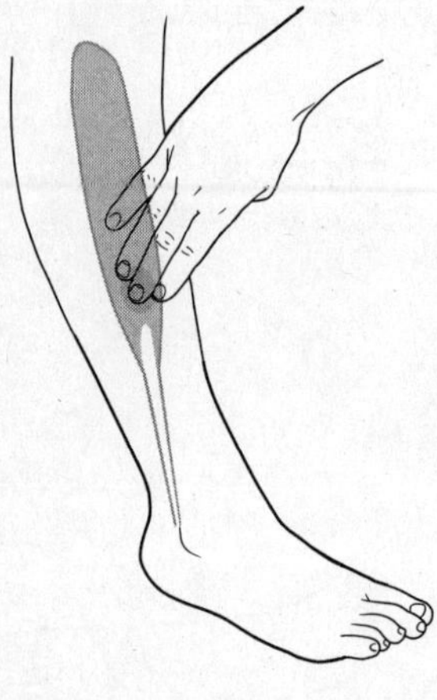

fig. 46

1. Rub your hands together to warm them; if you're using oil, rub a little between your hands.

2. Press firmly around the painful area and areas adjacent to it. Look for spots that are tender, or for bands of taut muscle, which may feel like rope **(fig. 45)**. These spots should cause some discomfort and even pain when you press on them; they may also send pain radiating outward to another location. These are the areas you want to focus on—those clenched muscles need to be worked before they'll release their grip.

3. Press your thumb or finger into the tender spot and hold it there firmly for a minute or two. If you can locate a taut band of muscle, use your thumb or fingertip to thrum back and forth against the grain **(fig. 46)**. Continue to check in the region for additional trigger points.

4. Have the person follow up by stretching the area. A hot pack might relax the muscles even further.

You'll need to work within the sufferer's tolerance level. She shouldn't be screaming in agony, but there should be a quality of "good hurt."

APPENDIX C

ACUPRESSURE MAPS

Acupressure employs firm, sustained fingertip pressure against certain sensitive points in the anatomy. Like massage, it works well for most disorders and has some kind of stress- or pain-relieving effect on almost everyone. While you may want to seek out professional treatment (see Chapter 10), you can also use acupressure on your own.

A few of the most commonly used acupressure points are mapped below. Use your fingertips or knuckles to apply firm pressure to a point for a minute or two. You can also try twisting your finger or knuckle as you press into the spot.

FOR HEADACHE AND NECK PAIN

Gall Bladder 20 and 21
Bladder 10 and 11
Small Intestine 15
Triple Heater 15

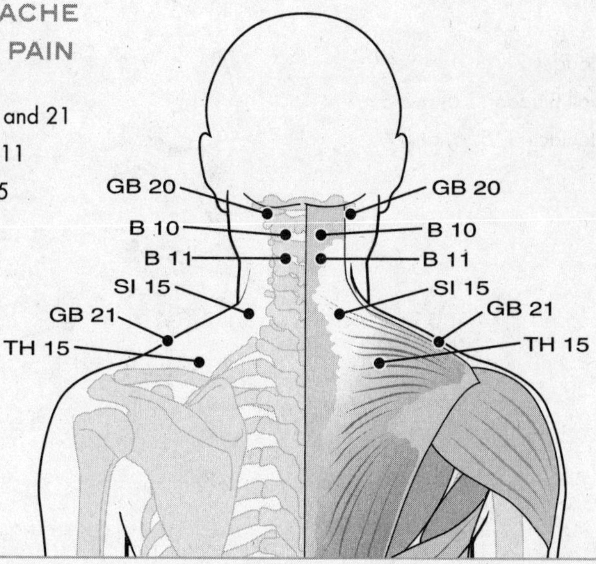

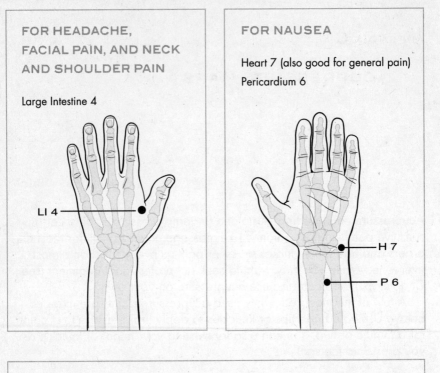

FOR HEADACHE, FACIAL PAIN, AND NECK AND SHOULDER PAIN

Large Intestine 4

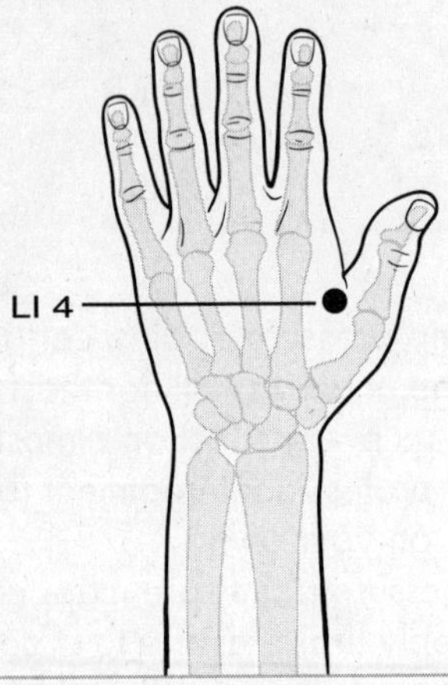

FOR NAUSEA

Heart 7 (also good for general pain)
Pericardium 6

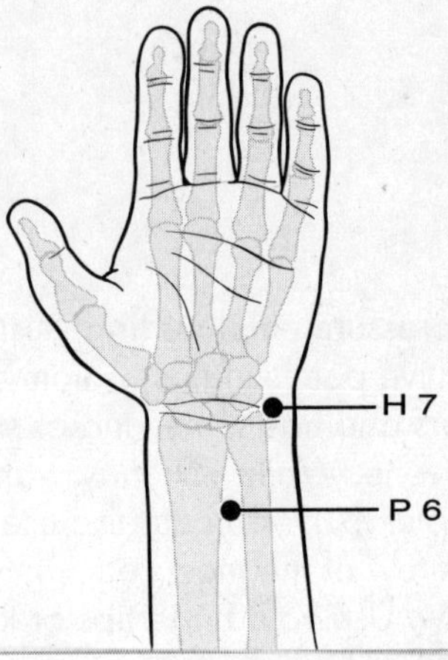

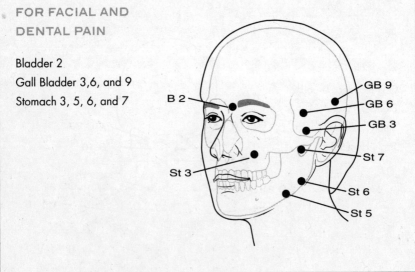

FOR FACIAL AND DENTAL PAIN

Bladder 2
Gall Bladder 3,6, and 9
Stomach 3, 5, 6, and 7

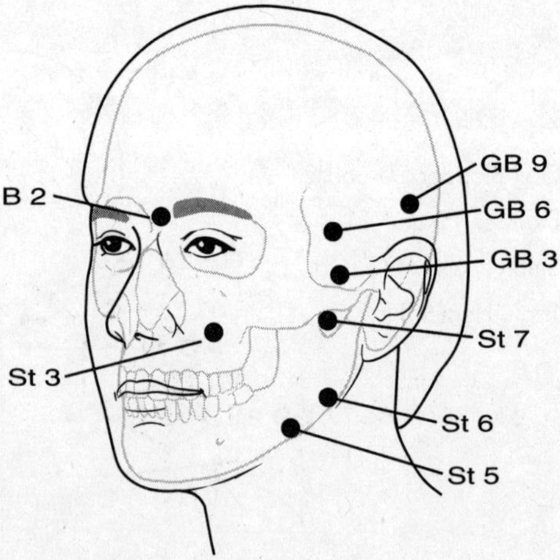

APPENDIX D

HOW TO WORK WITH YOUR INSURANCE PROVIDER

Insurance doesn't cover every kind of treatment for pain, but you may be surprised at how much your plan will pay for. Some insurance providers will, upon a doctor's request, cover prescription drugs that go over their stated caps, and a growing number will pay for certain alternative treatments, especially chiropractic, acupuncture, massage, biofeedback, and hypnosis. Here are some tips for getting the most from your plan.

▸ Know your policy. Health insurance is a product; as with any other purchase you make, you should know its terms and conditions. Read your policy, paying special attention to items regarding pain management, alternative therapies, limits on spending for prescription drugs, and durable medical equipment (found in what's known as a DME clause, which covers big-ticket items such as implanted pumps and stimulators). Be aware of what's excluded from coverage and if there are any exceptions to the exclusions.

▸ Investigate other health plans. If you buy your own insurance and are unhappy with your current plan, then you should shop around. Even if you are covered through your employer, you likely have a choice of plans, so inform yourself about the plan most likely to fit both your needs and your budget. Insurance that covers alternative medicine is increasingly available, although it is usually more expensive. You may also be able to purchase a rider to supplement your current plan.

▸ Consider a medical spending account. Medical spending accounts (sometimes known as flexible spending accounts) allow you and your employer to contribute money toward your health care costs, which you can then deduct from your taxes. Medical spending accounts usually allow for a wider range of services than insurance plans, but make sure you know the terms of the deal before you sign on.

▶ Make friends with your benefits administrator (BA). If you receive group insurance at work, your BA is the person at your company who is responsible for purchasing the plans—meaning that the insurer has a stake in keeping the BA happy. If you have a reasonable request for coverage, your BA might be willing to write a letter or make a phone call. Or you could ask your BA to offer a wider choice of insurance plans, including ones that cover alternative therapies and pain management. (Point out that alternative-medicine coverage is a relatively inexpensive way to attract and keep employees.)

▶ Enlist your doctor's help. It's part of your doctor's job to be your advocate with the insurance company, and frankly, your insurer is more likely to pay attention to a physician than to you. So ask your doctor if he will write letters or make phone calls on your behalf, and follow up to find out if he's done so.

▶ Know that many companies will go over stated caps for prescription drugs if you truly can't afford necessary medications. Ask your doctor to write a letter explaining your situation.

▶ When pursuing coverage for alternative therapies, make sure they are tied to a specific condition. Make it clear that you are receiving, say, acupuncture for irritable bowel syndrome, not for wellness or stress reduction. If you can document that the therapy is helping you—if you visit the emergency room less or if you have reduced medication—do so.

▶ If there is good medical evidence for a therapy that's not covered in your plan, you might be able to persuade your insurer to reimburse you for it. Look for articles in established medical journals (newsstand magazines, Internet sites, and advertisements don't count here). You or your doctor can submit these articles to your insurance company and ask if you can get coverage based on the evidence.

▶ When your plan covers a service but a plan-approved practitioner isn't in your area, the insurer may be willing to pay for treatment by someone else. Make sure the practitioner you have in mind has the appropriate credentials, and enlist your doctor's help.

▶ Does an alternative therapy cost less than conventional treatment? If regular massages allow you to stop medication that is more expensive than the massage therapy, ask your doctor to write a letter asking for coverage. But don't expect radically experimental or unproven treatments to be covered.

- Be persistent. Write your insurance company, then call, and call again, and again. Keep records of letters, and make notes of the dates and times you call and with whom you speak. If you can develop a relationship with someone inside the insurance company, usually a provider relations representative, all the better. Know the four stages of the appeals process (denial, appeal, grievance within the company, and grievance outside the company) and understand how your insurer handles them. As a very last resort, you can apply to the state body that overseas insurance providers. This measure is for use only when your case is really justified—the company refuses to cover a procedure that's listed in its policy, for example—but it will get your insurer's attention.

- Be realistic. In an ideal world, insurance would cover all necessary treatment as well as wellness measures such as exercise classes. But reality dictates that we have to accept that insurance is a business and that we need to work within its limits. Don't expect your insurer to pay for running shoes or for herbs that haven't been proven to work, and don't be shocked if a cheap plan doesn't cover many services.

- When all fails, you might need to pay up. If you've tried and tried and your insurance company still won't reimburse you for a therapy that really helps, *and* if you can afford it, you may wish to pay for that therapy out of pocket. For some people, this concept is difficult to accept: I've seen patients wearing $500 shoes who tell me that they can't afford acupuncture. That's their own decision to make, but sometimes I think that we're so used to the idea of free health care that paying for it ourselves seems unthinkable, even indulgent. But when it comes to your well-being, it might be necessary to make a shift in your priorities. Ask yourself is this is true for you.

APPENDIX E

ACCREDITATION SOCIETIES, PROFESSIONAL ORGANIZATIONS, AND SUPPORT GROUPS

ACCREDITATION SOCIETIES AND PROFESSIONAL ORGANIZATIONS

ALTERNATIVE MEDICINE (GENERAL)

American Pain Society
4700 West Lake Avenue
Glenview, Illinois 60025-1485
Phone: 847-375-4715
Fax: 877-734-8758
www.ampainsoc.org
A professional organization for pain specialists; also offers information to patients, including a directory of pain treatment centers.

The National Center for Complementary and Alternative Medicine at the National Institutes of Health
NCCAM Clearinghouse
P.O. Box 8218
Silver Spring, Maryland 20907-8218
Phone: 888-644-6226
TTY/TDY: 1-888-644-6226
Fax: 301-495-4957
http://nccam.nih.gov/
Tests complementary and alternative therapies and disseminates the results to physicians and consumers alike.

The Richard and Hinda Rosenthal Center for Complementary and Alternative Medicine
Columbia University, College of Physicians and Surgeons
630 West 168th Street, Box 75
New York, New York 10032
Phone: 212-543-9542
Fax: 212-543-2845
http://cpmcnet.columbia.edu/dept/rosenthal/
Devotes itself to research, education, and training in complementary and alternative medicine.

ACUPUNCTURE

American Academy of Medical Acupuncture
4929 Wilshire Boulevard, Suite 428
Los Angeles, California 90010
Phone: 323-937-5514
http://www.medicalacupuncture.org
General information is available, including acupuncture laws by state and a directory of practitioners.

National Certification Commission for Acupuncture and Oriental Medicine
11 Canal Center Plaza, Suite 300
Alexandria, Virginia 22314
Phone: 703-548-9004
Fax: 703-548-9079
http://www.nccaom.org
Certifies acupuncturists and Chinese herbologists. The Web site features a directory of practitioners.

ALEXANDER TECHNIQUE

North American Society of Teachers of the Alexander Technique
P.O. Box 60008
Florence, Massachusetts 01062
Phone: 800-473-0620 or 413-584-2359
http://www.alexandertech.com
Certifies practitioners of the Alexander Technique and offers a directory as well as further information.

BIOFEEDBACK

Biofeedback Certification Institute of America
10200 West 44th Avenue, #310
Wheat Ridge, Colorado 80033
Phone: 303-420-2902
Fax: 303-422-8894
http://www.bcia.org
Certifies biofeedback practitioners; offers general information and directory.

CHIROPRACTIC

American Chiropractic Association
1701 Clarendon Boulevard
Arlington, Virginia 22209
Phone: 703-276-8800
Fax: 703-243-2593
http://www.amerchiro.org
Has a directory of chiropractors, health tips, publications, and general information.

International Chiropractors Association
1110 North Glebe Road, Suite 1000
Arlington, Virginia 22201
Phone: 800-423-4690 or 703-528-5000
Fax: 703-528-5023
http://www.chiropractic.org
Offers a directory of chiropractors and general information.

FELDENKRAIS

Feldenkrais Guild of North America
3611 SW Hood Avenue, Suite 100
Portland, Oregon 97201
Phone: 800-775-2118 or 503-221-6612
Fax: 503-221-6616
http://www.feldenkrais.com
Trains and certifies practitioners; has a directory of practitioners available on its Web site as well as detailed information about Feldenkrais.

GUIDED IMAGERY

Academy for Guided Imagery
P.O. Box 2070
Mill Valley, California 94942
Phone: 800-726-2070 or 415-389-9324
Fax: 415-389-9342
http://www.interactiveimagery.com
Professional organization; Web site offers a store selling guided imagery audiotapes.

HELLERWORK

Hellerwork International
3435 M Street
Eureka, California 95503
Phone: 800-392-3900 or 707-441-4949
http://www.hellerwork.com
Certifies Hellerwork practitioners and offers a directory, articles, and general information.

HOMEOPATHY

Council on Homeopathic Education
801 North Fairfax Street, Suite 306
Alexandria, Virginia 22314
Phone: 212-560-7136
Fax: 212-737-2489
Accredits schools of homeopathy.

The National Center for Homeopathy
801 North Fairfax Street, Suite 306
Alexandria, Virginia 22314
Phone: 703-548-7790
Fax: 703-548-7792
http://www.healthy.net
Lists homeopathic services available by state.

HYPNOSIS

National Board for Certified Clinical Hypnotherapists, Inc.
111 Fidler Lane, Suite L1
Silver Spring, Maryland 20910
Phone: 800-449-8144 or 301-608-0123
Fax: 301-588-9535
Certifies hypnotherapists and offers a directory.

American Council of Hypnotist Examiners
700 South Central Avenue
Glendale, California 91204
Phone: 818-242-1159
Fax: 818-247-9379

http://www.sonic.net/hypno/ache.html
Certifies hypnotists and provides general information about hypnosis.

MASSAGE

American Massage Therapy Association
820 Davis Street, Suite 100
Evanston, Illinois 60201-4444
Phone: 847-864-0123
Fax: 847-864-1178
http://www.amtamassage.org/
Professional organization that offers information about therapeutic massage.

National Certification Board for Therapeutic Massage and Bodywork
8201 Greensboro Drive, Suite 300
McLean, Virginia 22102
Phone: 800-296-0064 or 703-610-9015
Fax: 703-610-9005
http://www.ncbtmb.com
Certifies massage therapists and other bodywork professions; provides a directory of professionals and a consumer's guide.

NATUROPATHY

American Association of Naturopathic Physicians
601 Valley Street, Suite 105
Seattle, Washington 98109
Phone: 206-298-0126
http://www.naturopathic.org
Lists qualified N.D.'s in your area; the Web site includes a searchable database of naturopathic physicians.

OSTEOPATHY

American Osteopathic Association
142 East Ontario Street
Chicago, Illinois 60611
Phone: 800-367-4895 or 312-202-8000
http://www.aoa-net.org
This professional organization will give detailed information about osteopathy; the Web site contains a directory of osteopathic doctors by state.

REIKI

International Association of Reiki Professionals
P.O. Box 481
Winchester, Massachusetts 01890
781-729-3530
http://www.iarp.org
A professional organization that provides information and a provider directory to consumers on its Web site.

ROLFING

The Rolf Institute
205 Canyon Boulevard
Boulder, Colorado 80302
Phone: 800-530-8875 or 303-449-5903
Fax: 303-449-5978
http://www.rolf.org
Certifies practitioners and offers a directory on their Web site.

THERAPEUTIC TOUCH

Nurse Healers Professional Associates, Inc.
1211 Locust Street
Philadelphia, Pennsylvania 19107
Phone: 215-545-8079
http://www.therapeutic-touch.org
Maintains a list of books and videos about Therapeutic Touch.

YOGA

American Yoga Association
513 South Orange Avenue
Sarasota, Florida 34236
Phone: 941-953-5859
http://www.americanyogaassociation.org
Educates consumers about yoga; the Web site contains suggestions for yoga practice.

SUPPORT GROUPS AND INFORMATION CENTERS FOR PAIN AND PAINFUL DISORDERS

PAIN (GENERAL)

American Academy of Pain Medicine
4700 W. Lake
Glenview, IL 60025
Phone: 847-375-4731
http://www.painmed.org
The primary organization for physicians practicing the specialty of pain medicine in the United States. Web site provides a searchable online member directory.

American Chronic Pain Association
P. O. Box 850
Rocklin, California 95677-0850
Phone: 916-632-0922
http://www.theacpa.org
An advocacy and consumer education group for people in pain.

American Pain Foundation
111 South Calvert Street, Suite 2700
Baltimore, MD 21202
Phone: 1-888-615-PAIN (7246)
http://www.painfoundation.org
An advocacy group and information resource for people in pain.

American Pain Society
4700 W. Lake Ave.
Glenview, IL 60025
Phone: 847-375-4715
http://www.ampainsoc.org
A professional organization seeking to advance pain-related research, treatment, and education.

Beth Israel Medical Center Department of Pain Medicine and Palliative Care
First Avenue at 16th Street
New York, NY 10003
Phone: 212-844-8970
http://www.stoppain.org
Center for the treatment of chronic pain, specializing in the creation of a better quality of life for pain sufferers,

including those who are unresponsive to treatment. Also home to the Jacob Perlow Hospice for end-of-life care.

International Association for the Study of Pain
909 NE 43rd St., Suite 306
Seattle, WA 98105-6020
Phone: 206-547-6409
http://www.iasp-pain.org
Professional organization dedicated to furthering research on pain and improving the care of patients with pain.

http://www.pain.com
A resource for both doctors and patients, including an "Ask the Doctor" column. Sponsored by the Dannemiller Memorial Educational Foundation.

ARTHRITIS

Arthritis Foundation
1330 West Peachtree Street
Atlanta, Georgia 30309
Phone: 800-283-7800 or 404-872-7100
Will supply written information and a list of arthritis specialists near you.

BACK PAIN

Back Pain Association of America
P.O. Box 135
Pasadena, Maryland 21122-0135
Phone: 410-255-3633
Fax: 410-255-7338
Offers referrals to specialists, a quarterly newsletter, and other written materials; sponsors support groups in the northeastern United States.

COMPLEX REGIONAL PAIN SYNDROME

Reflex Sympathetic Dystrophy Syndrome Association
Phone: 609-795-8845
http://www.rsds.org
Offers support groups nationwide, physician referrals, and written materials.

FACIAL, JAW, AND DENTAL PAIN

National Institute of Dental and Craniofacial Research
National Institutes of Health
Bethesda, Maryland 20892-2190
http://www.nidr.nih.gov
A source for physicians that includes patient information.

TMJ Association, Ltd.
5418 West Washington Boulevard
Milwaukee, Wisconsin 53213
Phone: 414-259-3223
Fax: 414-259-8112
http://www.tmj.org
A grassroots organization supporting multidisciplinary treatment of TMJ.

Trigeminal Neuralgia Association
P.O. Box 340
Barnegat Light, New Jersey 08006

Phone: 609-361-6250
http://www.tna-support.org
Offers written materials, support groups, and limited physician referrals.

HEADACHE

American Council for Headache Education
19 Mantua Road
Mount Royal, New Jersey 08061
Phone: 856-423-0258
http://www.achenet.org
Has a list of headache specialists; offers a newsletter and other written materials; sponsors support groups nationwide.

JAMA Migraine Information Center
The Journal of the American Medical Association
http://www.ama-assn.org/special/migraine/migraine.htm
A resource for you as well as your physician.

M.A.G.N.U.M. INC. Migraine Awareness Group: A National Understanding for Migraineurs
113 South Saint Asaph, Suite 300
Alexandria, Virginia 22314
Phone: 703-739-9384
http://www.migraines.org
A patient information group with a comprehensive Web site.

National Headache Foundation
428 West St. James Place, second floor
Chicago, Illinois 60614-2750
Phone: 1-888-NHF-5552
http://www.headaches.org
Provides a list of headache specialists and other written material; sponsors support groups nationwide.

IRRITABLE BOWEL SYNDROME

Irritable Bowel Syndrome Self Help Group
http://www.ibsgroup.org
An online group for IBS sufferers.

Mind Body Digestive Center
http://www.mindbodydigestive.com
Emphasis is on holistic, mind-body treatments for IBS and other digestive disorders.

PELVIC PAIN

American Foundation for Urologic Disease
300 West Pratt Street, Suite 401
Baltimore, Maryland 21201-2463
Phone: 800-828-7866
http://www.afud.org
Devoted to educating medical professionals, patients, and family members about urologic disorders, treatment, and the latest research.

Endometriosis Association
8585 North 76th Place
Milwaukee, Wisconsin 53223
Phone: 414-355-2200
http://www.endometriosisassn.org
A self-help group that offers brochures and other information and sponsors support groups nationwide.

Interstitial Cystitis Association
East Coast:
P.O. Box 1553
Madison Square Station
New York, New York 10159
West Coast:
P.O. Box 151323
San Diego, California 92115
Phone: 1-800-435-7422
http://www.ichelp.org
Offers information for patients and physicians, physician referrals, and support groups nationwide.

Interstitial Cystitis Network
5636 Del Monte Court
Santa Rosa, California 95409
Phone: 707-538-9442
Fax: 707-538-9444
http://www.ic-network.com
A resource for patients and physicians.

PERIPHERAL NEUROPATHY

Neuropathy Association
60 E. 42nd Street, Suite 942
New York, New York 10165
Phone: 212-692-0662
http://www.neuropathy.org
Supports education, public awareness, and research for neuropathies.

TERMINAL PAIN

The American Hospice Foundation
2120 L Street, NW, Suite 200
Washington, DC 20037
Phone: 202-223-0204
http://www.americanhospice.org
Advances hospice care and has publications and workshops.

VULVODYNIA

National Vulvodynia Association
P.O. Box 4491
Silver Spring, Maryland 20914-4491
Phone: 301-299-0775
Fax: 301-299-3999
http://www.nva.org
Offers a support network as well as a list of doctors interested in vulvar disorders.

APPENDIX **F**

RECOMMENDED READING

Alternative Medicine for Dummies, by James Dillard, M.D., D.C., C.Ac., and Terra Ziporyn, Ph.D. IDG Books, 1998.

Alternative Medicine: What Works, by Adriane Fugh-Berman, M.D. Williams and Wilkins, 1997.

Between Heaven and Earth: A Guide to Chinese Medicine, by Harriet Beinfield, L.Ac., and Efrem Korngold, L.Ac., O.M.D. Ballantine Publishing Group, 1991.

Choices in Healing: Integrating the Best of Conventional and Complementary Approaches to Cancer, by Michael Lerner. MIT Press, 1998.

The Culture of Pain, by David B. Morris. University of California Press, 1991.

Eating Well for Optimum Health: The Essential Guide to Food, Diet, and Nutrition, by Andrew Weil, M.D. Knopf, 2000.

Full-Catastrophe Living: Using the Wisdom of Your Body and Mind to Face Stress, Pain, and Illness, by Jon Kabat-Zinn, Ph.D. Delta, 1990.

Guided Imagery for Self-Healing: An Essential Resource for Anyone Seeking Wellness, by Martin Rossman, M.D. H. J. Kramer, 2000.

Healing Back Pain: The Mind-Body Connection, by John E. Sarno, M.D. Warner Books, 1991.

Healing from the Heart: A Leading Surgeon Combines Eastern and Western Traditions to Create the Medicine of the Future, by Mehmet Oz, M.D. E. P. Dutton, 1998.

Healing Visualizations: Creating Health Through Imagery, by Gerald Epstein, M.D. Bantam Doubleday Dell, 1989.

Kitchen Table Wisdom, by Rachel Naomi Remen, M.D. Riverhead, 1997.

Managing Pain Before It Manages You, by Margaret A. Caudill, M.D., Ph.D. The Guilford Press, 1995.

Manifesto for a New Medicine: Your Guide to Healing Partnerships and the Wise Use of Alternative Therapies, by James S. Gordon, M.D. Perseus Press, 1997.

The Mindbody Prescription: Healing the Body, Healing the Pain, by John E. Sarno, M.D. Warner Books, 1998.

Pain and Behavioral Medicine: A Cognitive-Behavioral Perspective, by Dennis C. Turk, Donald Meichenbaum, and Myles Genest. The Guilford Press, 1983.

Pain Free: A Revolutionary Method for Stopping Chronic Pain, by Pete Egoscue with Roger Gittines. Bantam Books, 1998.

The Relaxation Response, by Herbert Benson, M.D., with Miriam Z. Klipper. Wholecare, 2000.

Rituals of Healing, by Jeanne Achterberg, Ph.D., Barbara Dossey, R.N., and Leslie Kolkmeier, R.N. Bantam Doubleday Dell, 1994.

Soothing Your Child's Pain, by Kenneth Gorfinkle, Ph.D. Contemporary Books, 1997.

Spontaneous Healing, by Andrew Weil, M.D. Ballantine Publishing Group, 1995.

Touch Therapy, by Tiffany Field. Churchill Livingstone, 2000.

The Web That Has No Weaver: Understanding Chinese Medicine, by Ted J. Kaptchuk, O.M.D. Contemporary Books, 2000.

A Whole New Life, by Reynolds Price. Scribner, 1982.

Why People Don't Heal and How They Can, by Caroline Myss, Ph.D. Three Rivers Press, 1998.

Women's Bodies, Women's Wisdom, by Christiane Northrup, M.D. Revised edition, Bantam Books, 1998.

INDEX

Page numbers of main entries for therapies and conditions appear in bold type; page numbers of illustrations appear in italics.

B

E

H

I

ABOUT THE AUTHORS

JAMES N. DILLARD, M.D., D.C., C.AC., is formally trained in three health professions—acupuncture, chiropractic, and medicine. Dr. Dillard is an assistant clinical professor at Columbia University College of Physicians and Surgeons, and is on the medical staff of the New York-Presbyterian Hospital's Columbia Medical Center. He is also an attending physician at Beth Israel NY in the Department of Pain and Palliative Care, and at the Continuum Center for Health and Healing. He is the director of Complementary Medicine Services at University Pain Center in Manhattan. He also serves as clinical advisor to the Rosenthal Center for Complementary and Alternative Medicine, an NIH–NCCAM granted research and education center at Columbia University College of Physicians and Surgeons under the direction of Fredi Kronenberg, Ph.D. He is the founding medical director for the Oxford Health Plans Alternative Medicine program.

Dr. Dillard conducted research in spinal biomechanics with Gunnar Andersson, M.D., Ph.D., at Rush Presbyterian–St. Luke's Medical Center in Chicago while earning his medical degree at Rush Medical College. He also did cancer and transplantation immunology research at the University of California, Los Angeles, while earning his doctor of chiropractic degree from Cleveland Chiropractic College and attending California Acupuncture College.

Dr. Dillard is the author of *Alternative Medicine for Dummies,* published by IDG Books Worldwide. He served as the alternative-health content expert and columnist for the number-one health Web site in the world, OnHealth.com, from 1999 to 2001. He has been featured in such publications as *Newsweek, People, Outside, Mademoiselle, Shape, O,* and *Parenting*. He has appeared on *The Oprah Winfrey Show, Good Morning America, The View, The Today Show,* National Public Radio, and *The CBS Evening News,* among many other broadcasts.

LEIGH ANN HIRSCHMAN is a writer and editor. She lives in Chicago with her husband and daughter.